Tutorials in Clinical Surgery
Volume 2

Other books by F. G. Smiddy

Multiple Choice Questions in General Pathology
F. G. Smiddy/J. L. Turk

**Tutorials in Clinical Surgery in General
Volume 1**
F. G. Smiddy

For Churchill Livingstone:
Publisher: Peter Richardson
Copy Editor: Neil Pakenham-Walsh
Production Controller: Neil Dickson
Sales Promotion Executive: Caroline Boyd

Tutorials in Clinical Surgery in General
Volume 2

F. G. Smiddy MD CHM FRCS
Formerly Consultant Surgeon, The General Infirmary at Leeds and
Clayton Hospital, Wakefield, UK
Member of the Court of Examiners of the Royal College of Surgeons,
England, Examiner in Pathology

CHURCHILL LIVINGSTONE
EDINBURGH LONDON MADRID MELBOURNE NEW YORK
AND TOKYO 1993

CHURCHILL LIVINGSTONE
Medical Division of Longman Group UK Limited

Distributed in the United States of America by Churchill Livingstone Inc., 650 Avenue of the Americas, New York, N.Y. 10011, and by associated companies, branches and representatives throughout the world.

© F. G. Smiddy 1993

All rights reserved. No part of this publication may be reproduced, stored in a retrieval system, or transmitted in any form or by any means, electronic, mechanical, photocopying, recording or otherwise, without either the prior permission of the publishers (Churchill Livingstone, Robert Stevenson House, 1-3 Baxter's Place, Leith Walk, Edinburgh EH1 3AF), or a licence permitting restricted copying in the United Kingdom issued by the Copyright Licensing Agency Ltd, 90 Tottenham Court Road, London, WIP 9HE.

First published 1993

ISBN 0-443-04796-0

British Library of Cataloguing in Publication Data
A catalogue record for this book is available from the British Library.

Library of Congress Cataloging in Publication Data
A catalog record for this book is available from the Library of Congress.

The publisher's policy is to use paper manufactured from sustainable forests

Produced by Longman Singapore Publishers Pte Ltd
Printed in Singapore

Preface

The genesis of this book of tutorials lies in the needs and aspirations of the many candidates who are now taking the Fellowship of the Royal Colleges of Surgeons, which under the new regulations has become known as the Fellowship of Surgery in General. For this examination, the regulations inform us that the detailed knowledge of surgical techniques – except for those operations which the candidate has performed himself or at which he has assisted according to his operation book – is not required. Rather, the examination deals with the diagnosis and principles of surgery, and these tutorials have been written with this in mind.

The author is again reminded of one of the few mistakes made by the father of Leeds surgery, Lord Moynihan, who pronounced in the early 1930s that no further advances in surgery could be envisaged and that surgery had reached its apogee.

Great advances have been made in both the diagnosis and treatment of the surgical patient and it is with this in mind that this new edition has been written. From the observations I have made over the years, I consider that many candidates presenting themselves to their examiners lack the ability to express themselves clearly on paper or in speech when exploring a specific surgical problem, and it is also to help repair this defect that each topic dealt with has been explored in some depth.

I must express my thanks to my colleagues at the General Infirmary at Leeds who have helped with the development of the various sections and given so freely of their time, and I must also thank the librarians of the Leeds Medical School Library who have constantly helped me with references; and lastly, my editor, who has produced order out of chaos.

Leeds, 1992   F.G.S.

To my wife

Contents

SECTION ONE

1 Management of head injuries 3
  Injuries to the scalp
  Injuries to the skull
  Mechanisms of brain injury
  Clinical presentation
  Pathology
  Clinical management
  Operative treatment
  Late complications

2 Skin grafting 17
  Classification
  Advances in skin grafting technique
  Free skin grafts
  Full thickness grafts

3 Blood transfusion and haematological conditions of special interest to the surgeon 27
  Blood transfusion
  Haematological conditions of special interest to the surgeon

4 The 'surgical' parasites 45
  Hydatid disease
  Schistosomiasis
  Amoebiasis
  Ascariasis
  Filariasis

5 Diagnosis and management of acute abdominal pain 63
  Computer-assisted diagnosis

Investigations specifically related to the diagnosis
General management
Management of specific conditions

SECTION TWO

6 Fractures and the general principles of their treatment 81
Classification
Healing of fractures
Treatment of fractures

7 Common complications of fractures 91
Early local complications
Late local complications
Early general complications
Late general complications

8 Fractures of the cervical spine 103
Frequency and causation
Injuries due to flexion and hyperflexion
Injuries due to hyperextension
Compression fractures
Clinical features of cervical injuries
Treatment of cervical injuries

9 Lumbar disc lesions 113
Developmental anatomy
Aging and disc degeneration
Lumbar disc protrusion
Investigations
Treatment
Interventional procedures
Spinal stenosis

10 Principles involved in the treatment of tendon and nerve injuries, with special reference to the hand 123
Injuries to the flexor mechanism of the hand
Extensor tendon injuries
Nerve injuries

SECTION THREE

11 Benign prostatic hypertrophy 133
Aetiology
Anatomy

Pathology
Clinical presentation
Investigations
Medical management of prostatism
Prostatectomy

12 Prostatic cancer 143
Aetiology
Pathology
Clinical presentation
Staging
Histological confirmation
Treatment

13 Cryptorchidism 155
Embryology
Classification
Associated conditions
Treatment of the undescended testis

14 Swellings of the scrotum and testicular tumours 165
Cystic swellings
Solid swellings
Testicular tumours
Treatment of testicular tumours

SECTION FOUR

15 Common benign swellings of the breast 177
Developmental anatomy
Anatomy of the breast
Benign swellings

16 Breast cancer 185
Pathology
Clinical presentation
Diagnostic confirmation
Staging methods
Other factors influencing prognosis
Treatment of early breast cancer
Disseminated or recurrent disease

17 Malignant tumours of the skin 203
Basal cell carcinoma

Squamous carcinoma
Pigmented naevi
Malignant melanoma

SECTION FIVE

18 Enlargement of the parotid gland 213
Generalized parotid enlargement
Tumours of the salivary glands

19 Dysphagia 221
Aetiology
Pharyngeal pouch
Plummer-Vinson syndrome
Carcinoma of the oesophagus
Dysphagia associated with gastro-oesophageal reflux
Achalasia

20 Historical development of duodenal ulcer surgery 239
Gastroenterostomy
Partial gastrectomy
Vagotomy
Treatment of the uncomplicated duodenal ulcer

21 Gallstones 251
Classification
Biochemical composition of bile
Cholesterol stone formation
Pigment stones
Symptoms of gallstones
Treatment of uncomplicated biliary disease
Major complications of gallstones

22 Acute pancreatitis 275
Aetiology
Pathology
Clinical presentation
Classification of the severity of the disease
Investigations
Management

23 Chronic pancreatitis 289
Aetiology

Pathology
Clinical presentation
Investigations
Management

24 Crohn's disease 297
Aetiology
Pathology
Clinical presentation
Investigations
Management

25 Tumours of the large bowel and rectum 309
Aetiology
Pathology
Symptoms associated with colonic tumours
Investigations
Treatment of colonic cancer
Complications of colonic cancer and their treatment
Rectal tumours

26 Complications of colostomy and ileostomy 331
Complications of colostomy
Complications of ileostomy

27 Non-malignant conditions of the anal canal 337
Haemorrhoids
Fissure-in-ano
Fistula-in-ano

SECTION SIX

28 Chronic ischaemia of the lower limb: pathology, clinical features, and investigations 349
Atherosclerosis
Thromboangiitis obliterans (Buerger's disease)
Symptoms of ischaemia of the lower limb
Physical signs of arterial occlusion
Investigations
Acute occlusion

29 Chronic ischaemia of the lower limb: management 365
Lifestyle management
Medical treatment
Surgical treatment

Results of surgery
Lumbar sympathectomy

30 Acute ischaemia of the lower limb 377
Embolism
Clinical presentation
Treatment

31 Varicose veins and the postphlebitic limb 385
Anatomy of the venous system of the lower limb
Venous pressure in the lower limb
Treatment of uncomplicated primary veins
Complications of simple varicose veins
The postphlebitic limb

32 Amputation 395
Indications
Sites of lower limb amputation
Lower limb amputation in peripheral vascular disease
Technique of above-knee and below-knee amputations
Distal amputations
Amputations of the upper limb
Complications of major amputations

SECTION ONE

SECTION ONE

1. Management of head injuries

In the Western world the commonest cause of injury to the head remains the road traffic accident, although the incidence has fallen somewhat with the introduction of compulsory seat-belts. In areas of high alcohol consumption there is also a condition known as the 'moving pavement syndrome' due to drunkenness. In the majority of patients suffering from a head injury an associated injury is present, which may involve only the face, chest, an extremity, or the abdomen; in a large percentage of sufferers, however, the head injury is merely a small part of a complex injury situation.

In all patients suffering from an injury to the head the same general management must be applied as to any other type of injury. Care should be taken that the airway is adequate, bleeding must be controlled and the peripheral circulation must be maintained. Specifically, however, in patients in whom a period of unconsciousness has occurred, repetitive clinical assessment of the patient must be made and the results of such assessment carefully recorded. When the patient is first seen the Glasgow Coma Scale can be used to provide an accurate clinical assessment from which improvement or deterioration of the patient can be evaluated. This scale is based on the observation of three functions:

1. Eye opening.
2. Best motor response.
3. Best verbal response.

Each of these is subdivided in the following manner so that a numerate value can be placed on the clinical observation:

1. *Eye opening.* 4, spontaneous; 3, responding to command; 2, responding to pain; 1, no response.

2. *Best motor response.* 6, following commands; 5, localized painful stimuli; 4, complex arm movements (withdrawing to pain); 3, reflex flexor posturing; 2, reflex extensor posturing; 1, flaccid (no response to pain).
3. *Best verbal response.* 5, orientated; 4, confused; 3, inappropriate words; 2, incomprehensible words; 1, none.

Sequential recording of these observations are recorded at intervals during which the patient is under observation.

Using the Glasgow Coma Scale, Miller and Jones in 1985 found that, of 1919 admissions due to head injury, 84% were assessed as mild, score 13–15; 11% as moderate, score 9–12, and 5% as severe, score < 8. However, this study also showed that whereas severe injuries are relatively infrequent most patients developing signs of increasing intracranial pressure were classified as mild or moderately injured when first assessed.

INJURIES TO THE SCALP

From the surgical point of view the scalp consists of two layers, the dermis and the galea. The unyielding character of the scalp with the major vessels running between the galea and the dermis mean that injured blood vessels are held open, with the result that considerable haemorrhage normally occurs even following trivial head wounds. To control such bleeding direct compression of the wound against the skull may suffice or, in the accident and emergency department, artery clips can be applied to the edge of the galea and allowed to fall backwards over the dermis, after which the wound can be sutured at leisure taking care to include the divided galea within the sutures. If a lengthy wound has occurred, the attachment of the galea to the occipitalis and frontalis muscles means that the wound will separate. Thus wounds left open for more than 4–5 days may then require special methods for their closure.

INJURIES TO THE SKULL

Clinically a skull fracture indicates that a fracture of the vault or base of the skull has occurred. In the vault various types of fracture have been described, e.g. linear, stellate, comminuted or depressed. If the base of the skull has been involved it is termed basilar. If the fracture is associated with an injury to the scalp or to the paranasal sinuses, the fracture is compound. This is the most important distinction that can be made since in all compound or open injuries the possibility of infection of the brain exists; while the majority of closed fractures require no treatment (except some depressed fractures), compound fractures – because of the danger of infection – require immediate attention either by open operation or by treatment of the patient with antimicrobial agents.

MECHANISMS OF BRAIN INJURY

1. The commonest mechanism by which the brain is injured following a head injury is by the application of *acceleration, deceleration or rotational forces*. The significant aspect of this type of injury is that the subsequent brain damage is not necessarily limited to the point of impact. When the various forces are sufficiently severe the brain directly opposite to the point of primary impact is also damaged – the contrecoup injury.

Rotational forces applied to the head set up shearing forces, both within the brain and between the brain and its coverings, leading to neuronal and vascular damage. This type of injury is often associated with musculotendinous injuries to the cervical spine, the so-called 'whiplash' injury of the neck, and may occasionally be associated with an actual fracture; thus many surgeons refer to this type of head injury as a combined pathology and speak of the cranio-cervical injury.

2. *The static crush*. This injury is rare but tends to affect certain occupational groups such as miners, printers or railwaymen in whom, for example, the vault is crushed between buffers.

3. *Penetrating injuries*. These are rare in civilian life in the UK because the majority are caused by missiles. The damage to the brain may be much less than would appear from the external wound unless an explosive or high-velocity bullet has been used in which case the negative pressure wave which follows the bullet may produce extremely severe brain damage.

Clinical presentation

Rotational or acceleration/deceleration injury

This type of injury – if severe enough – is always associated with loss of consciousness, the degree and duration of which is proportional to the severity of the injury. In addition, there may be severe damage to the cervical spine and, often, varying degrees of injury to the face, involving fractures of the mandible, maxilla or zygomatic arches. The most severe facial injury is the Forte 3, which results in separation of the maxillary and malar bones from the base of the skull. This always produces deformity of the face, usually flattening and if the suture lines separate the face is also lengthened, whereas if the suture lines are impacted, the face is shortened.

Such extensive injuries are frequently associated with airway obstruction which of itself leads to deterioration of the cerebral condition.

Static crush injury

Such an injury, if severe, may lead to instantaneous death. In lesser injuries, however, the brain does not move until the compression forces have shattered the skull into splinters and, because of this, immediate loss of consciousness does not necessarily follow. As the skull is shattered, fracture lines extend from the vault to involve the base of the skull, finally involving the various foramina or sinuses. The clinical result is the development of multiple cranial nerve lesions together with rhinorrhoea and/or otorrhoea.

Penetrating injury

The clinical picture depends upon the instrument used, the site of injury and the magnitude of the cerebral damage. A stab wound of the head may, for example, lead to little disturbance, but should it penetrate the brain stem, there may be single or multiple cranial nerve lesions associated with upper motor neurone lesions involving the extremities. Massive injury such as that associated with high-velocity missiles is nearly always followed by death.

PATHOLOGY OF HEAD INJURIES

Closed and open

Clinically it is very important to distinguish between closed and compound or open injuries of the head because with open injuries infection of brain tissue may result. Compound injuries include all those that communicate directly with the exterior, or indirectly via the paranasal sinuses or ear.

Primary brain stem injury

The acceleration/deceleration injury results in shearing forces which not only disrupt vessels, but also disturb the function of the brain leading to unconsciousness which may last a variable length of time, producing post-traumatic amnesia. This is to be distinguished from retrograde amnesia, the loss of memory for events leading up to the injury. Damage to the brain may be focal when contusions or lacerations occur. These develop either beneath the point of impact or in the contrecoup position, where the brain is compressed against the skull diametrically opposite to the original blow or against the falx or tentorium. Thus the common sites at which contusions and lacerations occur are on the frontal poles, the orbital gyri, the temporal poles, and the inferior and lateral surfaces of the anterior halves of the temporal lobes. A contusion may be superficial and restricted to the crest of the gyri or extend more deeply, involving not only the overlying grey matter but also the underlying white matter. Old contusions may be represented by shrunken scars, which are golden-brown in appearance.

In addition to focal lesions, generalized neuronal damage may occur. This is brought about by the shearing strains set up within the brain by the forces of acceleration and deceleration. This is not necessarily associated with contusion. Histological preparations of the brain may show little if the patient dies rapidly after the injury. However, a sign that a sudden acceleration/deceleration injury to the brain has occurred is the presence of oedema and haemorrhagic areas in the corpus callosum and in the dorsolateral quadrant of the rostral brain stem adjacent to the cerebellar peduncles.

If severe, this type of injury may cause generalized cerebral oedema resulting in an increase in intracranial pressure, which itself may cause death by producing herniation of the brain stem through the foramen magnum. If the patient survives, the principal histological change which develops in the brain is a Wallerian type of degeneration of the nerve fibres in the cerebral and cerebellar hemispheres. Although referred to as primary brain stem injury it must be appreciated that such damage as has been described may affect the whole brain.

Secondary brain stem injury

This term implies that an event has followed the initial injury causing an increase in the volume of the contents within the skull. This increase is most frequently due to bleeding, which may be extradural, subdural, subarachnoid or intracerebral. Alternatively, cerebral oedema may develop with only slight superficial damage to the surface of the brain.

When 'space-occupying' lesions develop, the brain is displaced or the ventricles deformed. Since the skull itself is rigid, movement of the brain can only take place in the following directions:

1. The medial aspect of the cerebral hemisphere is pushed downwards and medially beneath the falx cerebri.

2. The temporal lobe is displaced downwards through the tentorium cerebelli, which causes pressure on and elongation of the 3rd oculomotor nerve leading to paralysis of the superior rectus, the medial and inferior recti and the inferior oblique muscle of the eye, together with the sympathetic fibres to the sphincter pupillae and the ciliary muscles of the globe, resulting in a fixed dilated pupil on the side of the lesion.

3. Herniation of the lower cerebellum through the foramen magnum, which produces 'coning'; as this increases in severity, so the medulla is compressed, producing bradycardia and periodic respiration.

CLINICAL MANAGEMENT

In the absence of a compound fracture of the skull which requires careful debridement, elevation of the depressed fragments and repair of the dura if this is torn, the chief concern at the initial examination is to determine the level of consciousness and to assess the patient as a whole, knowing that in severe head injuries associated injuries elsewhere in the body occur in nearly 50% of patients. Of particular importance is airway obstruction or an associated chest injury since both conditions aggravate hypoxia and hypercarbia, the latter being particularly important since it induces cerebral vasodilation and consequently increases intracranial pressure. Assuming that a careful examination of the patient reveals no other injury, the level of consciousness can be assessed using the Glasgow Coma Scale and thereafter repeated observations must be made at frequent intervals, recording in addition the pupillary reactions, blood pressure and respiratory rate. The integrity of the brain stem is assessed by examination of the various brain stem reflexes, which include:

1. *Pupillary reaction to light*. This permits evaluation of the optic and oculomotor nerves, and the midbrain. However, even a head

injury of minimal severity may cause a temporary derangement of the pupils. If, however, repeated observations confirm the presence of a dilated pupil not reacting to light, it is highly suggestive of a secondary brain stem injury on the ipsilateral side, this sign being even more valuable if it is associated with external signs of damage on the same side as the pupillary changes.

2. *Corneal reflex.* This is absent if pontine damage has occurred.

3. *Oculocephalic reflex.* This consists of conjugate eye deviation contralateral to the direction of rotation of the head. This reflex depends on intact connections between the vestibular apparatus, the gaze centre in the pons, the brain stem nucleus of the 6th nerve located in the pons, and the 3rd nerve nucleus also in the pons. If the neck has been injured and rotation is impossible, the function of the pontine gaze centre and its connections with the 6th and 3rd cranial nerves can be evaluated by caloric testing – the oculovestibular reflex. In an unconscious patient the expected response to cold water injected into the auditory canal is conjugate deviation of the eyes towards the irrigated ear.

4. *Cough and gag reflexes* also provide assessment of medullary function.

In addition, a rising blood pressure suggests increasing cerebral compression. Similarly, a fall in the pulse rate, respiratory rate or hyperpyrexia all indicate brain stem damage.

Clinical diagnosis of secondary brain stem lesion

The clinical diagnosis of a secondary brain stem lesion is made on the evidence of a deteriorating conscious level, usually in association with developing lateralizing signs.

Causes of secondary brain stem lesions include:

1. *Extradural haematoma.* In the classical syndrome associated with an extradural haematoma the patient does not lose consciousness at the time of the initial injury or, having lost consciousness, rapidly regains it only to deteriorate slowly after a symptom-free interval. This so-called lucid interval is, however, present in only about 30% of patients who develop this complication. Extradural haematomata are rare in infants and older people.

2. *Acute subdural haematoma.* This is the commonest extracerebral intracranial lesion. The signs of an acute subdural haematoma usually appear within hours. They arise from the cortical veins torn as they traverse the subdural space and they are commonly associated

with severe brain contusion or lacerations, which complicate the subsequent management. Subdural haematomata are not infrequently bilateral. Symptoms develop when the layer of blood is 0.5–1 cm in thickness.

3. *Subarachnoid haemorrhage.* This occurs due to disruption of the small pia-arachnoid blood vessels and bridging vessels crossing the subarachnoid space.

4. *Contusion.* This is the most common parenchymal post-traumatic injury and consists of a mass of macerated haemorrhagic tissue, most commonly involving the superficial cortex.

5. *Intracerebral haemorrhage.* This complication is usually associated with other lesions. It complicates approximately 1% of closed head injuries and occurs in 10% of severely injured patients. This lesion is attended by a poor prognosis.

6. *Cerebral oedema.* This is always a manifestation of severe head injury. It appears shortly after the injury and causes a rapid deterioration in conscious level. If the oedema is unilateral, lateralizing signs will be present, whereas if it is generalized there will be no lateralizing signs, although signs of raised intracranial pressure will develop.

Investigations

Plain X-ray of the skull

It is customary to perform a plain X-ray of the skull in all head injuries and if injury to the neck is also suspected the cervical spine should be included. The positive information that may be obtained from a plain X-ray is as follows:

1. Fracture lines may be found. It is important to note the position of the lines and the involvement or otherwise of the paranasal sinuses. If the fracture is depressed this has considerable importance in regard to management.
2. The position of the pineal body. If this is calcified, a lesion of one side of the brain may produce shift.
3. The presence or absence of an aerocele. This lesion can only appear if the dura mater has been torn at the time of the initial injury and the fracture line communicates with a paranasal sinus.

Special investigations

Special investigations that have been used, but which have now been surpassed by the development of computerized axial tomography, include:

a. Arteriography.
b. Echoencephalography.
c. Intracranial pressure monitoring.

Intracranial pressure monitoring may be conducted by: insertion of ventricular catheters introduced via a burr hole; extradural catheters, which are also introduced via a burr hole, but recording may be difficult; or metallic devices, which are snuggly screwed into a small burr hole and can be used for either extradural or subdural pressure recordings and may be left in place for not longer than 10 days.

Whichever monitoring system is used, the catheter is normally connected to an external pressure transducer. The normal intracranial pressure is approximately 10 mmHg and any rise may indicate one of the complications listed above.

Computerized axial tomography

This investigation has completely revolutionized the evaluation and management of head injuries. The following are the chief findings:

1. *Subdural haematomas.* These may be found situated over the convexity of the cerebrum, in the interhemispheric fissure, and along the floor of the middle cranial fossa, and are quite commonly bilateral. Their appearance varies with their size, the time after injury, the haemoglobin level, the presence of membrane formation, and whether bleeding has recurred.

Their density decreases as a function of time and the attenuation coefficient is directly related to the haemoglobin concentration in the haematoma and more specifically to the protein component of the haemoglobin. The majority presenting within 7 days of the injury are hyperdense; isodensity is variously reported to occur within 30–90 days, in which case one must look for the secondary signs of the mass effect, including subfalcial shift, compression of the ipsilateral ventricle, pineal shift, or enfacement or medial displacement of the ipsilateral convexity sulci.

2. *Extradural bleeding* is rare and the commonest site is in the middle cranial fossa. Extradural bleeding tends to remains more localized than subdural bleeding because of the dural attachments.

3. *Brain contusion.* If the area affected is merely one of scattered petechial haemorrhage it may not be seen, but if somewhat larger a contusion appears as a homogeneous area of high or low absorption value.

4. *Intracerebral haematomas*. These appear as homogeneous, relatively rounded collections of increased density, the brain parenchyma being surrounded by a zone of low absorption representing the surrounding oedema and macerated tissue.

5. *Oedema*. This may result in a normal scan, in which case one must look for compression of the ventricles or cisterns.

OPERATIVE TREATMENT

When bleeding is suspected because of a deteriorating conscious level or the development of lateralizing signs, the skull should be explored by burr holes, even if its presence cannot be confirmed by investigation. In general, the first burr hole should be made over the site of any external injury or radiologically demonstrable fracture. If no such injury is apparent, temporal, frontal and occipital burr holes should be made.

The whole head should be prepared and draped. The temporal burr hole should be made 2.5 cm above the zygoma and 1.5–2.0 cm in front of the ear, the frontal burr hole in line with the pupil and 2.5 cm within the hairline, and the parietal burr hole over the point of maximum convexity of the skull.

Possible findings

An extradural clot is exposed as soon as the burr penetrates the inner table. If this space is dry, a bluish tense dura indicates the presence of subdural bleeding. If there is no discoloration but the dura is tense, there is either an intracerebral clot or cerebral oedema. To distinguish these two conditions the brain tissue should be explored with a brain needle.

Cerebral oedema

If the diagnosis of cerebral oedema has been made an attempt is commonly made to reduce the rise in intracranial pressure. In some centres this would be attempted by the use of mannitol and in others by the administration of frusemide. If mannitol is used it is administered intermittently intravenously in a 20% solution giving 0.5–1 g/kg. Attention is paid to the plasma osmolality, which should not be allowed to rise above 320 mosmol/l since if this occurs there is a considerable risk of renal damage or increasing cerebral oedema.

The use of dexamethasone 10 mg every 6 hours has proved of considerable value in the treatment of cerebral oedema associated with cerebral tumours but it does not appear to be effective in reducing the rising intracranial pressure associated with the severe oedema of a head injury.

Some centres also advocate the use of controlled hyperventilation with muscle paralysis and, in addition to measures used to control the intracranial pressure, would also administer hypnotic agents such as the barbiturates in order to reduce cerebral metabolism.

Communicating injuries

The risk of meningitis and/or cerebral abscess in the presence of an open injury is approximately 10% if there are no overt signs, and about 25% if there is rhinorrhoea.

For this reason sulphadiazine 4 g daily in divided doses together with ampicillin 250 mg four times daily, should be given.

Death following severe head injury

90% of all deaths from head injury occur within the first 7 days.

The criteria of brain death are as follows:

- Unconscious patient
- Fixed dilated pupils
- Absence of any spontaneous respiratory effort
- Absence of both superficial and deep reflexes
- Hypothermia
- Negative calorimetric test (performed by introducing ice-cold water into the external ear)
- Flat electroencephalogram.

LATE COMPLICATIONS

The ultimate result following any head injury is difficult to forecast. However, the duration of post-traumatic amnesia (PTA), i.e. the time from the injury until the patient has a clear, continuous memory of events, is of particular importance. In ascending order of severity based on the duration of PTA, head injuries can be classified as: very mild, PTA < 5 minutes; mild, PTA 5–60 minutes; moderate, PTA 1–24 hours; severe, PTA 1–13 days; or very severe, PTA beyond 14 days. Following very severe injuries in which the duration of post-traumatic amnesia extends over several weeks only a small percentage of patients will return to full employment, especially if the latter requires intense intellectual involvement.

Specific sequelae

Chronic subdural haematoma

When bleeding occurs into the subdural space the blood becomes surrounded by a fibrous membrane. As the erythrocytes break down so fluid is pulled into the haematoma by osmosis, causing an increase in volume of the space-occupying lesion. This may cause further bleeding from tears in the membrane or rupture of other traversing veins. Chronic subdural haematomas occur at any age but are commonest in infancy and old age. The causative injury may be so trivial that the patient does not recall it. The symptoms usually commence 4–6 weeks after the injury with deterioration of the mental state and level of consciousness. Simple drainage without removal of the membrane appears to be the treatment of choice.

Epilepsy

Early traumatic epilepsy, defined as epilepsy developing within 1 week of injury, is more frequent in children than in adults and may occur after comparatively trivial injuries. Adults, on the other hand, have early fits only after substantial brain damage, as evidenced by an associated depressed fracture, the development of a haematoma, or coma.

Late epilepsy developing after the first week can occur even in patients who have apparently made a good recovery, but it is more likely in patients who have (a) developed early epilepsy; or (b) suffered a depressed fracture, in which case the incidence of epilepsy is related to the duration of the post-traumatic amnesia, dural injury, focal signs or pre-existing early epilepsy.

In patients in whom neither a depressed fracture nor an intracranial haematoma has occurred the risk of epilepsy is low.

Cranial nerve injuries

The optic and olfactory nerves are the most commonly injured. The axons of the olfactory nerve occupy the foramina of the ethmoid bone on either side of the crista galli. Crossing the subarachnoid space the axons enter the olfactory bulb. The very thin structure of the cribriform plate predisposes to easy injury to the nerve fibres. Unfortunately loss of sense of smell also has an adverse effect on taste. Injury to the optic nerve leads to field defects, while injury to nerves governing eye movements may cause squint or double vision.

Hearing loss may occur as a result of damage to the auditory nerve as it passes through the temporal bone.

Facial palsy may also occur, due to damage to the nerve as it passes through the temporal bone.

Mental defects

These include changes in behaviour patterns, changes in personality and impaired cognitive performance. Measured by means of various tests, the score of some patients may be well within the limits set for the population as a whole but this may be far removed from the patient's own normal ability as assessed from his previous employment or performance.

In 1975 Jennett described the Glasgow Outcome Scale based on a survey of 1000 patients in whom the minimal severity of injury was measured by coma lasting at least 6 hours and a post-traumatic amnesia of at least 6 days. In this group of patients a 50% mortality occurred and of the remainder Jennet and his co-workers examined 150 survivors who were divided into four groups:

1. *Good recovery* – a group capable of normal physical and mental activity
2. *Moderately disabled* – a group independent but disabled
3. *Severely disabled* – a group conscious but dependent
4. *Vegetative state* – in which no evidence of meaningful response was apparent although spontaneous eye movements may occur.

The nature of the disabilities were classified as either physical or psychological, and Jennett and his coworkers found that the latter contributed the most to severe disability.

Another pertinent finding was that 90% of patients making a good recovery at 12 months had achieved maximal improvement at 6 months and that improvement beyond this period took place in only 10% of patients.

2. Skin grafting

CLASSIFICATION

Biological

According to their origin skin grafts may be classified as:

- Iso- or autografts when skin is removed from one part of the body to another in the same individual.
- Homo- or allografts when skin is transferred from one individual to another.
- Hetero or xenografts when skin is transferred from one species to another.

In the human an allograft can survive indefinitely only in certain biological situations:

Where the graft is between identical twins.
Where grafts are performed between genetic chimeras in whom a crossed placental circulation in utero leads to each pregnancy having a mixed cell population.
In patients suffering from agammaglobulinaemia.

The duration of survival and the speed of rejection of skin allografts varies in different species. In the rabbit, for example, skin allografts are abruptly rejected on or about the fifth day, the change in skin colouration and texture which marks rejection taking place within a few hours, whereas in the human the rejection phenomenon is a much more indolent process, slower to develop and less intense. A skin graft obtained from a close relative, e.g. mother, may not be rejected by her baby for as long as 300 days.

Anatomical

So far as iso- or autografts are concerned, these may be classified as:

17

- *Free*, indicating the graft is separated completely from its donor site before being transferred to the recipient area. The most commonly used free graft is of partial thickness but it is also possible to graft small areas of full thickness skin and skin plus other tissue as in the composite graft, e.g. a wedge-shaped segment of ear skin together with cartilage can be used to repair a defect in the nasal alar rim. The term 'free' can also be applied to full thickness grafts in which the blood supply is first 'cut off' and then immediately restored by the use of microvascular techniques.
- *Flap* or *pedicle* grafts, which may be subdivided according to their blood supply into:
  a. Random pattern skin flaps.
  b. Axial pattern flaps.

ADVANCES IN SKIN GRAFTING TECHNIQUE

Three significant advances in skin grafting technique have recently been made:

1. The development of *microvascular surgery* so that the vascular supply and in some cases the nerve supply of a free graft can be directly anastomosed to the corresponding structures in the recipient area.

2. The introduction of *myocutaneous flaps* based on the principle that in most regions of the body the skin derives its blood supply from multiple small blood vessels passing to the skin from the underlying muscle. Thus one may take an entire unit of muscle with its overlying fascia and skin anticipating that it will survive so long as there is a dominant vascular pedicle. Examples of myocutaneous flaps which have been used include gracilis, the upper part of trapezius, latissimus dorsi, the upper and lower segments of the rectus abdominis which can be used as island flaps, and the rectus femoris.

3. *Tissue expansion.* This technique, first described by Radovan, is based on the fact that skin and subcutaneous tissues will stretch under the influence of gradually increasing pressure, an obvious example being the abdominal skin of the pregnant woman. To simulate this state in reconstructive surgery a distensible plastic bag in a collapsed state is placed in the subcutaneous tissues as near as possible to the defect that requires closure. Over a period of several weeks the bag is slowly expanded by means of saline injected into a self-sealing reservoir, thus expanding the overlying skin. When sufficient expansion has been achieved the expander is removed and the adjacent defect closed by transposition of the expanded skin.

FREE SKIN GRAFTS

The thickness of a free graft can vary from partial to full thickness. Partial thickness grafts include the epidermis and a variable amount of dermis and such grafts can be subdivided into thin, medium and thick depending on the amount of dermis included in the graft, whereas full thickness grafts include the entire epidermis and the dermis.

Partial thickness grafts may be harvested from the surface of all the limbs and if necessary from the abdomen and chest wall thus allowing large areas to be covered. Full thickness free grafts are only applicable to the closure of small defects and in taking such grafts the surgeon must be aware that the donor defect must be closed by either suture of the resulting wound or by applying a partial thickness graft from another area.

It was once thought that partial thickness skin grafts must be taken through the level of the dermal–epidermal undulating interface so that small islands of the cells of the stratum germinativum would remain to re-epithelialize the denuded surface, but it has now been recognized that epithelial cells migrate out of the deep glands and hair follicles to heal the resulting defect.

Partial thickness grafts should not be used under the following circumstances:

a. When gross infection is present with either *Streptococcus pyogenes* or *Pseudomonas aeruginosa*.
b. On bone denuded of periosteum.
c. On tendon denuded of paratenon.
d. On cartilage denuded of perichondrium.
e. Areas denuded of skin as result of previous irradiation.

The advantages of a partial thickness graft are:

1. The thinner the graft, assuming that it is not wholly composed of the epidermis alone, the greater the percentage of 'take' which can be expected. The graft laid on the recipient site is cemented into position by plasma exuding from the surface of the wound, which coagulates to form fibrin. Endothelial loops then invade the graft and on or about the fourth or fifth day fibroblasts replace the layer of leucocytes at the graft–recipient interface. The vital period during which the life of the graft is in danger is between 2 and 5 days.
2. Any donor skin in excess of immediate requirements can be readily and easily stored in saline-soaked gauze for up to 3 weeks at a temperature of 4°C.

The disadvantages of thin partial thickness grafts are:

1. They are always abnormal in appearance and function since a degree of contracture and deformity occurs as they mature. In fact, as soon as the graft is separated from the donor site its area is reduced by almost 50% due to shortening of the elastic fibres and after 'take' secondary contraction can continue for as long as 6 months.
2. They can be rendered valueless in the presence of infection.
3. They tend to become pigmented on exposure to the sun.

In contrast, thick partial thickness grafts do not tend to contract so much but as with thin grafts tend to become pigmented, so their exposure to the sun should be also avoided.

Technique of cutting partial thickness grafts

A partial thickness graft can be cut by a variety of free-hand knives, or by a dermatome. Commonly used knives are the Watson and the Humby. The latter consists of a guarded disposable blade, which is pressed against the donor site and advanced with firm back-and-forth strokes. The guard can be adjusted to assist in determining the thickness of the graft.

The skin selected as the donor site is first lubricated and then flattened and kept taut between two flat boards. The operator normally holds one board in his left hand just in advance of the knife whilst the assistant exerts tension on the skin in the opposite direction. As the skin is removed, punctate bleeding ensues but if fat lobules appear in the donor site the pressure on the cutting edge is relaxed, the angulation of the blade adjusted or the instrument recalibrated.

The donor area can be reused, at least once, after 3 weeks, the interval before the second cut being determined by the initial thickness of the skin removed.

Technique of application

The dermal side of the graft must be in complete contact with the recipient area and if possible fixed in position by means of interrupted sutures, the long ends of which are tied firmly over proflavine wool lightly impregnated with paraffin or a synthetic foam stent cut to the required size. Normally a series of small puncture wounds are made in the graft to allow fluid under the graft to escape. If a greater area of coverage is required the graft can be 'meshed' by a series of parallel cuts which, when the graft is put under tension, open out to increase the surface area covered. Applied to a 'clean' donor site the wound should be left without inspection for some 5 to 6 days unless symptoms or signs of infection develop, e.g. local pain, swelling, odour, purulent discharge, or unexplained fever.

When grafts are applied to the lower limb the treated limb should be elevated for the first week, after which firm pressure with elastic bandages should be applied for up to 3 weeks.

The donor area should be carefully dressed to allow re-epithelialization to occur from the remaining sweat glands and hair follicles of the dermis.

FULL THICKNESS GRAFTS

These are composed of the total thickness of the skin. They may be free grafts or flap grafts.

Free grafts

Such grafts include the epidermis and all levels of the dermis. Favoured donor sites are the postauricular skin, the supraclavicular fossa, the naso-labial area, the submammary fold and the inguinal crease. When using such grafts all the subcutaneous tissues should be removed from their undersurface to ensure a successful take. Furthermore such grafts should be carefully shaped to exactly fit the defect they are designed to fill. Tie-over dressings should be applied to keep the graft firmly in place whilst the donor site is covered by a partial thickness graft.

Flap grafts

Skin flaps are classified according to their blood supply, into:

1. *Random pattern skin flaps.* In this type the flap receives its blood supply from segmental anastomotic or axial arteries which lie deep to the muscle sending perpendicular perforating musculo-cutaneous arteries at the flap base to the interconnecting dermal–subdermal plexus of the skin. The surviving length of such a flap is related to the vessels' perfusion pressure. Such flaps can be made somewhat longer by using delaying techniques described below.

2. *Axial pattern flaps.* These flaps receive their blood supply through a direct cutaneous artery arising from a segmental, anastomotic or axial artery, often by way of a short perforating artery. Such flaps include the iliofemoral island flap receiving its blood supply from the superficial circumflex iliac artery, the lateral forehead flap receiving its blood supply from the superficial temporal artery, and the deltopectoral island flap receiving its blood supply from the 2nd, 3rd and 4th perforating branches of the internal mammary artery, the term island indicating that such a flap is connected to its base by a direct cutaneous artery and vein but with no skin bridge. Also included in this group is the omental graft, which is sustained by the right and left gastroepiploic vessels.

The simplest form of a random pattern skin flap is the advancement flap (Fig. 2.1) which can be used where the soft tissues are loose and abundant and where the long axis of the wound corresponds to the lines of minimal tension, the edges of the wound are approximated without tension, sutures maintaining this position during healing. If an elliptical wound is situated in an area of the body in which the surrounding tissues are under tension, then approximation may be facilitated by undermining the skin edges of the wound through the subcutaneous tissues, thus releasing the superficial tissues from their deep attachments. The inherent elasticity of the skin permits a certain amount of advancement but under no circumstances should the flap formed by outlining three sides by means of incisions be stretched like a rubber band.

To facilitate advancement, triangles of skin may be excised at the base (as shown in Fig. 2.1), a method first described in 1838.

In contrast to mere advancement, flaps may be rotated, transposed or interpolated. All these various methods of closing a defect by means of a flap have in common a pivot point and an arc through which the flap is rotated. The simplest is the rotation flap (Fig. 2.2) which is frequently used to advance skin from the neck to the cheek. A rotation flap will normally stretch into a wound if the flap is so cut that the curvilinear perimeter is at least four times greater than the distance to be advanced. Advancement is facilitated by a back cut which is really the excision of the Burrow triangle.

The survival of all flaps depends on the meticulous control of the blood supply to the flap. At all times the blood supply should be adequate. The length of a flap in relation to its base depends to a large degree on the profuseness of the vascular supply in the area from which the flap has been fashioned. For example, in the facial

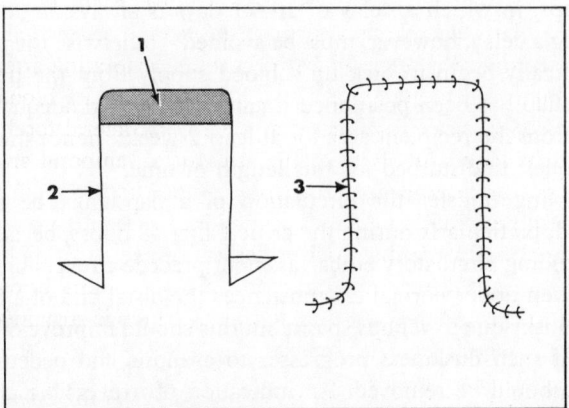

Fig. 2.1 Skin graft: forward advancement.
1, Skin defect; 2, Line of incision; 3, Finished effect.

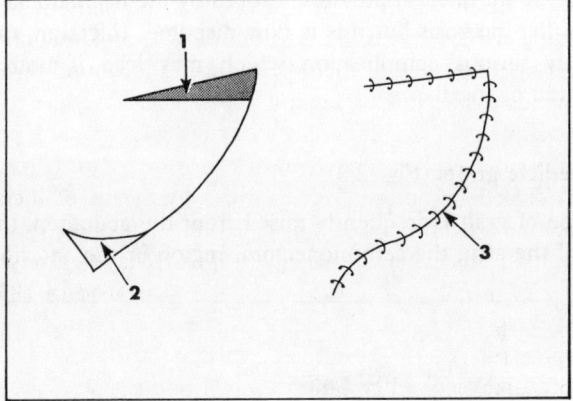

Fig. 2.2 Skin graft: rotation flap.
1, Skin defect; 2, Triangle excised; 3, Finished effect.

and cervical region a flap may be raised in which the length is three times the width whereas without delaying techniques a flap fashioned on the lower limb should be no longer than its width. The blood supply to a flap can be improved by *delaying* the flap. This is achieved by partially raising the flap from its bed and then replacing it in situ, a manoeuvre which ensures the flap obtains its blood supply from the pedicle and one particularly useful when dealing with lower limb flaps, in which a delay of 10–21 days is always an advantage. Too long a delay, however, must be avoided – otherwise the graft will automatically begin to pick up a blood supply from the periphery. Once a flap has been positioned it cannot obtain an adequate blood supply from the recipient area for at least 2 weeks, hence the pedicle must be left undisturbed for this length of time.

Following transfer the circulation of a flap must be carefully observed, particularly during the critical first 48 hours, because signs of impending circulatory embarrassment precede irreversible thrombosis. Even under normal circumstances the distal end of a flap may appear dusky due to venous spasm but this should improve over a few hours. If such duskiness progresses to cyanosis and oedema a few sutures should be removed. An indication of irreversible change is the development of a sharp line of demarcation caused most commonly by venous thrombosis rather than arterial insufficiency. Should a haematoma develop in a flap it must be immediately evacuated and haemostasis obtained. It was originally considered that the increase in 'internal pressure' caused by the haematoma was the cause of flap necrosis but this is now disputed. Infection, too, is an extremely serious complication which may lead if untreated to destruction of the flap.

Tube pedicle grafts (Fig. 2.3)

This type of graft is frequently raised from the abdomen, the inner aspect of the arm, the acromiopectoral region or the anterior aspect

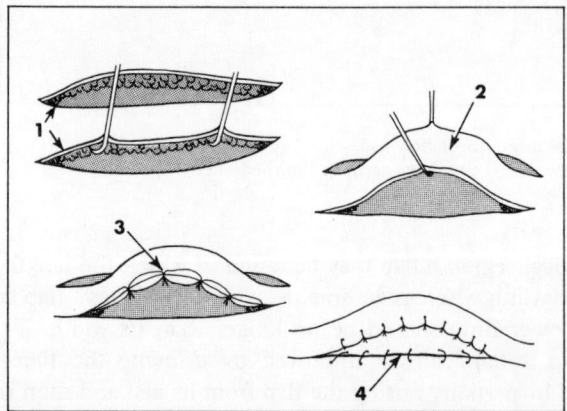

Fig. 2.3 Limits of pedicle graft construction (Gillies): 18 cm long if at least 5 cm wide.
1, Parallel incisions; 2, Flap raised; 3, Tube completed; 4, Skin defect closed.

of the thigh. In general the length of the tube should be not greater than twice its width at the time of its formation. Furthermore, the long axis of the tube must be parallel to the direction of cutaneous and subcutaneous vasculature. The advantages of a tube pedicle graft are its resistance to infection and the final cosmetic appearance of the recipient area.

The most important feature of a tubed pedicle graft is that it is the ideal way of delaying before transfer. Normally, movement of the tube should be carried out 3 or more weeks after its formation. Such a tube may be moved over considerable distances; for example, a tube raised on the abdomen can first be attached to the wrist and then brought down to the lower limb or upwards to the face. Because most people are right-handed the left wrist is normally used. The complications of a tube pedicle graft immediately after its formation are usually those asociated with haemorrhage; as with a recently positioned flap such a complication must be dealt with immediately, otherwise the viability of the tube may be compromised. If a haematoma develops in a tube it must be removed, otherwise it may severely compromise the blood supply of the tube and at worst cause necrosis.

Axial flaps

Axial flaps are better vascularized than random flaps and hence the length:base ratio plays less part in their construction.

The commonly used axial flaps are:

1. The forehead flap used to resurface intraoral defects.
2. The deltopectoral flap used to reconstruct head and neck wounds.
3. The groin flap used to cover hand and forearm wounds.
4. Omental grafts which can be used to fill a defect in the abdominal wall or chest. It is then itself covered by a split thickness graft.

Muscle flaps and myocutaneous flaps

A muscle flap consisting of pectoralis major was first used by Ombredonne of Paris in 1906 for the reconstruction of a breast, the muscle itself being covered by a partial thickness graft. However the use of myocutaneous flaps was not widely accepted until the mid-1970s.

Muscle flaps complete with their blood supply can be used to repair defects, covering the exposed muscle with a partial thickness skin graft. Thus the temporalis muscle, which can be detached from the side of the skull, can be used to reconstruct defects of the upper face, the muscle after detachment being rotated over the zygoma and into the orbit or an area of exposed dura, after which the skin graft is applied immediately.

Myocutaneous flaps are based on the principle that in most regions of the body the skin derives its blood supply from multiple small blood vessels passing to the skin from the underlying muscles. Thus one may take an entire unit of muscle with its overlying fascia and skin and expect it to survive as long as there is a dominant vascular pedicle.

The advantages associated with this type of flap are:

1. Transfer to the recipient site can be achieved at a single operation thus avoiding the repetitive operations necessary in the case of tube pedicles.
2. Since the transposed tissue is well-vascularized tissue it can be expected to survive in difficult situations, for example in areas where the blood supply has been jeopardized by previous irradiation.
3. If necessary a myocutaneous flap can incorporate a segment of bone for osseous reconstruction, e.g. a rib for reconstruction of the jaw.

The only disadvantages of muscle flaps and myocutaneous flaps are their possible bulk and absence of sensory innervation. So far as the former is concerned the bulk of such a flap rapidly diminishes with the passage of time, since detachment of a muscle from its origin or insertion leads to the almost immediate loss of 50% of its bulk, and with denervation almost complete atrophy occurs.

The commonly used myocutaneous flaps are derived from the pectoralis major, latissimus dorsi, the upper part of the trapezius, the rectus abdominis, tensor fascia lata and gastrocnemius.

Free flaps

The advent of microvascular techniques has made feasible the anastomosis of arteries and veins of 1 mm or even less in diameter, the anastomosis being performed with some 7–9 interrupted sutures of 10/0 nylon for the arterial and some 6–7 sutures for the venous. However, since both continuing experience of microvascular techniques is required, free flaps have a limited use. However, the technique is applicable not only to skin but also to muscle bellies which are supplied by a specific artery and drained by a specific vein, as for example the latissimus dorsi.

3. Blood transfusion and haematological conditions of special interest to the surgeon

BLOOD TRANSFUSION

The hazards associated with blood transfusion are fortunately rare. Some which were previously commonplace, such as thrombophlebitis and sepsis at the site of administration, have disappeared as disposable plastics have replaced rubber donor sets. Similarly, air embolus, once an ever present danger when bottled blood was used, has also disappeared due to the use of plastic bags.

Prior to any blood transfusion, however urgent, blood should be taken for cross-matching. If a very urgent transfusion is required Group O blood can be given, followed as rapidly as possible by ABO RhD group specific blood. In a woman of childbearing age RhD negative blood should be used from the start. The replacement of Group O with ABO group specific blood is made in order to minimize the volume of Group O plasma. ABO and RhD matched blood can be given following the completion of emergency grouping and an immediate spin-saline cross-match against the recipient's serum.

Specific hazards

Overtransfusion

The circulation can easily be overloaded by too great a volume of tranfused blood in the neonate with a relatively small blood volume, or in a patient suffering from cardiopulmonary disease. When a patient is grossly anaemic and surgical intervention is imperative, blood with a packed cell volume of 65-75% should be used within 24 hours of the removal of the excess plasma.

Overtransfusion results in heart failure and the development of pulmonary oedema and, later, peripheral oedema.

Prevention. This complication can be avoided by continuous monitoring of the central venous pressure. When pulmonary oedema inadvertently occurs during or soon after a transfusion, it should be treated by diuretics and aminophylline and, if necessary, venesection.

Febrile response

A febrile response to blood transfusion is still relatively common although the use of disposable plastics and filters has reduced their incidence and severity.

The causes of a febrile response are:

1. Transfusion of incompatible blood.
2. After multiple transfusions, the development of antibodies to platelet, white cell or plasma protein fractions.
3. Use of infected blood.

In patients in whom repeated transfusions are required a small dose of hydrocortisone and chlorpheniramine will reduce the response.

Incompatible transfusion

Cause. An incompatible blood transfusion occurs when:

a. Donor cells are administered to a recipient whose plasma contains isoantibodies capable of damaging them. This is the typical 'mismatched' transfusion that may be due to technical error or poor labelling of donor blood or recipient.
b. Donor blood itself contains sufficient antibodies to haemolyse recipient cells.
c. Red cells of reduced viability, usually due to poor storage conditions, are administered.

Any of these situations leads to haemolysis, which may be intravascular if brought about by antibodies that are haemolytic in vitro, or extravascular when caused by antibodies that cannot haemolyse in vitro.

Intravascular haemolysis leads to an increase in the circulating haemoglobin, which is bound by the plasma protein, haptoglobin, until the amount exceeds 100 mg/100 ml, after which the excess circulates in the bloodstream and is excreted in the urine. Haem separated from the haemoglobin molecule combines with albumin to form methaemalbumin.

Clinical syndrome. *Symptoms.* An incompatible blood transfusion usually gives rise to symptoms within 20 minutes. A feeling of warmth may spread up the limb into which the transfusion is being administered, followed by rigors, flushing and fever. Tightness develops in the chest and severe hypotension may occur. The cause of the constricting pain in the chest is unknown but two explanations have been advanced: first, that agglutinates block the pulmonary blood vessels; second, that histamine-like substances constrict the pulmonary vessels and bronchioles.

Renal effects. The effect of a mismatched transfusion on the kidney depends upon its condition before the transfusion. Organic renal disease or the presence of gross physiological disturbance produced by severe dehydration, hypovolaemia, hypotension or anoxaemia may result in haemoglobin or its degradation products producing a severe renal lesion.

Although haemoglobin itself may block the tubules, a major factor causing renal damage appears to be the stroma of the damaged red cells. There is an antigen–antibody reaction in the kidney which produces renal ischaemia, later followed by renal failure.

Transmission of diseases

Hepatitis B. Hepatitis B is conveyed by blood transfusion and has an incubation period of 50–180 days (cf. 15–20 days for Hepatitis A, otherwise known as infectious hepatitis, which is chiefly spread by contaminated water and food, notably shellfish). Infection with hepatitis B virus leads to the presence of several antigens in the serum: the Dane particle is probably the complete virus – both surface and core particles – hepatitis B surface antigen (HB_sAg), and hepatitis core antigen (HB_cAg). There is also a fourth, HB_eAg, whose presence strongly indicates that the acute condition may progress to a chronic hepatitis and cirrhosis with all its attendant complications.

HB_cAg can be detected in the serum before hepatitis is clinically suspected but 80–90% of patients clear the antigen from the blood within 2 months of the disease. In the remainder the antigen persists to be associated with a chronic active hepatitis, and in 1–2% eventual cirrhosis develops. For this reason all blood is now tested for the antigen and, if found positive, is discarded. The Australia antigen has gained a sinister reputation in dialysis units, but its significance is probably related to the diminished resistance to infection of patients requiring dialysis, and the exposure of staff to large quantities of blood. Nevertheless, stringent precautions to prevent contamination with blood from patients requiring dialysis should be taken.

Cytomegalovirus (CMV). The virus is named from the histological appearance of the infected cells, which become large and contain a large intranuclear inclusion. CMV is a major cause of congenital abnormalities, producing cytomegalic inclusion disease. The virus was isolated in 1956 from human embryonic fibroblasts. Its replication produces a variety of abnormalities, including hepatitis, chorioretinitis and progressive sensorial deafness. The baby may be born with hepatomegaly and prolonged jaundice.

Acquired immune deficiency disease (AIDS). This condition is due to the retrovirus human T-cell lymphotrophic virus, which specifically attacks and destroys OKT4 (helper) T-cells. Three-quarters of all cases of AIDS in the UK occur in homosexual or bisexual men, but other groups at risk are intravenous drug users and patients transfused with infected blood. In recent years a number of haemophiliacs in the UK were infected by contaminated factor VIII obtained from the US.

Progress from asymptomatic carriage of HIV to AIDs has been associated with a depletion of the helper T-cell population and other abnormalities in the numbers of immunocompetent cells and their functions.

The presenting picture of AIDS itself is varied but may consist of:

1. Several months of general malaise associated with loss of weight.
2. Pneumonia caused by the multiflagellate protozoa, *Pneumocystis carinii*, complicated by infection with other opportunistic infections.
3. Generalized lymphadenopathy.
4. Kaposi's sarcoma, otherwise known as multiple idiopathic haemorrhagic sarcoma. Particularly on the distal parts of the lower limbs bluish red nodules develop, which may lead to lymphoedema and may ulcerate.
5. Oropharyngeal candidiasis.

In 1000 cases of AIDS in New York the median survival time was 35 weeks in patients with AIDS and Kaposi's sarcoma, 61 weeks in those with Kaposi's sarcoma and pneumocystis pneumonia, and 125 weeks in those with pneumocystis pneumonia alone.

Malaria. The malarial parasite is able to survive for days or weeks in blood stored at 4°C. Therefore, the only positive way to prevent transmission is to avoid using as blood donors any person who has lived in an endemic area or to screen donors carefully.

Syphilis. Spirochaetes cannot survive at blood-bank temperatures of 2–6°C for longer than 3–5 days. This alone reduces the incidence of transfusion syphilis. In addition, blood is routinely tested by one or other of the serological techniques, although this is not necessarily a complete safeguard because about 35% of individuals suffering from primary syphilis are seronegative.

Transfusion for massive blood loss

Definition

A massive transfusion is arbitrarily defined as the transfusion of a volume in excess of the patient's own blood volume in less than 24 hours. If immediate transfusion is not available, prolonged hypotension may result predisposing to the development of intravascular coagulation and ARDS (see vol. 1, p. 133). Patients with severe head injuries may also be at risk of cerebral oedema if the plasma oncotic pressure has been allowed to fall excessively.

Problems

Thrombocytopenia. Blood stored for more than a few days is devoid of functioning platelets and because of this a dilutional thrombocytopenia may occur, although clinical problems do not arise until at least 1.5 blood volumes have been transfused (7–8 l in an adult). Platelet counts should be maintained above $50 \times 10^9/l$ to achieve effective haemostasis when platelet function is normal.

Coagulation factor deficiency. Although theoretically possible, this situation is uncommon because stored blood contains adequate quantities of all the coagulation factors except Factors V and VIII, which decay during storage, but Factor VIII is rapidly synthesized and released in patients subjected to trauma and stress. If disordered haemostasis develops it is much more likely to be due to the onset of disseminated intravascular coagulation.

Hypocalcaemia. The citrate of anticoagulant fluids binds ionized calcium and potentially lowers the plasma calcium level. This is a lesser problem, however, than might be expected on theoretical grounds because a healthy adult can metabolize citrate at a rate equal to 1 unit of blood transfused every 5 minutes. The major consequences of a lowered calcium level are due to its synergism with a high potassium level; together they may produce disturbances of cardiac function. If the ECG suggests hypocalcaemia is developing 5 ml of 10% calcium gluconate should be given at 5-minute intervals until the ECG changes are reversed.

Hyperkalaemia. The plasma potassium content of stored blood increases so that concentrations as high as 30 mmol/l may be reached, but in practice hyperkalaemia is not a common problem as long as renal function is normal or rapidly returns to normal.

Acid-base disturbance. Since red cell glycolysis produces lactic acid the arterial pH should be monitored. However, normally the acidosis of the hypoxic shocked patient is generally relieved by transfusion because of the improved tissue perfusion.

Hypothermia. When blood is transfused at greater volumes than 1 unit every 10 minutes, the blood should be warmed as hypothermia slows citrate metabolism, potentiates the harmful cardiac effects of hyperkalaemia and a low calcium level, and reduces oxygen release from haemoglobin. If blood is not immediately available, the following may be of assistance after taking a sample for cross-matching: Ringer lactate solution, synthetic colloids or 4.5% human albumin. All are valuable alternatives. Platelet concentrates are indicated if the platelet count is falling below $50 \times 10^9/l$, and fresh frozen plasma provides a broad spectrum of coagulation factors.

HAEMATOLOGICAL CONDITIONS OF SPECIAL INTEREST TO THE SURGEON

Haemophilia

Until the work of Bullock and Fildes in 1911 the term haemophilia was used to describe any inherent haemorrhagic condition. In 1936 Patek and Taylor demonstrated that the essential factor missing from the blood was associated with neither platelets nor fibrinogen.

The condition is normally inherited as a sex-linked recessive characteristic, the male exhibiting the disease and the female acting as a carrier and transmitting the disease to the next generation. The female heterozygote is usually unaffected because she is protected by the normal allele on her second X chromosome. In the male, however, the heterozygote is affected since the Y does not carry the allele. The disease may occur in the female, but only following the mating of an affected with a female carrier. Approximately one-third of all cases occur in the absence of a family history, suggesting that spontaneous mutation may occur.

Haematological defect

The essential haematological defect in haemophilia is a deficiency in the procoagulant activity of Factor VIII, which can be as low as 1-2% of normal. A protein recognized immunologically as 'Factor VIII-related antigen' is always present but without coagulant activity. A similar deficiency in Factor IX causes the much rarer Christmas disease, sometimes called haemophilia B to distinguish it from the classical haemophilia, often referred to as haemophilia A. The latter is ten times commoner than the former but it is still a rare condition affecting only about 6 in 100 000 of the population, hence about 3000 cases exist in the United Kingdom.

A third variant is von Willebrand's disease, a condition in which both sexes are equally affected and in which the bleeding time is prolonged because of a platelet defect accompanied by abnormal platelet adhesion and aggregation plus a Factor VIII deficiency.

Severity of haemophilia

The severity of haemophilia is determined by measurement of the reduced Factor VIII activity. In families in which many members are involved the severity of the condition appears to be the same in all those affected.

The unit of measurement used to assess the disease is the international unit of Factor VIII; one international unit is based on the activity of 1 ml of average fresh normal plasma, also described as having 100% activity. In a normal individual, Factor VIII activity varies from 60-75% of the mean. Individuals with levels of 26-40% are, in practice, unlikely to bleed unless subjected to major surgery or trauma; 6-25% indicates mild haemophilia with a tendency to bleed only if injured. If, however, the level reaches 1-5%, bleeding will follow minor trauma and haemarthroses are likely; below this level the disease is particularly severe and spontaneous bleeding can be expected.

Symptomatology and pathological features

Haemophilia is commonly diagnosed in early childhood when either excessive bruising or persistent bleeding following minor injury is usually the presenting feature. In more severe forms of the condition deep painful haematomas develop. In the neck such an episode may produce asphyxia and in the soft tissues in general the regional vascular or nervous supply may be compromised by the increase in tissue tension. Severe bleeding followed by organization and fibrosis ultimately leads to deformity, e.g. in the lower limb an equinus deformity may follow bleeding into the posterior compartment and in the upper limb a Volkmann's contracture may follow bleeding into the forearm.

Bleeding into joints is also a characteristic feature of severe haemophilia. Severe pain may occur due to stretching of the joint capsule, and a large haemarthrosis will be extremely painful, tender to touch, and swollen and warm; therefore, in the absence of any previous history, the condition must be distinguished from a septic arthritis. Blood mixed with synovial fluids acts as an irritant to the synovial membrane with the result that, eventually, when large quantities of haemosiderin have been deposited in the subsynovial tissues, a reactive granulation tissue develops and forms a pannus, which gradually extends over and absorbs the articular cartilage. At the same time the deposition of iron in the cartilage itself leads to degeneration, the cartilage becoming soft and yellowish and unable to withstand stress. This results in breakdown and irregularity of the cartilage, which develops a map-like appearance, and the subchondral cortex tends to thin out and form cysts. The hyperaemia in the growth period causes enlargement of the epiphyses of the affected joints, commonly in an asymmetrical fashion, so that gross deformities develop. The overall rate of growth may be either increased or retarded. In addition to actual haemarthroses, subperiosteal haemorrhages may lead to pseudo-tumours. Ill-advised aspiration, biopsy of either joint or haematoma may lead to infection. The joints most commonly affected are the knees, ankles, elbows, and hips in that order, and while the acute stage may last for days or weeks the chronic synovitis that follows the haemarthrosis may persist for weeks or months.

When considering the alleviation of pain in the haemophiliac it must be remembered that many of the common analgesics and antiinflammatory drugs inhibit platelet aggregation and prolong bleeding time, hence the use of aspirin to prevent deep venous thrombosis. Thus, aspirin and indomethecin should be avoided and the relief of pain sought in pentazocine, or in one of the narcotic group of drugs if the pain is very severe.

Retroperitoneal bleeding also occurs and may follow mild abdominal trauma or even strenuous exercise. The ability of the retroperitoneal space to hold large quantities of blood may result in the development of haemorrhagic shock and the appearance of

Cullen's or Grey Turner's signs, both of which are commonly associated with acute haemorrhagic pancreatitis or a ruptured abdominal aortic aneurysm.

Diagnosis

The diagnosis of haemophilia should always be suspected in a patient with a bleeding tendency and a classical family history in whom the platelet count and the bleeding and prothrombin time are normal. Further investigation will show that the activated partial prothrombin time is prolonged and that reduced levels of Factors VIII or IX are present.

Treatment

The indications for surgical intervention in the haemophiliac are precisely the same as in a normal individual except for those patients in whom antibodies to Factor VIII have developed due to previous treatment. Basically, should the haemophiliac suffer a major bleed or require surgery then the defective level of AHG should be made good by replacement therapy so that the level exceeds the 30% level. It was first demonstrated in 1955 that the condition could be controlled by the use of fresh blood or plasma, 1000 ml of the latter raising the AHG from 0 to 15%. However, following the administration of a given dose of Factor VIII, approximately half of the initial post-transfusion activity disappears from the plasma within 4 hours. This disappearance is thought to be due for the most part to diffusion from the intravascular space. The period of equilibration extends for about 8 hours, after which only about 25% of the initial level remains. Thereafter the slope is less steep, but after 24 hours only about 10% of the administered activity remains.

One unit of Factor VIII activity is defined as that amount present in 1 ml of fresh normal plasma, and is expressed as a percentage in that 100 IU/100 ml = 100%, although the range of normal varies from 40–180%. Thus, assuming that the initial concentration of AHG was zero, to achieve a level of 30% of normal, using fresh plasma, a volume of plasma equal to 30% of the estimated plasma volume would be needed and, because of the natural loss already described, at least half of the initial volume would need to be administered every 12 hours. Such volumes are excessive, and the use of fresh plasma or fresh frozen plasma has now been replaced by the use of cryoprecipitate or AHG concentrate. Cryoprecipitation was developed from observing that a cold precipitate of plasma was rich in AHG. Fresh plasma is snap frozen and then thawed at 4°C, when a stringy precipitate, the cryoprecipitate, is left in the plasma. This contains appproximately 50% of the AHG of the original material but still contains very variable amounts of AHG.

The supernatant plasma is removed and the cryoprecipitate is then frozen. AHG concentrate in a lyophilized state is the material of choice administered by most haemophilia authorities to haemophiliac patients bleeding or requiring major surgery. It has the advantage over cryoprecipitate in that the amount of AHG administered is known exactly, as the batches of AHG concentrate have been assayed for Factor VIII content. These materials come in vials containing about 250 units of Factor VIII and are stable for many months at 4°C. For use, the material is dissolved in 10–20 ml of sterile water, enabling effective haemostatic doses to be injected in a small volume.

The formula for the amount of Factor VIII to be administered, as recommended by Biggs, is as follows:

$$\text{Total units of Factor VIII required} = \frac{\text{weight (kg)} \times \text{desired Factor VIII rise (\%)}}{k}$$

where $k = 1.5$. (The same formula may be used for Factor IX, in which case $k = 1.7$.)

The dose required and the frequency with which it should be given are determined by the type of operation, the weight of the patient, and the fact that half-life of Factor VIII is about 12 hours. In a surgical setting, the initial level of Factor VIII should first be assayed so that adequacy of the calculated dose can be determined and throughout the course of treatment the assay should be repeated at intervals. The aim of treatment, particularly if the patient is to undergo major surgery, is to obtain an initial plasma level above 0.8 IU/ml (80% of normal) and then maintain the level above 40% for about 7–10 days by repeated administration of AHG at 12-hourly intervals.

Complications of therapy

　1. Serum hepatitis.
　2. Development of inhibitors that neutralize AHG activity. Their presence should be suspected when an apparently adequate dose of Factor VIII raises the plasma level only slightly, transiently, or not at all. Various workers have found the incidence of inhibitors

to be 5-21%. Their development makes treatment of the individual exceedingly complicated, if not impossible.

Bovine and porcine preparations have also been used, but these also stimulate antibody formation in the majority of patients. Should, however, antibodies to human AHG be present in a life-threatening situation animal preparations can be used. Recent reports suggest that activated Factor IX concentrates are of considerable value when high concentrations of inhibitor prevent the use of AHG. The basis of such therapy is that these concentrates contain certain activated factors which may bypass the point of action of Factor VIII in the haemostatic process and thus make the presence of antibody of no consequence.

3. Allergic reactions. These also are relatively rare. The reaction usually occurs during or within 1-2 hours. The symptoms may consist of headaches, backache, urticaria, rigor, fever and tightness in the chest and, rarely, pulmonary oedema. Minor reactions may be treated by antihistamines, and major reactions accompanied by bronchospasm with subcutaneous adrenaline and intravenous hydrocortisone.

4. Acquired immune deficiency syndrome (see p. 30)

Factor IX deficiency (Christmas disease, haemophilia B)

Christmas disease is clinically indistinguishable from Factor VIII deficiency and was recognized only in 1952. It is, however, a much less common condition than Factor VIII deficiency and affects only approximately 1 per 1 000 000 of the population. Like haemophilia A, Christmas disease is inherited as a sex-linked recessive characteristic; it mimics haemophilia A so closely that it can be differentiated only by a direct assay of Factor IX.

Recently, Factor IX concentrates have become available in most haemophiliac centres for clinical use.

Von Willebrand's disease

This condition, first described by von Willebrand in the inhabitants of the Aland Islands in the Baltic Sea, has aroused considerable interest.

The disease is inherited as an autosomal dominant trait and, therefore, appears in consecutive generations affecting both males and females equally.

Clinical presentation and pathology

The condition is characterized by bleeding from mucous membranes, haemarthroses, and postoperative haemorrhage.

The three abnormal haematological features are a prolonged bleeding time, reduced platelet adhesiveness, and a diminished Factor VIII activity which, although always present, is never as great as in classic haemophilia. Also, whereas in the latter the AHG level, whatever its concentration, tends to remain constant, in patients with von Willebrand's disease it seems to vary appreciably from time to time. Similarly, although a prolonged bleeding time is nearly always present it, too, various considerably.

Aetiology and treatment

Von Willebrand's disease is due to a deficiency of 'Factor VIII-related antigen'. In this disease, once this factor is transfused into a patient, he or she can then produce Factor VIII procoagulant activity. Within 4–6 hours post-transfusion, the activity of Factor VIII can rise by a factor of 5–8 and this synthesis may continue for a period of 25 hours. This response can be obtained even following the transfusion of haemophiliac plasma because the haemophiliac has the 'Factor VIII-related antigen'. In summary, therefore, haemophilia A has a reduced procoagulant activity but the Factor VIII-related antigen is normal, whereas in von Willebrand's disease the procoagulant activity is normal but the Factor VIII-related antigen is reduced.

Bleeding associated with liver disease

Complex changes in the haemostatic mechanism occur in liver disease. The liver is the site of all protein production, with the exception of the immunoglobulins. Therefore in liver failure the biosynthesis of fibrinogen, vitamin K-dependent factors – factors V, VIII–C, XI, XII and XIII – as well as plasminogen and various inhibitors, is reduced or ceases.

In severe liver disease haemostatic defects characteristic of DIC may be found, possibly due to necrotic hepatocytes being a source of procoagulants and the failure of the reticuloendothelial cells of the liver to clear endotoxins derived from the gut.

To the gastrointestinal surgeon, however, the most common disturbance causing difficulty is the presence of *obstructive jaundice*.

Absence of bile salts from the lumen of the small intestine leads to failure of absorption of the fat-soluble vitamin K, with the result that the synthesis of vitamin K-dependent factors is blocked. The low plasma levels of these factors causes a marked prolongation of the prothrombin time which must be corrected prior to operation by the parenteral administration of vitamin K_1 (phytomenadione).

In patients suffering from *severe liver disease* such as hepatic necrosis or severe alcoholic cirrhosis, not only the vitamin K-dependent factors but also Factor V and the fibrinogen level may be disturbed. Such patients represent a severe haemostatic risk and require not only vitamin K but also fresh blood, fresh frozen plasma, and platelet concentrates.

Disseminated intravascular coagulation (DIC)

Synonyms: defibrination, consumption coagulopathy, intravascular coagulation with fibrinolysis and abnormal proteolytic activity.

This condition is associated with breakdown of all haemostatic mechanisms, i.e. the vessel walls, platelets, coagulation sequence, fibrinolytic mechanisms, inhibitors, kinin and complement systems.

Pathogenesis

Disseminated intravascular coagulation develops when the coagulation mechanism is activated within the circulation. The effects are catastrophic only when certain modifying factors, the most important of which are blockage of the reticuloendothelial system, pregnancy or liver disease, are also present. The severe disorder of the whole haemostatic mechanism results in the consumption of coagulation factors, platelets, the activation of fibrinolysis and lastly, fibrin deposition in the microcirulation which leads to multiple organ failure. The depletion of the various coagulation factors and platelets leads in severe cases to a bleeding tendency.

The major mechanisms which trigger intravascular coagulation are:

1. The direct activation of prothrombin (Factor II) or Factor X (the Stuart-Prower factor) by proteolytic enzymes, commonly by amniotic fluid embolism, acute pancreatitis and certain snake venoms.

2. Activation of the Hageman factor (Factor XII) and the intrinsic system by conditions leading to widespread endothelial damage as in anoxia, acidosis, viraemia and situations in which antigen-antibody complexes are present in the circulation.

3. Activation of the extrinsic system following the release of tissue thromboplastin, commonly by massive injury, septicaemia and the presence of necrotic tumours.

All the cellular elements of the blood play an important part in triggering intravascular coagulation. Endotoxins are potent destroyers of leucocytes which are a source of a procoagulant material with the properties of tissue thromboplastin. Red cell stroma released by the destruction of erythrocytes also has potent thromboplastic activity and thus may trigger coagulation in acute haemolytic states. Platelet damage may provoke intravascular clotting although these elements are not necessary to the production of DIC since experimentally the syndrome can be produced in thrombocytopenic animals.

In a normal individual any activated clotting factors or fibrin monomer complexes are removed by the reticuloendothelial system which can also, if functioning normally, remove a triggering mechanism such as the endotoxin of Gram-negative shock.

In severe cases of disseminated intravascular coagulation the following changes take place within the circulation:

1. The concentration of fibrinogen, prothrombin and factors V, VIII-C, XIII, and to a lesser extent X is reduced. Fibrinogen and factors V and VIII: C may be virtually absent with partial degradation of prothrombin and reduced levels of plasma prothrombin.

2. Degradation and precipitation of fibrin occurs and soluble fibrin–fibrinogen complexes can be found within the circulating blood.

3. Fibrin deposition, the site and extent of which depends upon several interrelated features. These include thrombin–fibrinogen and plasmin–fibrin interactions, the stage of the condition and various factors affecting the localization of the fibrin deposition.

4. Secondary fibrinolysis. This again depends upon a variety of factors, e.g. the trigger which initiates intravascular coagulation may itself activate the fibrinolytic sequence, the activated form of Factor XII induces fibrinolysis simultaneously with activation of the intrinsic pathway. Proteases, other than plasmin, derived from damaged cells may produce fibrinolysis.

The disorganized haemostatic mechanism in disseminated intravascular coagulation causes:

1. *A bleeding tendency* due to the consumption of coagulation factors, platelets and the effects of secondary fibrinolysis. If a patient develops a severe bleeding tendency the mortality reaches 100%,

while moderate or minimal bleeding is associated with a mortality of 50%. The bleeding may arise from puncture sites, it may be the result of severe bruising, or it may come from a wound, a peptic ulcer or the uterus.

2. *Multiple organ damage.* This is caused by either bleeding or intravascular clotting, or by a combination of both factors.

a. Because of the rich microvasculature of the kidney which enables it to act as an efficient sieve, acute renal failure may occur.
b. The deposition of fibrin thrombi in the capillary and venules of the dermis causes a variety of skin lesions including petechiae, purpura, gangrene and acrocyanosis. In a classical lesion the affected vessel and the surrounding tissues exhibit necrosis and haemorrhage without accompanying inflammation.
c. Pulmonary lesions leading to the adult respiratory distress syndrome, otherwise known as shock lung. The bases of the pathological changes in the lung which may lead to severe disturbances of pulmonary physiology are, first, the deposition of platelet-rich microthrombi which, following the destruction of the platelets, leads to the formation of fibrin-rich thrombi. At a later stage still, hyaline membranes are deposited both intravascularly and extravascularly in the alveoli and ductuli alveolares. Pulmonary bleeding may also occur leading to increasing respiratory failure and haemoptysis.
d. Disturbance of the central nervous system, due to thrombosis causing focal ischaemia or bleeding, leading to more severe disturbance.
e. Red cell fragmentation within the loose fibrin network which is deposited may cause severe anaemia, so-called microangiopathic anaemia.

Clinical presentation

The most common initial presentation of disseminated intravascular coagulation is bleeding, which varies in severity according to the underlying cause of the condition. Thus septicaemia, severe shock, extensive injury and burns nearly always present with severe bleeding whereas less severe bleeding may occur in chronic DIC in which thrombotic manifestations may predominate, as in disseminated malignancy or liver disease. Should the patient survive the immediate crisis, in severe cases multiple organ failure may develop followed by oliguria or pulmonary distress.

Diagnosis

The diagnosis of disseminated intravascular coagulation is confirmed by various measures of coagulation, the most important of which are:

1. *Platelet count* (normal, $150-400 \times 10^9/l$) is grossly reduced.
2. *Prothrombin time* (normal, 13–16 s) is prolonged due to the consumption of Factor V.
3. *Activated partial thromboplastin time* (normal, 32–46 s) is prolonged due to the consumption of Factor VIII.
4. *Fibrinogen* (normal, 2–4 g/l) is reduced by virtue of its breakdown by plasmin. This results in the appearance of fibrin degradation products (normal, <5 µg/ml); extremely high concentrations occur in DIC.
5. *Thrombin time* (normal, 13–17 s) is prolonged due to the reduction in fibrinogen.

In addition the density of the clot is poor. Once the diagnosis is established the course of the disease can be monitored by remeasuring the various parameters described.

Treatment

See volume 1, page 162.

Idiopathic thrombocytopenic purpura

In this condition spontaneous symptoms rarely occur if the platelet count is $>50 \times 10^9/l$, but purpura due to minor trauma may occur if the platelet count is $30-50 \times 10^9/l$. Severe bruising usually reflects a count below $30 \times 10^9/l$. Severe bleeding from mucosal surfaces is rare unless the count is less than $5-10 \times 10^9/l$, or patients are on medication which diminishes platelet function, such as aspirin.

The condition can be rectified by giving immune globulin, which blocks the reticuloendothelial system: 4 g/kg/day for 5 days produces a rapid response.

In 70% of patients suffering from ITP complete remission occurs after splenectomy and an additional 10% will achieve safer platelet counts, i.e. greater than $30 \times 10^9/l$.

Sickle cell anaemia

Sickle cell syndromes are due to the inheritance of a gene producing a structurally abnormal β-globin chain subunit.

HbS can be found in the heterozygous state (HbAs or sickle cell trait), or in the homozygous state (HbSS, sickle cell anaemia or sickle cell disease).

The condition is most prevalent in black persons of Africa or North Americans of negro ancestry, but it also occurs in Mediterraneans, Greeks, Scandinavians and Indians. The highest gene frequency is in equatorial Africa, where it confers some protection against malaria.

The sickle cell syndromes result from the aggregation of HbS molecules inside the erythrocytes, which causes the red cell to be much less deformable and therefore alters flow characteristics. This results in:

1. Chronic and progressive tissue damage.
2. Acute, painful vaso-occlusive crises.
3. Chronic haemolytic anaemia.

Polymerization only occurs when the HbS molecule is in the deoxy conformation; when HbS is in the oxy conformation it has essentially normal physicochemical properties.

The common screening test used to diagnose this condition, which should be performed in all the above groups, is to mix the blood with a solution of sodium metabisulphate. The latter totally deoxygenates the blood and induces sickling, which can be seen under the microscope.

4. The 'surgical' parasites

HYDATID DISEASE

Geographical distribution

The highest incidence of this disease occurs in those geographical areas that are most densely populated by the intermediate host of the parasite, the sheep. This disease, therefore, is most commonly found in Australia, New Zealand and southern Africa. In Britain, the disease is somewhat commoner in Wales than elsewhere.

Causal agents

Hydatid disease is caused by the tapeworms, *Echinococcus granulosus* and *E. multilocularis*. The latter, which is much less common, is found only in the colder climatic conditions of Alaska and Russia, and neither can infect man in any area unless personal hygiene is substandard.

Life cycle (Fig. 4.1)

Man is infected by the worm only by accident since the natural cycle is between the dog and the sheep, the latter acting as the intermediate host. This natural cycle stems from the domestic dog eating sheep offal contaminated by hydatid cysts. The scolices within the cysts adhere to the wall of the small intestine and develop into the adult tapeworm, which consists of only four segments including the head on which are two rows of hooklets and four sucking pads. These enable the worm to adhere to the wall of the bowel. An adult worm is 3–5 mm in length and the gravid terminal segments are shed by the worm (Fig. 4.2). The dog's faeces adhere to its fur and generally contaminate the environment.

45

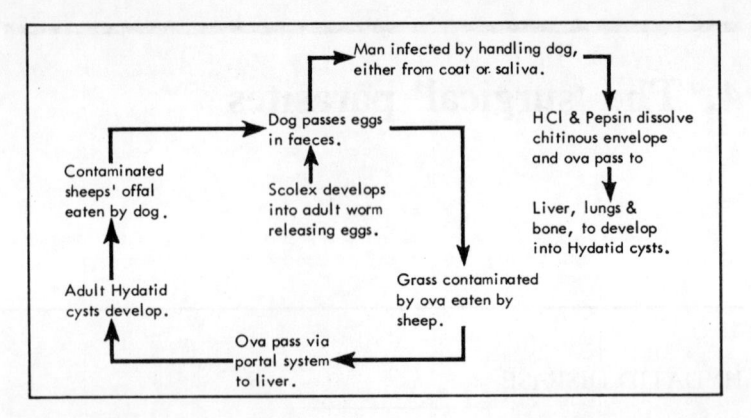

Fig. 4.1 Life cycle of *Echinococcus granulosus*.

The life cycle is normally completed when sheep eat the eggs or gravid segments. Dissolution of the chitinous coat liberates a hexacanth embryo which then burrows into and through the wall of the intestine. In a similar manner the human is infected by eating materials contaminated by the excreta of dogs, an incident most likely to occur in childhood when hygienic standards are at their lowest.

Once through the mucosa, the hexacanth embryo invades the capillaries and is carried by the portal blood, first to the liver, where about 70% of all hydatid cysts develop or, passing through the sinusoids of the liver, the embryos proceed via the right side of the heart to the lungs where they are caught up in the pulmonary circulation and give rise to pulmonary cysts. Still fewer ova, approximately 5%, escape from the pulmonary capillaries to reach the systemic circulation and give rise to cysts in areas such as the spleen, brain and bone. Unlike *E. granulosus*, *E. multilocularis* does not produce the characteristic cysts of the former.

The danger facing man is that once a hydatid cyst has developed it continues to grow until the lining germinal epithelium dies. Furthermore, if the cyst wall is broken, the germinal epithelium and/or the cyst contents may be carried to new sites in which further cysts may then develop.

Pathology of the cyst (Fig. 4.3)

The cyst developed from the embryo is composed of three layers:

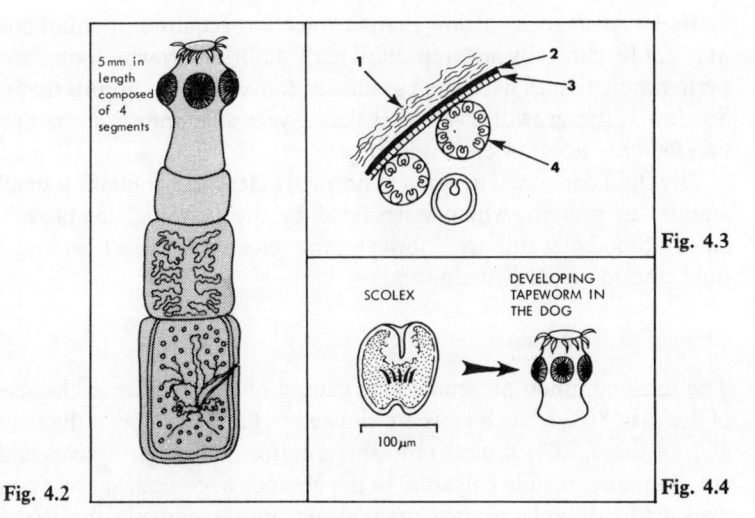

Fig. 4.2 Adult tapeworm developed in dog's intestine.

Fig. 4.3 Hydatid cyst developing in man or sheep.
1, adventitious wall derived from host; 2, external laminated layer; 3, internal germinal layer; 4, brood capsule containing scolices.

Fig. 4.4 Developing tapeworm in intestine of dog.

a. The outer adventitial layer or ectocyst derived from host tissues, which may eventually calcify.
b. The intermediate or laminated layer.
c. The inner or germinal layer forming the brood capsules from which the scolices are developed.

The brood capsules form from nodes of multiplying cells in the germinal layer, which becomes vacuolated and pedunculated. Scolices develop from a thickening of the lining of the brood capsule and eventually indent it. As the brood capsules increase in size so their attachment to the germinal layer becomes progressively thinner until, finally, the capsule bursts, releasing the scolices into the fluid of the cyst. Alternatively, a fertile hydatid daughter cyst may bud off externally and become separated, forming a secondary cyst. A scolex (Fig. 4.4.) has suckers, hooklets and a body; ingested by the dog it is able to adhere to the mucosa of the small intestine and develop into an adult tapeworm.

The majority of embryos reaching the liver excite a host reaction which is sufficient to kill them, after which they are removed by phagocytosis. Only a minority survive and, in man, growth of the cystic larval stage is so slow that an infection acquired in childhood may not be clinically apparent until early adult life by which time the periparasitic tissues have been gradually converted into fibrous tissue. So slow is the growth of the cyst that 1 year after infection the cyst may be only about 4 cm in diameter.

The fluid contained in a cyst is normally clear and contains a small amount of protein, which is secreted by the germinal membrane. After a brood cyst ruptures, however, the released scolices float in the fluid, the so-called hydatid sand.

Clinical presentation

The most common presentation is caused by an increase in the size of the cyst. 80% of such cysts are situated in the right lobe of the liver and, of these, 70% project onto the anterior or inferior aspects and are, therefore, readily palpable. In the absence of complications a cyst may gradually enlarge over many years until eventually the larvae die, after which the cyst contents become a putty-like mass and the wall of the cyst calcifies.

On clinical examination a cyst of the liver must be distinguished from other swellings in the upper quadrant of the abdomen. These would include conditions such as hydronephrosis and mucocele of the gallbladder.

Hydatid disease affecting bones is uncommon. There is a peculiar diverticulated type of growth which results in the production of semisolid buds of hyaline tissue in which little or no fluid is produced. Clinically, bone involvement may result in bone enlargement, paraosseous abscesses or even spontaneous fractures.

Diagnosis

1. *Plain X-rays* may reveal hepatomegaly. In some cases calcification of the cyst wall makes the diagnosis obvious. The diaphragm is often grossly distorted and a pleural effusion may be present.

2. *Ultrasonography* demonstrates the presence of a 'cystic' space-occupying lesion (see Vol 1, p. 285).

3. *Casoni's test*. This intradermal test becomes positive because the capsule is semipermeable and allows the protein containing hydatid fluid which is antigenic to leak into the general circulation. The test, therefore, is performed by injecting a little hydatid fluid intradermally into the patient under investigation, the presence of antibodies being revealed by the rapid development of a skin reaction.

4. *Aspiration*. Aspiration followed by microscopic examination of the contents of the cyst is helpful if scolices or hooklets can be found in the aspirate. This investigation, however, may lead to leakage of hydatid fluid from the cyst and be followed by an anaphylactic reaction.

Treatment

Until recently the only definitive treatment of hepatic cysts was surgical removal. Recently, however, optimistic reports have appeared in the literature indicating that the drug mebendazole may produce complete regression of intrahepatic cysts. This drug is an anthelminthic effective against threadworms, roundworms, whipworms and hookworms. In the treatment of hydatid cysts the drug is given in increasing doses up to 400–600 mg t.d.s. for 21–30 days in up to nine courses. Should this treatment be ineffective, operation is required.

The liver is exposed, the cyst is partially emptied by aspiration, and the contents are replaced by 10 ml of pure formalin in order to kill any contained scolices, although the daughter cysts remain unaffected. The operation field is then packed with gauze soaked in 10% formalin and the whole of the cyst contents are removed by suction. The liver substance is then divided and the cyst gently removed by dissection in the plane between the hyaline and adventitial layers.

Cysts in the lung may be treated in the same fashion when they are situated at the periphery. Occasionally, when they are situated in a deep parabronchial position, they undergo natural cure by expectoration.

Complications

a. *Rupture*. Rupture of a cyst may cause hydatid anaphylaxis accompanied by an erythematous urticarial rash.
b. *Infection*. Infection may occur in either a dead or a living cyst.

SCHISTOSOMIASIS

Causal agents

Three species of schistosome, or blood fluke, infect man and are responsible for the chronic disease known as schistosomiasis:

1. *Schistosoma haematobium*, common throughout the African continent and the Middle East and in endemic foci in Egypt, and West and East Africa.
2. *S. mansoni*, common in South America and Africa.
3. *S. japonicum*, confined to the Far East.

The schistosome is a blood fluke which lives in the vascular system, *S. haematobium* favouring the venous channels of the lower ureters; *S. mansoni* and *S. japonicum* are associated with the venous tributaries of the gut. In endemic areas such as Egypt the extension of irrigation systems has solved the problem of water shortage but increased the overall danger of infection by the schistosome.

Schistosoma haematobium

Life cycle and pathology (Fig. 4.5)

The intermediate host of *S. haematobium* is the freshwater snail, *Bulinus globosus*, which is infected by free-swimming miracidia liberated from eggs passed in the urine of an infected human. In the snail's liver the miracidia develop into sporocysts in which the fork-tailed cercariae form. These tiny hair-like creatures, about a millimetre in length, leave the snail in thousands, usually during daylight hours. The definitive host, man, is infected by the cercariae penetrating the skin. This usually occurs when the host is wading or bathing in water that contains the cercariae, which have only a lifespan of about 12 hours.

Penetration is marked by an urticarial reaction which lasts 1–2 days. Once through the skin, the cercariae shed their tails and invade the lymphatic system and so eventually gain access to the bloodstream. Carried to the liver the cercariae settle in the portal system and there mature into either male or female flukes. This is followed by a secondary migration to the site of election during which a generalized allergic reaction may occur. *S. haematobium* passes to the venules of the bladder and surrounding pelvic viscera, and in the perivesical venules the female, gripped in the gynaecophoral groove of the male, lays her eggs. The nonoperculate eggs, which possess spines (the position of which reflects the species), penetrate the walls of the venules and pass into the substance of the bladder wall.

At this stage there are two possibilities:

1. The egg may lyse its way through the wall of the bladder and slowly develop into the miracidial stage, ready to hatch once the egg has been passed in the urine, or
2. The egg will be retained in the bladder wall and ultimately die.

THE 'SURGICAL' PARASITES   51

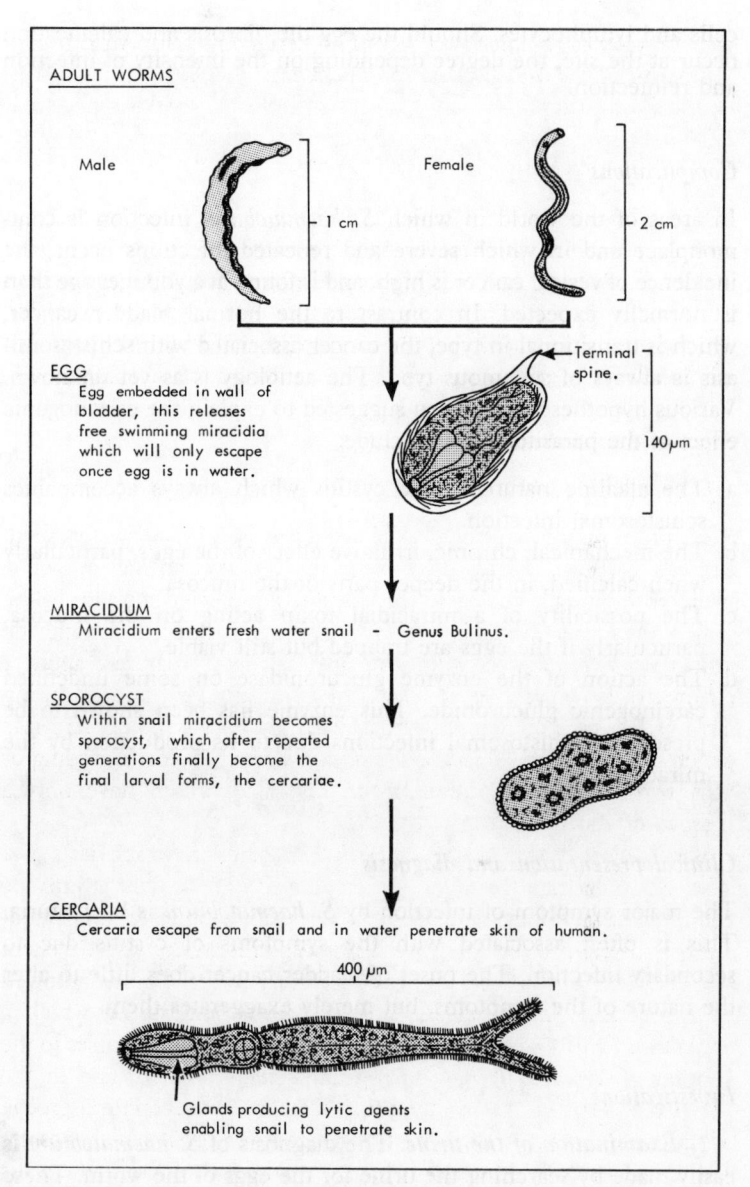

ADULT WORMS

Male — 1 cm

Female — 2 cm

EGG
Egg embedded in wall of bladder, this releases free swimming miracidia which will only escape once egg is in water.

Terminal spine — 140 μm

MIRACIDIUM
Miracidium enters fresh water snail – Genus Bulinus.

SPOROCYST
Within snail miracidium becomes sporocyst, which after repeated generations finally become the final larval forms, the cercariae.

CERCARIA
Cercaria escape from snail and in water penetrate skin of human.

400 μm

Glands producing lytic agents enabling snail to penetrate skin.

Fig. 4.5 Life cycle of *Schistosoma haematobium*.

Whatever occurs, the eggs always excite a granulomatous reaction in the affected tissues. The typical lesion consists of a focus of epithelioid cells, fibroblasts, and giant cells surrounded by plasma cells and lymphocytes. Should the egg die, fibrosis and calcification occur at the site, the degree depending on the intensity of infection and reinfection.

Complications

In areas of the world in which *S. haematobium* infection is commonplace and in which severe and repeated infections occur, the incidence of vesical cancer is high, and is found at a younger age than is normally expected. In contrast to the normal bladder cancer, which is transitional in type, the cancer associated with schistosomiasis is always of squamous type. The aetiology is as yet unknown. Various hypotheses have been suggested to explain the carcinogenic effect of the parasite. These include:

a. The alkaline nature of the cystitis which always accompanies schistosomal infection.
b. The mechanical, chronic, irritative effect of the eggs, particularly when calcified, in the deeper parts of the mucosa.
c. The possibility of a miracidial toxin acting on the mucosa, particularly if the eggs are trapped but still viable.
d. The action of the enzyme glucuronidase on some undefined carcinogenic glucuronide. This enzyme has been shown to be present in schistosomal infections due to its production by the miracidia.

Clinical presentation and diagnosis

The major symptom of infection by *S. haematobium* is haematuria. This is often associated with the symptoms of cystitis due to secondary infection. The onset of bladder cancer does little to alter the nature of the symptoms, but merely exaggerates them.

Investigations

1. *Examination of the urine.* The diagnosis of *S. haematobium* is easily made by searching the urine for the eggs of the worm. These have a characteristic appearance, the hook of this particular species being in a terminal position on the somewhat ovoid egg.
2. *Cystoscopy.* This may reveal a number of changes according to the degree and duration of the infection. These include hyperaemia, oedema, granulations, ulceration, fine sandy patches, polypi, or

carcinoma. A biopsy should be performed on any visible lesion. If the specimen is positive, the eggs will be seen surrounded by varying degrees of reaction and, of course, in the latter stages of the disease squamous cancer may be identified.

3. *Intravenous pyelography.* A variety of deviations from normal may be seen including:

a. filling defects on the cystogram which are due to the acute proliferating granulomatous lesions, blood clot, or to actual carcinoma
b. hydronephrosis caused either by obstructive lesions of the lower ureters or contraction of the bladder
c. gross calcification of the bladder and lower ureters
d. non-functioning kidneys.

Treatment

The drug of choice for the treatment of *S. haematobium* is metriphonate, which is an organophosphorus insecticide used in agriculture. Administered in a dose of 7.5 mg per kg of body weight on three occasions at 2 weekly intervals, an overall reduction in the egg count has been reported in 95% of infected children and cure in 50%. Another effective drug is niridazole. Both drugs, in young patients, may cause the resolution of the schistosomal granulation tissue and thus relieve obstruction at the lower end of the ureters with a return to normal of renal function.

Surgery is only required when chronic or repeated infection has led to severe structural changes in the urinary tract. Once carcinomatous degeneration has occurred in the bladder the disease is commonly inoperable and resort must be made to radiotherapy or chemotherapy, but whatever the treatment the prognosis is extremely poor.

Schistosoma mansoni

Life cycle

The life cycle of *S. mansoni* is similar to that of *S. haematobium* except that the ova of the former are deposited in the venules of the inferior mesenteric vein so that the subsequent pathological lesions develop in the large bowel.

Pathology

The pathological lesions caused by *S. mansoni* are very similar to those of *S. haematobium* in that granulomata and papilloma form in the bowel wall, after which mucosal ulceration leads to secondary infection and eventually the bowel wall increases in thickness due to advancing fibrosis. Strictures, however, rarely occur.

Malignant degeneration

It is still in doubt whether *S. mansoni* can induce malignant change. The conclusions of various authorities have been somewhat different. Shindo (1976), who reviewed 276 cases of adenocarcinoma of the colon associated with schistosomal infection, found a significant difference between it and carcinoma unassociated with such infection in regard to age, sex ratio, symptoms and histopathological findings, and suggested in consequence that the schistosome could induce malignancy.

Clinical presentation

Symptoms. The initial symptoms associated with *S. mansoni* are commonly intermittent abdominal pain and attacks of mucus diarrhoea. When there has been mucosal ulceration, blood and pus are found in the stools and the clinical picture resembles ulcerative colitis, which is an extremely uncommon disease in the native African, or carcinoma of the colon, which is also rare because of the relatively low age at death, or lastly, amoebic colitis, which is common.

Signs. Physical examination may reveal the easily palpable thickened loops of bowel, and if the rectum is severely involved, rectal prolapse may occur or fistula in ano.

In severe cases the ova are carried in the portal system to the liver, in which periportal fibrosis develops, later to be followed by portal hypertension. Portal hypertension is naturally accompanied by increasing splenomegaly.

Medical treatment

The drug of choice in the treatment of *S. mansoni* is oxamniquine, which has no effect on *S. haematobium*. The adverse side-effects include severe pain at the site of injection, and abdominal and muscular pain. The dose recommended is one or two doses of 7.5–30 mg/kg by deep intramuscular injection, or 10–15 mg/kg by mouth. Cure rates as high as 95% have been reported.

Surgical treatment

Surgical treatment is usually reserved for those cases in which medical treatment fails to halt the progress of the disease and bowel complications have occurred. Portal hypertension may demand surgical treatment if bleeding occurs from the enlarging oesophageal varices.

Schistosoma japonicum (Katayama disease)

S. japonicum mainly affects the small bowel and the proximal part of the large bowel. The pathological changes are similar to those found after infection with *S. mansoni* but tend to be more severe and extensive because of the greater number of ova produced by this parasite. Changes also occur at an early stage in the liver and spleen and the mesentery and omentum become so thickened and fibrotic that they may so constrict the colon that the intestine becomes obstructed.

AMOEBIASIS

Causative agent

The protozoa, *Entamoeba histolytica* is small, measuring 10–40 μm. On a warm stage, the cell is constantly active, erupting from the surface pseudopodia which contain a hyaline cytoplasm. In the living cell little intracellular detail can be made out although, in a case of active dysentery, ingested red cells can be recognized within the parasite.

Life cycle (Fig. 4.6)

Primary development occurs in the lumen of the large intestine in which the amoebae thrive, feeding on bacteria and reproducing by binary fusion. Invasion of the mucosa leads to necrosis and ulceration and from this site the protozoa may spread to form abscesses in other tissues, particularly the liver, and less commonly the lung or brain.

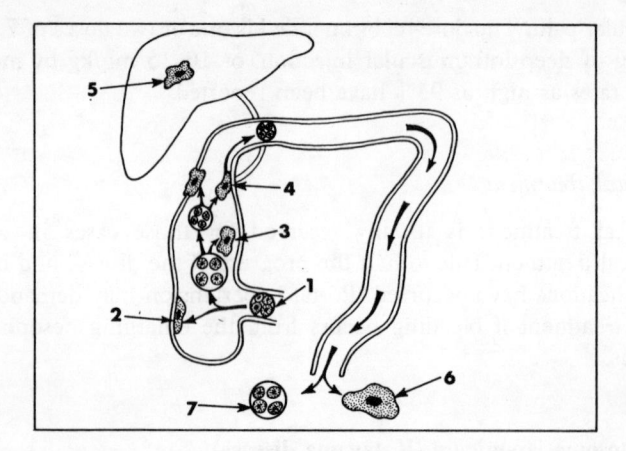

Fig. 4.6 Life cycle of *Entamoeba histolytica*.
1, Swallowed cyst about to enter colon; 2, Invasive amoeba producing ulceration of bowel wall; 3, Commensal amoeba; 4, Invasive amoeba passing into portal blood stream; 5, Amoebic abscess filled with 'anchovy sauce'; 6, Trophozoite which dies; 7, Cyst capable of infecting further individuals.

In favourable conditions the amoebae encyst. A living cyst has the appearance under the microscope of an air bubble or oil droplet. Within it there may be small refractile rods, the chromatoid bodies, which are thought to be aggregations of ribosomes, and, on reaching maturity, four nuclei.

The cysts are passed in the faeces of the host and may remain viable for several weeks. Once ingested the cyst becomes active, and in the small intestine the contained cytoplasm begins to squeeze through the cyst wall until the whole amoeba is finally free in the lumen. At this point each of the four nuclei divide, followed by the cell itself, so that eight small amoebae are produced from a single cyst. Amoebae passed in the stools survive only for 2–3 days and are not infective because they are destroyed in the stomach.

Distribution

Amoebiasis is of worldwide distribution and infection in man is nearly always contracted from a human source, the infection spreading from man to man by the faecal–oral route. The disease is commonly spread by carriers who themselves have few or no symptoms and who may give no history whatsoever of a previous attack of dysentery.

The spread of infection is linked to factors such as poor personal hygiene, food handling by carriers, and contamination of food by flies or, in the case of uncooked vegetables, the use of human excreta as fertilizer.

The relationship between the parasite and clinical dysentery is, however, unclear. The large *E. histolytica*, indigenous in Britain although morphologically identical with the invasive tropical strains, is non-pathogenic. Some strains appear to be more invasive than others and it has been suggested that the bacterial flora of the gut may predispose to invasion of the mucosa.

Intestinal amoebiasis

Pathology

Penetration of the intestinal mucosa by the trophozoite is followed by ulceration, most commonly in the caecum, sigmoid colon, and rectum. The parasite, having penetrated the mucosa, appears to spread in the submucosal tissue rather than in the mucosa itself, producing the classic 'flask-shaped' lesion. In the absence of secondary infection little more than a mild mononuclear reaction occurs. Occasionally, bacterial infection causes the formation of a granulomatous lesion known as an amoeboma, or perforation of the bowel occurs which leads to a localized pericolic abscess or general peritonitis.

Clinical presentation

The onset of symptoms following infection by *E. histolytica* may be almost immediate or be delayed for months or even years. The dysenteric symptoms may also vary in severity, in mild cases only three or four loose stools being passed per day, whereas in severe attacks the stools may be liquid and contain copious quantities of mucus and blood. Such attacks may last for a few days or weeks before remission occurs. Mild attacks are associated with no general symptoms and few physical signs whereas in very severe cases the patient is prostrated, suffering from a swinging fever, chills, sweating and dehydration.

Remission following a mild attack may last for days, months or years but at any time an amoebic abscess may develop and does so in about 20% of untreated patients, whilst in severe cases gross haemorrhage or perforation followed by an amoebic peritonitis may occur.

Occasionally the patient may develop a mass, most commonly in the caecum, due to gross thickening of the intestinal wall. This is known as an amoeboma and is commonly associated with the symptoms of intestinal obstruction. The mass itself is indistinguishable on clinical examination from a neoplasm in this region, hypertrophic ileocaecal tuberculosis, a mycetoma or an appendix abscess.

Diagnosis

1. *Stool examination.* Microscopic examination of fresh stools on a warm stage, if positive, will reveal motile amoebae, some containing engorged red cells. In asymptomatic patients or during remission, cysts may be found containing one or more bar-shaped chromatoid bodies, one to four nuclei, and a glycogen mass. Repeated stool examinations are required before a negative diagnosis can be assumed in the presence of typical symptoms.

2. *Sigmoidoscopy.* Amoebic ulceration is common in the rectum and sigmoid. The classic appearance of amoebic colitis is one of discrete mucosal ulceration. Each ulcer produces a slight elevation of the mucosa accompanied by a small central depression which contains a minute discrete yellow slough whilst the mucosa between remains normal.

3. *Serological tests.* A number of serological tests are now available, including indirect immunofluorescence, gel diffusion and countercurrent electrophoresis.

Treatment

Medical. A number of antiprotozoal drugs are now available for the treatment of amoebiasis. These include metronidazole given orally in a dose of 800 mg t.d.s. for 5 days or 400 mg t.d.s. for 10–14 days. Tinidazole, another nitroimidazole derivative, appears to be even more effective, cure rates using this drug being as high as 97% in patients passing trophozoites, and 93% for those passing cysts. The adverse effects of both drugs are the same, both commonly causing gastrointestinal upset. Neither should be given in pregnancy. Emetine hydrochloride, an alkaloid of ipecacuanha, is also effective in both intestinal and hepatic amoebiasis. This drug can be administered either subcutaneously or intramuscularly. The dose should never exceed 60 mg per day, it should never be given continuously for more than 10 days, and any course should not be repeated at an interval of less than 6 weeks. The most serious adverse reaction to emetine is myocardial degeneration and it should, therefore, never be used in individuals suffering from heart disease.

Other effective drugs include diolaxamide furorate and di-iodo hydroxyquinalone.

Indications for surgical intervention. Uncomplicated intestinal amoebiasis never requires surgical treatment. However, surgical intervention may be necessary in:

1. *Acute fulminating disease* uncontrolled by medical treatment, which results in:
   a. Toxic colonic dilatation associated with severe systemic upset and abdominal tenderness.
   b. Severe bleeding.
2. *Perforation of the colon.* Whilst any segment of the bowel may be affected, the common sites of perforation include the caecum, ascending colon and sigmoid. Whilst perforation is normally associated with fulminating disease it may occur in the absence of acute dysentery.
3. *Hepatic amoebiasis* (see below).

Hepatic amoebiasis

Pathology

In severe infections the amoebae invade the portal system and are carried to the liver. If these are few in number each amoebic embolus becomes surrounded by an acute inflammatory reaction, and death of the invading trophozoites occurs. During this period the liver may swell and become tender.

When, however, large numbers of amoebae reach the liver, some survive, multiply and produce liquefaction. The liquified and necrotic liver tissue form the so-called 'amoebic abscess', which is not in fact a true abscess because it contains no pus. The feebleness of the inflammatory response may lead to rapid enlargement of the cavity which is surrounded by relatively little fibrosis. Approximately 80% of amoebic abscesses develop in the right lobe of the liver, possibly because blood from the right side of the colon flows into this lobe. The contents of a mature amoebic abscess are classically described as 'anchovy sauce' because of the necrotic liver tissue within the cavity.

Invasion of the liver produces tenderness and enlargement of the organ, but if the infection is limited it will be defeated and the organ will return to normal within a few days.

If an amoebic abscess develops, there is fever and the liver enlarges rapidly, but jaundice only occurs if a large intrahepatic bile duct is occluded.

The chief danger associated with an amoebic abscess is the frequency with which rupture may occur. This may then be complicated by the development of an empyema or lung abscess, generalized peritonitis, or the development of a communication between the abscess cavity and the biliary tract, the skin or the colon.

Examination usually reveals a hepatomegaly, a high, swinging fever and night sweats.

Diagnosis

1. *Chest X-ray.* This may demonstrate a raised immobile diaphragm, some collapse of the lung, and a pleural effusion.
2. *Blood count.* A polymorphonuclear leucocytosis is always present.
3. *Liver scan.* A filling defect in the liver will be present if an abscess has become established.
4. *Aspiration.* This diagnostic measure is now less frequently used than in the past. It is normally performed under local anaesthesia using a wide bore needle mounted on a syringe with a two-way tap. A successful aspirate reveals the typical anchovy sauce contents of the cavity.

Treatment

The majority of abscesses respond to treatment with metronidazole or emetine, and in areas in which amoebiasis is commonplace early medical treatment rather than repeated attempts at aspiration is now the treatment of choice.

ASCARIASIS

Infection with the roundworm, *Ascaris lumbricoides*, can cause surgical complications.

Life cycle

The life cycle of this worm is extraordinary. The larvae emerging from the eggs that have been swallowed by man burrow into the intestinal mucosa and are then carried by the blood stream to reach the capillaries of the pulmonary circulation. Here they moult to the third stage, and after a short time burst into the alveoli where they undergo a further moult. The larvae, now in the fourth stage, migrate upwards in the bronchial tree and finally reach the back of the throat where they are once more carried down into the digestive tract by the simple act of swallowing. In the small intestine they undergo one final moult to become adult worms some 10 to 20 cm long. The eggs produced by the adult female can live for a considerable period of time after being passed in the faeces and are able to withstand disposal in advanced sewage systems, desiccation, and low temperatures.

Clinical presentation

The presence of a few worms has probably little or no effect on general health. However, during the passage of a large crop of larvae through the lungs, a cough, bronchospasm and eosinophilia may occur and plain radiographs of the chest may show the presence of multiple, soft, mottled opacities.

Of greater importance to the surgeon is the mechanical effect of a bolus formed by a large number of worms entwining, which may result in intestinal obstruction. Furthermore, the adult worms tend to migrate and their entry into the common bile duct may result in biliary obstruction, jaundice and even a suppurative cholangitis, while migration into the pancreatic duct may result in acute pancreatitis. Once lodged in these ducts the worm usually dies and may even become calcified.

Treatment

Although the roundworm can be killed by the piperazine salts, reinfection is commonplace in areas in which personal hygiene is poor. Surgery is required to deal with obstruction or to remove dead worms lodged in the common bile or pancreatic ducts.

FILARIASIS

The filarial worms of greatest importance to man include the *Wucheria bancrofti* and *Brugia malayi*, which cause elephantiasis and loa loa, the eye worm. The former are widely distributed in tropical areas although the distribution of the worms is limited by the vectors, i.e. the mosquito.

Life cycle

The adult nematodes of *W. bancrofti* live in the lymphatic system, in which the female lays the first stage larvae enclosed in an elongated eggshell. The larvae migrate via the lymphatic system to the bloodstream where they can inadvertently infect the mosquito, which is the intermediate host. In the arthropod the larvae develop in the haemacele of the labium and, when the mosquito bites, the larvae emerge and enter the wound. Once within man the parasite completes its development by moulting twice and migrating through the tissues into the lymphatic system, there to produce the first stage larvae, or microfilariae, approximately 1 year after infection.

Clinical presentation

The adult nematodes spend their lives in the lymph nodes of the body, most commonly those of the inguinal region, in which, by their presence, they cause a slowly progressive sclerosing inflammation which ultimately causes obstruction of the lymphatics and lymphoedema, popularly called elephantiasis.

Prior to the development of elephantiasis the affected nodes are enlarged, rubbery, and painless. Although the lower limb is commonly involved, other parts of the body are occasionally affected. The scrotum and its contents may be affected, the scrotal skin may become thickened, bilateral hydroceles and bilateral epididymitis may occur.

Any affected area is liable to secondary bacterial infection, usually with the streptococcus, the repeated attacks of infection hastening the onset of lymphoedema and producing attacks of so-called 'filarial fever'.

Diagnosis

The disease should be suspected by the presence of the rubbery, hard lymph nodes. Confirmation may be obtained by the identification of microfilaria in the blood, specimens of which should be taken at night during which period the larval forms flood into the peripheral circulation; they withdraw into the pulmonary capillaries and great veins by day. It is possible to identify the microfilariae in a wet specimen or, alternatively, they can be stained by Leishman or Giemsa's stain.

5. Diagnosis and management of acute abdominal pain

The medical causes of acute abdominal pain have been described in Volume 1, Chapter 27, and whilst many of these conditions are rare they should always be borne in mind, especially the possibility of viral infections and diaphragmatic pleurisy in children, acute myocardial infarction in the adult, and sickle cell anaemia in patients of negro extraction. The majority of patients suffering from acute abdominal pain who are admitted to hospital, however, are suffering from one of three conditions: non-specific abdominal pain, in which no obvious cause can be found following investigation and even laparotomy; acute appendicitis; or intestinal obstruction. Several large series have now been reported in the literature showing this to be so, non-specific abdominal pain accounting for approximately 35% of admissions, acute appendicitis approximately 20% and intestinal obstruction 15%. In terms of frequency, gallbladder problems (biliary colic or acute cholecystitis) and renal problems account for a further 10%; after this, all other conditions are relatively rare. For example, in a group of nearly 1200 patients reported by Irvin only 1% were suffering from a ruptured aortic aneurysm.

Perforated peptic ulceration, once a relatively common surgical emergency, has become a rarity; whilst perforated duodenal ulcers used to be five times more common in males than in females and were nearly always due to chronic ulceration, the sex ratio is now almost equal and the majority of perforations are caused by acute ulcers – the result of medical treatment with either steroids themselves or non-steroidal anti-inflammatory agents.

The first step in the diagnosis of the cause of acute abdominal pain is to elicit a clear history and perform a thorough physical examination. The importance of this step can be illustrated by consideration of the two most common causes of admission of patients suffering from acute abdominal pain, i.e. acute appendicitis and non-specific abdominal pain. Failure to differentiate between these two conditions is the commonest cause of the unnecessary exploration of the abdomen followed by removal of the appendix.

Consider six aspects:

1. *Pain.* Whereas the pain of acute appendicitis nearly always begins in the periumbilical region and moves to the right iliac fossa, usually within hours of its commencement, the pain of non-specific abdominal pain (NSAP) either begins in the right iliac fossa or is diffuse from the start.

2. *Pain on movement.* In acute appendicitis, especially when the parietal peritoneum is involved, movement aggravates the pain; if the appendix is lying on the psoas, extension of the hip will aggravate the pain; if the patient is suffering from NSAP, movement causes no greater discomfort.

3. *Anorexia, nausea and vomiting.* Suffering from acute appendicitis a progression of these symptoms occurs: first loss of appetite, then increasing nausea, and finally vomiting. In NSAP these symptoms are rare.

4. *Specific tenderness.* In acute appendicitis palpation of the abdomen normally reveals a specific point of maximum tenderness, commonly over or about McBurney's point if the appendix is lying in the right iliac fossa or above and posterior to the right anterior superior iliac spine if the appendix is retrocaecal in position, whereas in NSAP the tenderness is more diffuse.

5. *Guarding and rebound tenderness.* These physical signs are nearly always present in acute appendicitis, except when the appendix lies behind the ileal mesentery. In NSAP, however, both are absent.

6. *Rectal examination.* This examination should be performed on every patient suffering from acute abdominal pain. In acute appendicitis the patient will normally exhibit tenderness on the right side, whereas in NSAP the tenderness is minimal or more diffuse.

As the number of positive or negative symptoms and signs increases, so the probability of one or other diagnosis becomes more certain. Thus, of the six features described, if four are present appendicectomy is indicated on clinical grounds alone.

COMPUTER-ASSISTED DIAGNOSIS

Efforts to increase the accuracy of clinical diagnosis in patients suffering from acute abdominal pain have been made by computer analysis. A leading protagonist of this methodology is de Dombal of St James University Hospital, who wrote his first paper on this subject in 1971. This has meant the development of structured data sheets on which the clinical history and the physical signs are recorded. This can be achieved by merely ringing the appropriate data number, e.g. male 01, female 02; site of pain at onset 11, right upper quadrant 19, central 20; site of pain when seen, right lower quadrant 26. These features are thus recorded, together with various other symptoms, including a description of the pain suffered, e.g. intermittent, colicky, etc., attendant symptoms such as jaundice or blood in the stools and, lastly, aggravating factors or urinary symptoms – as well as physical signs elicited on examination. In all, the World Congress of Gastroenterology (ONGE) studies used 136 features to fully describe the clinical picture in a patient suffering from abdominal pain. The data thus obtained are then fed into a computer primed with a database produced by the examination of data previously obtained from patients in whom an accurate diagnosis of the cause of their symptoms has been achieved. Furnished with the entry of the details of the – as yet – undiagnosed patient, the computer then performs what is known as a Bayesian analysis.

Although widely known for some time, the application of Bayes' theorem to statistical analysis has been extremely limited by controversy over the necessary assignment of the 'prior probabilities', but although controversy remains, increasing use of the method is being made. Essentially the theorem is as follows. Suppose we have a set of possible alternative diagnoses $D_1, D_2, D_3 \ldots D_n$ for a given patient A, one of which will be 'nothing wrong', and of which one and only one will be correct. Before a given medical examination E, suppose the associated respective probabilities, known as the prior probabilities, are $p_1, p_2, p_3 \ldots p_n$, then $p_1 + p_2 + p_3 + p_n = 1$. Now suppose that E reveals a set S of signs, let l_1 denote the probability or likelihood that disease D_1, when known to be present, will give rise to sign S with similar likelihoods $l_2, l_3 \ldots l_n$ for the alternatives, then after examination E, Bayes' rule gives the final probabilities, $w_1, w_2, w_3 \ldots w_n$, called the posterior 'post-examination' probabilities that $D_1, D_2, D_3 \ldots D_n$ are correct as:

$$w_1 = \frac{p_1 l_1}{T} \quad w_2 = \frac{p_2 l_2}{T} \quad W_n = \frac{p_n l_n}{T}$$

where $T = p_1 + p_2 l_2 + \ldots p_n l_n$

Example

Suppose a child A has been admitted with abdominal pain and the diagnosis suspected lies between one of non-specific abdominal pain, acute appendicitis, mesenteric adenitis, or intussusception.

Then n, the number of possible diagnosis, is 4, so:

D_1 is 'non-specific abdominal pain'.
D_2 is 'acute appendicitis'.
D_3 is 'mesenteric adenitis'.
D_4 is 'intussusception'.

Taking figures at random, suppose that before examination it is 30% probable that the child has non-specific abdominal pain, 10% probable that he has acute appendicitis only, and only 1% probable that he has mesenteric adenitis:

Then $p_1 = 0.30$, $p_2 = 0.10$, $p_3 = 0.01$, so that $p_4 = 1 - (p_1 + p_2 + p_3) = 0.59$. That is, the prior probability that an intussusception is present is 0.59.

Now, let S denote the physical signs of a particular type observed during examination E. Suppose:

90% of those children suffering from non-specific abdominal pain exhibit S ($l_1 = 0.9$). 50% of those suffering from acute appendicitis exhibit S ($l_2 = 0.5$) 99% suffering from mesenteric adenitis exhibit S ($l_3 = 0.99$) 10% suffering from intussusception exhibit S ($l_4 = 0.10$)

Then T being equal to $p_1 l_1 + p_2 l_2 + \ldots p_n l_n =$
$(0.3 \times 0.9) + (0.1 \times 0.5) + (0.01 \times 0.99) + (0.59 \times 0.10) = 0.3889$

$$w_1 = \frac{0.3 \times 0.9}{0.3889} = 0.69$$

$$w_2 = \frac{0.1 \times 0.5}{0.3889} = 0.1286$$

$$w_3 = \frac{0.01 \times 0.99}{0.3889} = 0.0225$$

$$w_4 = \frac{0.59 \times 0.10}{0.3889} = 0.1517$$

with $w_1 + w_2 + w_3 + w_4$ equal to unity is correct. In other words, examination and the elicitation of the physical signs of disease has pushed up the probability of non-specific abdominal pain from 30%

to 69% while that of acute appendicitis has increased only fractionally from 10 to 13%.

The probability of mesenteric adenitis has more than doubled, but is still small at 2.5% and the chances that an intussusception is present has fallen from 59 to 15%.

The doubt hanging over the Bayes' theorem is the requirement of allotting the prior probabilities $p_1, p_2 \ldots p_n$ and until this is resolved Bayes' rule is unacceptable to the purist.

Nevertheless, the theorem has been made to work in the field of surgical diagnosis provided the database is built from a large enough number of representative cases and the clinical history, examination and subsequent investigations of the patient are accurately recorded. In the majority of systems that have been described, following entry of the information into the computer, a printback of the case history precedes the computer printout of the diagnostic probabilities.

Of equal importance using computer-aided diagnosis is the finding by de Dombal and many others that, when this system is introduced, the initial data fed into the computer has of necessity to be recorded with complete accuracy, and the actual clinical diagnostic accuracy of the clinician in first contact with the patient, whatever his position in the medical hierarchy, also increases – only to diminish once again if for any reason the system is temporarily abandoned. In other words the discipline imposed by the accurate collection of data is itself extremely valuable.

The ability of the computer to assess the probability of a given disease results in a clinician being able to reconsider his management of the patient. This is of considerable importance in, for example, making a distinction between acute cholecystitis and acute pancreatitis because many surgeons are adopting a more aggressive attitude to the former, advocating immediate cholecystectomy in the acute stage, whereas in the early stages of acute pancreatitis the treatment in the absence of gallstones remains conservative.

INVESTIGATIONS SPECIFICALLY RELATED TO THE DIAGNOSIS

Emphasizing once again the importance of the clinical history and careful physical examination in reaching the correct diagnosis, it should be appreciated that what really matters is whether or not the patient requires emergency surgery. In some cases a precise anatomical diagnosis may be of assistance in the management of the patient; for example, if a diagnosis is made of acute large bowel obstruction due to a cancer proximal to the splenic flexure, the most acceptable surgical option is resection, whereas immediate resection of left-sided tumours causing acute obstruction is followed by mortality rates in excess of 40% in most recorded series.

The commonest investigations that may assist in accurate diagnosis are non-invasive, e.g. haematological, ultrasonography, plain X-rays of the abdomen, and biochemical. Many surgeons have also shown that laparoscopy is helpful, particularly in differentiating non-specific abdominal pain from acute appendicitis and pelvic inflammation, thus avoiding the chief cause of unnecessary appendicectomies. The contraindications to this investigation include previous abdominal surgery and suspected intestinal obstruction, in both of which there is a danger of perforating the bowel.

In acute abdominal pain following trauma, peritoneal lavage may be of great assistance (see Vol. 1, p. 180) but this investigation is of little value in patients suffering from constitutional disease except in patients suspected of having acute pancreatitis, where the results of lavage may give some indication of the severity of the condition. Nevertheless papers have been written describing how fine-catheter aspiration cytology of the peritoneal cavity is of value in the diagnosis of both acute appendicitis and pelvic inflammatory disease in women. When the diagnosis is uncertain a polymorphonuclear neutrophil percentage count of greater than 50% indicates the need for either appendicectomy or, if pelvic inflammatory disease is suspected, laparoscopy.

Haematological investigation

Since blood counts in most laboratories are now automated, en bloc results are obtained.

In the majority of acute abdominal conditions knowledge of the precise haemoglobin concentration is of little or no value in reaching a correct diagnosis, although in suspected haemorrhagic conditions associated with bleeding, such as a ruptured abdominal aneurysm, knowledge of the haemoglobin concentration is helpful, not as a diagnostic measure but as an indicator of the severity of the condition and the necessity for transfusion.

Whilst it is a reasonable assumption that the total white count will rise in any patient suffering from an infective lesion within the peritoneal cavity, this investigation seldom reflects the severity of the underlying pathological condition. Thus, for example, in patients suspected of suffering from acute appendicitis the chance that this is so only becomes a near certainty when the count is above $15 \times 10^9/l$.

Ultrasonography

This investigation is now widely used in patients with acute abdominal pain. It is non-invasive, and is rapidly and easily performed without discomfort to the patient. Its chief use is in conditions not affecting the gut. Thus it is useful in: (a) the diagnosis of stones in the biliary tract, including patients suspected of acute cholecystitis, where specific ultrasonic signs may be found such as a hyperechogenic thickened gallbladder wall interspersed with a discontinuous hypoechogenic layer (the latter being specific but inconstant); (b) in detecting changes in the pancreas in acute pancreatitis; (c) in detecting calculi or dilatation of the urinary tract; and (d) in diseases of the pelvic organs in the female.

Plain radiology of the abdomen

A plain X-ray of the abdomen will reveal in only approximately 50% of patients suffering from acute abdominal conditions classic changes allowing a definitive diagnosis to be made on the evidence of this investigation alone. However, nearly every acute condition affecting the abdominal contents is on occasion accompanied by radiological changes specific for the condition. These classical changes are listed below.

Acute appendicitis

There may be a local ileus restricted to the distal loops of the ileum and caecum. Also, an increase in the density of the soft tissue of the wall and base of the caecum may be present, caused by the presence of inflammatory oedema in the periappendicular tissues. Rarely the entire small bowel is distended, leading to an appearance markedly similar to that observed in small bowel obstruction. This appearance may be associated with acute obstructive appendicitis alone or may follow the development of general peritonitis, such radiological changes indicating the presence of an ileus. Other features include: lumbar lordosis with convexity to the left, caused by spasm of the psoas; loss of the psoas shadow; presence of a faecolith in the right iliac fossa.

Intestinal obstruction

In most cases of intestinal obstruction the diagnosis is obvious from the clinical history and the physical signs. The aim of radiological investigation is to establish if possible the level of obstruction prior to operation. A plain X-ray in the erect position in nearly every patient suffering from small bowel obstruction shows the classic ladder pattern, but it must not be forgotten that the same radiological appearances also occur in non-mechanical obstruction caused by a paralytic ileus, the result most commonly of a general peritonitis.

The level of the obstruction can often be identified by observing the position of the distended bowel and the presence or absence of plicae. The latter are most marked in the upper reaches of the small bowel in which regular and complete cross-hatching occurs, because these mucosal folds are stretched; in the lower ileum the mucosal folds disappear, causing a distended and featureless bowel.

The commonest site of large bowel obstruction is the descending colon, the commonest cause being a carcinoma of the sigmoid. The diagnostic radiological feature is visible dilatation of the colon proximal to the site of obstruction, which may be most obvious in the caecum. The large bowel is distinguished from the small by its position at the periphery of the abdominal cavity and by the presence of haustra, which can be seen as incomplete transverse bands in the ascending and transverse colon. When the ileocaecal valve remains competent the caecum may be grossly distended, whereas the small bowel remains relatively normal in calibre for some time.

Rarer forms of intestinal obstruction produce quite classic signs; for example, volvulus of the sigmoid causes a grossly distended loop containing a double fluid level, and in caecal volvulus gross distension of the caecum and/or right colon develops in which one, or less commonly two, fluid levels may be seen.

Occasionally, radiology has a therapeutic part to play, as in intussusception in infancy, a condition most commonly seen at about 6 months. In this condition a carefully performed barium enema not only shows a crescentic filling defect or meniscus, but sometimes an incomplete cylindrical shell of barium passing between the receiving and returning layers. If the barium then flows onwards it can be assumed that reduction is occurring but, whereas the early stages of reduction are usually easy to interpret, the appearance of an oedematous ileocaecal valve after total reduction may be extremely difficult to distinguish from a partially reduced lesion. The use of a barium enema as a therapeutic measure was first described by Retan in 1927, and in 1955 Zachary of Sheffield showed that in 70% of infants the condition could be successfully treated in this fashion if the lesion had been present for less than 24 hours, whereas after 24 hours the method was successful in only 25%.

Acute pancreatitis

There are no specific radiological signs of this condition, although the following may be seen:

1. A sentinel loop seen in some 40% of all patients suffering from this condition. This appearance is caused by a single dilated segment in the upper abdomen.
2. Gallstones.
3. Generalized dilatation of the small bowel.

Perforation of the bowel

Peptic ulcer. The chief radiological sign of a perforated peptic ulcer is pneumoperitoneum, leading to gas under the diaphragm in majority of patients. The incidence of this physical sign is dependent on the number and manner in which the films are taken. The presence of gas is undoubtedly more common after perforation of a chronic gastric ulcer than a chronic duodenal ulcer, possibly because the former are nearly always associated with an ulcer crater twice the diameter of the latter. In the erect film, small quantities of air cause a sickle-shaped translucency to develop between the diaphragm above and the liver below. On the left this must obviously be distinguished from gas in the fundus of the stomach or the splenic flexure. Gas in the former is at a lower level and always overlies a horizontal fluid level whilst the latter is always inferolateral in position.

Oesophageal perforation. The majority of perforations of the oesophagus follow instrumentation with a rigid oesophagus. Therefore, since the introduction of fibre-optic instruments, the frequency of this condition has diminished. Nevertheless, spontaneous rupture can occur as a result usually of a suppressed attack of vomiting. A longitudinal tear at the lower end of the oesophagus produces severe pain in the lower chest or upper abdomen. Radiologically a careful inspection of the abdominal or chest film will show mediastinal emphysema around the lower end of the oesophagus, and if the condition has remained untreated for several hours the emphysema extends upwards; commonly a pleural effusion develops.

Perforation of the colon. This is rare and the plain X-ray is seldom diagnostic, but some radiological signs may be apparent:

1. A soft tissue mass in the left iliac fossa due to the presence of a pericolic abscess, most frequently caused by either diverticulitis or a carcinoma of the sigmoid.
2. Distension of the colon proximal to the perforation.
3. A small bowel 'ladder pattern' due to ileus.
4. Gas in the pericolic and retroperitoneal tissues.

Ruptured aortic aneurysm

Aneurysmal rupture usually causes sudden, severe, agonizing pain in the abdomen, which rapidly spreads to the back. The abdomen is tender and guarding may be present, preventing the clinician from palpating the expansile pulsation typical of aneurysmal dilatation. However, hypovolaemic shock usually develops at an early stage due to blood extravasating into the retroperitoneal tissues. There are no pathognomonic features on a plain X-ray which indicate that an aneurysm has bled, only features indicating the presence of the aneurysm itself. In the majority of patients a calcified curvilinear shadow lies on one or both sides of the lumbar spine. The size of the aneurysm, as measured by the calcified rim, is of some importance when considering the possibility of rupture, since Crane reported that rupture causing death occurred in only 4% of aneurysms less than 4 cm in diameter as compared to 82% when the sac was larger than 7 cm.

Overall opinion as to whether plain X-rays of the abdomen should be taken in every patient suffering from acute abdominal pain differs among various centres. There can be little doubt that if the history and physical signs suggest the presence of a perforated viscus, intestinal obstruction, or biliary or renal colic, plain X-rays may be of great assistance both in diagnosis and management.

Biochemical investigations

In any patient who has a history of severe vomiting the sodium and potassium levels should be estimated. In intestinal obstruction the fluid loss is of the order of 3 l/day and the peripheral blood pressure may remain normal, even when the ECF volume loss is of the order of 30%, although in such patients the CVP may well be zero. In general, a loss of 300–500 mmol of sodium produces clinical evidence of dehydration indicated by a dry mouth, sunken cheeks, furred tongue, loss of skin turgor, thirst and oliguria. If clinical dehydration is present immediate steps should be taken to correct it, and if the CVP is low it should be restored to normal prior to operation.

Specific biochemical tests are of value when the clinical diagnosis of acute pancreatitis has been made. In this condition the serum amylase rises to abnormally high levels, often exceeding 1000 Somogyi units (normal 80–150 units). Unfortunately the magnitude of this biochemical abnormality does not necessarily reflect the severity of the disease; in the milder oedematous form the elevated level falls to normal within 48 hours, making a retrospective diagnosis virtually impossible. However, the serum amylase may also increase in other conditions in which acute abdominal pain is the primary symptom, e.g. perforated peptic ulcer, acute cholecystitis and intestinal obstruction, although the level attained is never that normally associated with acute pancreatitis.

Also, in acute pancreatitis the serum calcium may fall due to the ionic calcium component of the plasma combining with the fatty acids formed by the hydrolysis of fat. The severity of the resultant hypocalcaemia is related to the severity of the disease; if the fall approaches 30% of the normal value (2.25–2.60 mmol/l) the attack can be considered severe.

GENERAL MANAGEMENT

In all patients the general conditon must be carefully assessed and note made of any concomitant illness which requires medical treatment, e.g. diabetes or heart failure. In all reported series both the operative and perioperative mortality, i.e. deaths occurring within 28 days of operation, increase with advancing age, partly because of increasing incidence of cardiorespiratory disease and also because increasingly lethal conditions prevail, e.g. ruptured abdominal aortic aneurysm and malignant disease. In all patients in whom an inflammatory lesion is suspected or the bowel may be opened, prophylactic antibiotic therapy should be commenced to reduce the incidence of postoperative infective complications (see Vol. 1, p. 43).

MANAGEMENT OF SPECIFIC CONDITIONS

Appendicitis

In the Western world the treatment of acute appendicitis is appendicectomy, access to the abdominal cavity being achieved, if a definite diagnosis has been made, by a classical McBurney incision centred over the point of maximum tenderness. If difficulty is encountered in removing the appendix through this limited access the incision can be enlarged either by dividing the outer fibres of the sheath of the rectus abdominis or by dividing the internal oblique and transversus abdominis muscles at right angles to the line of their fibres.

In an adult where a mass is present in the right iliac fossa at the time of the initial examination and a diagnosis of appendix abscess is made, the classical treatment is to manage the patient conservatively, observing the mass daily. In the vast majority of patients the mass usually begins to diminish in size to finally resolve in a matter of days, and thereafter an interval appendicectomy is performed some 3 months after the initial attack. The indications for surgery in this small group of patients are an expanding mass or, very rarely, rupture of the abscess producing general peritonitis – an extremely rare event. Recently, with the development of ultrasonography, the progress of an abscess can be watched with great precision, and if a pus-containing cavity develops it is now possible for an interventional radiologist to aspirate the abscess with a fine catheter.

In children, even in the presence of a palpable mass, appendicectomy is advisable since the short omentum of the child makes containment of the inflammatory process less effective than in the adult, so that the risk of general peritonitis is greater.

The morbidity following acute appendicitis arises from the infective complications and these have been much reduced by the use of prophylactic antibiotics and particularly by the introduction of metronidazole.

Intestinal obstruction

Small bowel

Whilst the diagnosis of intestinal obstruction can be readily made by the history alone, the problem in the obstructed patient is to distinguish between simple mechanical obstruction and a strangulating obstruction in which the blood supply of the bowel wall and hence its integrity is endangered. Clinically the distinction can be made in part on the history alone, for in simple obstruction the patient complains of colicky abdominal pain during the strong peristaltic contractions, but the pain disappears as these diminish in intensity, whereas when the obstruction is due to strangulation the patient is left with a constant background pain even when the colicky pain subsides. Regarding the physical signs, in a strangulating obstruction an area of peritoneal irritation is usually found as the gangrenous bowel abuts against the parietal peritoneum, best exemplified by the tenderness present in a strangulated external hernia.

Causation

Simple mechanical obstruction. The majority of simple obstructions are caused by adhesions following previous surgery or inflammatory conditions of the peritoneal cavity and less commonly by a bolus, especially in countries in which *Ascaris lumbricoides* is common. In the aging adult the commonest cause of simple obstruction is a carcinoma of the colon.

Strangulating obstruction. The commonest causes of strangulating obstruction are external or internal hernia, and volvulus – either of the small bowel around a congenital band, e.g. a Meckel's diverticulum, which may remain attached to the anterior abdominal wall, or of the large bowel, more commonly of the sigmoid but occasionally of the caecum. It must, however, be appreciated that if a simple obstruction is allowed to progress, ultimately the blood supply to the bowel wall may become compromised.

In the infant an intussusception may occur, most commonly at about 6 months of age.

Treatment

In all patients in whom intestinal obstruction is suspected the stomach should be decompressed by means of an indwelling gastric tube, and blood taken for estimation of the electrolyte content. The passage of a nasal tube is of great importance, for in patients suffering from severe obstruction the first critical moment is during the induction of anaesthesia; stomach distension prior to the passage of the endotracheal tube may lead to regurgitation and aspiration, the patient either dying forthwith or later developing severe pulmonary problems.

In patients suffering from simple obstruction, decompression may relieve the situation completely allowing a later, more accurate assessment of the cause followed if necessary by definitive surgery. However, if suction brings no relief laparotomy is indicated in order to ascertain the cause of the obstruction and deal with the matter.

Malignant obstruction of the large bowel

Approximately 15% of all colonic neoplasms present with acute intestinal obstruction requiring some form of surgery. The site at which obstructing growths develop varies somewhat according to the series examined. Thus in a study of 713 patients reported by Phillips and others in 1985 as part of the Large Bowel Carcinoma Project, the site of the obstructing growth was in the splenic flexure in no less than 45% of patients. The precise cause of the obstruction has not been established. Several factors are probably responsible: the area of the growth becomes oedematous; the area becomes infected; the faeces become more solid; and the gut proximal to the obstructing lesion becomes atonic.

In all reported series, however, it would appear that the long-term outlook in patients presenting with acute obstruction is poorer than in patients who are treated by an elective operation. Thus Phillips found that the 5-year survival in patients presenting with obstruction was 25% as compared to a 5-year survival of 45% for those patients undergoing an elective procedure.

All are also agreed that the in-hospital and perioperative mortality is greatly increased in obstructed patients.

Treatment

There is no dispute concerning the treatment of patients in whom the tumour is situated in the right side of the colon or even in the transverse colon, as far as and including the splenic flexure. In all these patients a right hemicolectomy or extended colectomy should be performed, even in the presence of gross obstruction.

The difficulty arises when the obstructing tumour is situated in the left colon. Resection with an immediate anastomosis, if successful, reduces the duration of hospital stay but is associated with a high percentage of clinically manifest anastomotic leaks, and when this occurs further surgery may be required. Therefore high mortality rates are reported following this type of surgery, as high as 50% in some reported series.

However, examination of various series in which a defunctioning colostomy is performed followed later by resection and, at a third stage, closure of the colostomy, also reveals a high mortality even though the percentage of anastomotic leaks falls to around 6%. The mortality in this group arises from the fact that many of these patients are elderly and unable to withstand the trauma associated with three operations. It is, therefore, very much a matter of opinion and experience as to precisely what the surgeon should do when confronted with an obstructive left-sided tumour, a decision which may largely depend on the degree of dilatation of the proximal colon, gross dilatation making a primary anastomosis difficult because of the disparity in luminal size.

If the tumour is at the rectosigmoid junction, one option is to perform a Hartmann operation, removing the tumour, closing the upper end of the rectum and constructing a terminal colostomy in the left iliac fossa. An old operation, the Paul Mikulicz procedure, may also be suitable for some patients when the tumour is situated in the sigmoid colon, bringing out the colon, excising the tumour and constructing a double-barrelled colostomy which will later be closed. However, this operation is only satisfactory when at laparotomy distant metastases are found, since it can in no way be regarded as a radical procedure.

Acute cholecystitis

In the past the treatment of this condition, once diagnosed, was conservative, but over the past 25 years a growing number of surgeons have advocated an immediate cholecystectomy. The author himself found that this was a relatively easy technical operation to perform and that the mortality was limited to the elderly patient but that in this group conservative treatment carried just as high a mortality. An alternative approach which can be used in the frail elderly patient is to perform a cholecystostomy and remove the obstructing calculi. If this is done, in the great majority of elderly patients no further action is necessary.

Perforated duodenal ulceration

As previously stated, the natural history of peptic ulceration has been altered by the introduction of the H_2 blocking agents, and so whilst in the past it was recommended that simple suture should be abandoned in favour of definitive gastric surgery, this view is now no longer tenable because in the majority of perforations seen the ulcer is acute and precipitated by medication. Thus if there is no previous history together with a history of the administration of ulcerogenic drugs it seems reasonable to suggest that simple suture followed by the administration of H_2 blocking agents is all that is required. It is also possible to treat perforated acute simple ulcers merely by nasal suction and intravenous fluids, but if this method is adopted a careful watch must be kept on the extent of the 'guarding' since if this extends after admission this is an indication for immediate surgery.

SECTION TWO

SECTION TWO

6. Fractures and the general principles of their treatment

CLASSIFICATION

Type

Fractures may be classified as *open* or *closed*.

Open fractures may be produced by a small spicule of bone puncturing the overlying skin or, alternatively, massive skin loss may have been sustained because of external or internal forces at the time of the injury. Once the skin has been punctured, no matter what the size of the external wound, bacterial contamination of the wound, soft tissues and bone may occur.

In closed injuries no such risk occurs.

Stress fractures

This type of fracture is found in bones subjected to repeated minor trauma, e.g. march fracture of the metatarsals.

Pathological fractures

These are found when bones have been weakened by disease, in which case the force required is insufficient to break a normal bone. The commonest causes are postmenopausal osteoporosis, secondary metastases and osteopenia. In aging women fractures of the lower radius and neck of the femur are several times commoner than in the male because of osteoporosis.

Pattern of the fracture line

The specific pattern of the fracture line or lines is determined by:

- The forces that caused the bone to break.

81

- The internal structure of the involved bone.

The latter varies from the dense cortical bone of the shafts of long bones to spongy or cancellous bone found in the metaphyses of long bones, the body of short bones and in flat bones.

Common terms applied to fracture lines are transverse, oblique or spiral, comminuted, compression, greenstick, epiphyseal fracture separation, avulsion and osteochondral.

Deformity

The subsequent deformity at the fracture site is described by a variety of terms such as angulation, shortening, distraction and rotation.

HEALING OF FRACTURES

Long bones

Immediately a bone is fractured the torn periosteum and the small blood vessels traversing the broken Haversian canals bleed and form a fracture haematoma. Repair cells derived from the endosteum and the periosteum invade the haematoma to produce both external and internal callus, which is at first radiolucent because it contains no calcium.

As time passes, the callus becomes firmer as it becomes more cellular. Some osteogenic cells differentiate into chondroblasts and a variable amount of cartilage is normally formed in the early callus, which is later removed. At the same time new bone of the woven type is formed, first at a distance from the fracture line where there is least movement.

Later the woven bone is reabsorbed by osteoclasts and slowly replaced by lammellar bone. The healing process ends when gradual remodelling of the bone has restored the normal architecture, a process known as consolidation.

Cancellous bones

Cancellous bone, which consists of a sponge-like lattice of interconnected trabeculae, heals primarily through internal or endosteal callus formation, which spreads across the fracture.

Healing is usually much faster than in long bones because there is minimal bone destruction at the fracture site and, usually, a greater blood supply.

Factors influencing healing time

Age

Healing followed by final remodelling is always quicker in the young. Note Perkins' formula (p. 97).

Blood supply

An adequate blood supply is essential for healing, so cancellous bone, which has a greater vascular network than cortical bone, heals more quickly. If there is gross displacement in a fractured long bone the blood supply to one or several fragments may be jeopardized by damage to the nutrient artery. When this happens the blood supply to the fragments is dependent on the periosteum which, in turn, derives part of its blood supply from the attached muscles. Because of these factors fractures of the lower third of the tibia are much slower to heal than are fractures of the upper third, because the former have no muscles attached to the periosteum. In certain fractures, notably of the scaphoid and head of the femur, avascular necrosis occurs because of the peculiarities of the blood supply. Thus, in fractures through the middle of the scaphoid, avascular necrosis of the proximal fragment occurs because the greater part of the blood supply enters the distal half of the bone. In subcapital fractures of the femur all the blood supply to the head is interrupted with the exception of the vessels running in the ligamentum teres.

Avascular necrosis produces a 'relative' increase in density of the affected area of bone on plain X-rays because, usually, there is osteoporosis in the surrounding bone. The first radiological signs of this complication may appear as early as 6 weeks after injury.

Configuration of the fracture

In general, if there has not been soft tissue interposition, long oblique fractures heal more rapidly than do transverse ones. Associated with configuration is the initial displacement, and if the fragments are undisplaced they may have an intact periosteal sleeve, in which case healing from endosteal callus only is needed.

Infection

A fracture site may become infected because of the contamination of a compound fracture at the time of injury, or it may be a complication of the open reduction of a closed fracture. Commonly, acute infection is due to *Staphylococcus pyogenes*, but there can also be low-grade infections with Gram-negative organisms such as *Pseudomonas aeruginosa, Escherichia coli* and *Proteus mirabilis*. Infection delays or prevents healing, particularly if it is severe enough to give rise to acute or chronic osteomyelitis.

In addition to the types of infection already noted, the puncture wound overlying a compound fracture may form the point of entry for the two dangerous *Clostridia* infections, i.e. tetanus and gas gangrene, particularly if the wound is deep and heavily contaminated with soil or debris.

Apposition

If there is a gap between the bone ends, delayed healing or non-union is likely because callus can extend only over a few millimetres. One of the major aims of the surgeon is to produce reasonable bony apposition by reducing fractures in which apposition of the fragments has been lost.

In some fractures, successful reduction and apposition are frustrated by soft tissue interposition which cannot be overcome without open operation on the fracture site. Although apposition and reduction are usually associated with immobilization, the latter may not be necessary. Fractured ribs heal without immobilization, as also do fractures of the shaft of the humerus.

TREATMENT OF FRACTURES

The aims of treatment are:

- To relieve pain.
- To assist bony union and thus the recovery of function.
- To minimize deformity, which may of itself cause later degenerative changes in adjacent joints.
- To prevent or delay the development of degenerative changes in which fracture lines have run.

Apart from the relief of pain all these aims are attained if the fracture is reduced, the aim of reduction being to bring the ends or segments of fractured bone into apposition, after which the bone must be immobilized until healing has occurred. Not all fractures need to be reduced nor can all fractures be immobilized; for example, reduction is unnecessary for compression fractures of the thoracolumbar spine, impacted fractures, crush fractures of the distal phalanx and fractures of the ribs.

The commonest method of achieving reduction is by manipulation using either local or general anaesthesia, after which the fracture is immobilized by either external or internal fixation. Such methods fail if the fracture is spiral or comminuted. If a local anaesthetic agent is used it might be injected directly into the fracture site or used to produce a regional block.

External immobilization can be achieved by the use of:

1. Moulded casts of plaster of Paris or fibreglass.
2. External fixation.
3. Continous traction.

Moulded casts

Prior to applying the cast the fracture is manipulated, reversing the path of the original displacement.

Plaster consists of anhydrous calcium sulphate incorporated into a bandage which solidifies after hydration, setting in minutes but not completely drying for between 36-48 hours.

Fibreglass has the following advantages:

a. It is fast setting – within 29 minutes it is weightbearing.
b. It is light.
c. It has great strength.
d. It is radiolucent.

Its one great disadvantage is that it does not mould as well as plaster to the contours of the limb. It is most commonly used for lower limb plasters, its use in the upper limb being generally restricted to fractures of the scaphoid.

Prior to the use of either material the affected limb is enclosed in stockinette and then padded with wool, which should be applied in the form of a bandage from above downwards with an overlap of 50%, taking care especially of the bony prominences.

The use of either plaster or fibreglass is not without hazard, the most serious of which is the development of vascular insufficiency in the limb due to unrelieved swelling. Unrelenting and increasing pain in an enclosed limb should be investigated by splitting the cast with parallel cuts on either side of the extremity; not only should the cast, but also the underlying padding should be divided since dried blood soaked padding can itself be as equally resistant to expansion as can plaster or fibreglass. It is to prevent this complication that the cast is split immediately after its application if further swelling is anticipated.

Localized pain in an enclosed limb usually occurs over a bony prominence and may be followed by skin necrosis. An appropriate window should be cut in the cast and hollowed out, after which the window should be closed either by padding or by cutting a piece of orthopaedic felt to the same size as the opening.

In general, casts should immobilize the joints above and below the fracture. Fractures that include the ankle are extended to the base of the toes to prevent oedema and irritation of the forefoot. In the lower limb the knee is usually held at an angle of 170°, the ankle at an angle of 90° and the tarsus and forefoot in a neutral position. In the upper limb the position of the splinted joints varies with the fracture; where the fracture is near a joint, usually only that joint is included, but the joint above and below should also be included if rotation cannot otherwise be controlled.

Fashions in external immobilization by means of plaster are not constant. For example, fractures of the lower third of the tibia, which are notoriously slow to unite, were commonly treated by a full length plaster, but in 1967 Sarciento recommended the use of the so-called patella weightbearing plaster leaving the knee joint free to move.

A modification used by some in the treatment of supracondylar fractures of the femur or fractures of the tibial plateau is cast bracing. After manipulation of the fracture and traction for some weeks until the fracture is 'sticky' the limb is released and a series of plaster casts are applied. The first and upper segment is weightbearing on the ischial tuberosity; this extends to just above the knee joint allowing sufficient space between it and the plaster surrounding the leg to contain a knee hinge, which is then fitted into the two plaster casts. A less commonly used method of fixation is the use of pins attached to a rigid outrigger. This method was first described by Lambotte in 1907 and improved by Anderson in 1934. The method is particularly suitable for the treatment of tibial shaft fractures and the protagonists of the method state that it is particularly valuable when associated nerve, blood vessel or extensive soft tissue injury has occurred.

Much more commonly used is continuous traction to maintain position and immobilization.

Traction

Traction can be exerted by:

1. *Ventfoam* applied to the skin held by two crepe bandages. A cord is attached which can be tied to a Thomas splint or to weights led over a pulley. A maximum weight of 8–10 pounds (3.6–4.5 kg) is all that should be applied, otherwise the skin may be damaged or the fracture distracted. Ordinary adhesive tape should not be used since, being impervious to moisture, the skin becomes sodden and excoriated. In general, skin traction is used as a temporary measure.

2. *Skeletal traction.* Skeletal traction is applied by inserting either a Steinmann pin or Kirschner wire (usually the former) across the distal femoral shaft, proximal tibia or talus onto which is bolted a traction bow to which, via cords, weights can be attached.

Traction can be *fixed* or *balanced*. An example of the former is the treatment of a fracture of the shaft of the femur by tying extension tapes over the end of a Thomas splint, the counterthrust being exerted by a padded ring encircling the thigh and pushing against the ischium.

Balanced traction implies the use of a system of splints, cords, weights and pulleys. Used in the treatment of fractures of the femoral shaft it allows the patient to bend the knee whilst traction remains exerted on the femoral shaft itself thus helping to avoid stiffness of the knee.

Closed reduction with external immobilization or fixation has to be abandoned in the following circumstances:

1. When soft tissue interposition has occurred.
2. When experience indicates that closed reduction and external immobilization will be ineffective, e.g. a fracture involving both forearm bones.
3. When articular surfaces are fractured or displaced, e.g. fractures of the tibial condyles or medial malleolus.
4. In the presence of multiple fractures, multiple injuries or concomitant gross soft tissue injury.
5. If prolonged bed rest is undesirable.

The alternative to external immobilization is internal skeletal fixation by nails, screws, plates and screws or wires.

The use of intramedullary nails was introduced by Hey Groves in World War One but he was defeated by the poor metals then available. The method was revived by Küntscher in 1940. The Küntscher nail is clover-leafed in shape and is used especially for femoral shaft fractures. It may be inserted blindly using an image intensifier to guide the nail, but in most centres an incision is made over the site of the fracture and a guide wire introduced into the medullary cavity at the lower end of the proximal fragment. This is driven upwards in the medullary cavity until finally it protrudes in the buttock with the hip flexed and in adduction. The nail is then driven down along the wire and on reaching the distal fragment the wire is withdrawn to be reinserted from above into the upper end of the distal fragment to act as a guide as the nail is punched home into the distal segment.

Other nails in common use have been designed to deal with tibial shaft fractures and the Rush nail is used for smaller long bones. Screws, screws and plates and also wire can be used to hold fractures together. The commonest screw used in orthopaedics is the machine screw, a screw threaded from head to tip with a blunt end. Screws may be self-tapping, or prior tapping before insertion may be required. The predominant factor in determining the holding power of a screw immediately after its insertion is the diameter of the screw thread. One modification which gained a considerable following in recent years, particularly on the Continent, was the AO System developed by the Swiss with the dual object of making the fixation so stable that external spintage was unnecessary and making movement of the joints above and below the fracture possible immediately, thus avoiding atrophy, osteoporosis and joint stiffness. To achieve this type of fixation interfragmental compression is produced by lag screws and axial compression by plates under tension. This method has never gained in popularity in the UK, where the majority of orthopaedic surgeons prefer to think of a plate as a suture and not as an aid to union.

Treatment of open fractures

The treatment of an open fracture depends in large measure on the time interval between the injury and the beginning of treatment and the extent of the soft tissue injury. When the injury is seen within 8 hours, immediate primary closure of the skin, either by suture or by skin graft, can be attempted. When the wound is extensive, heavily contaminated, or seen late, debridement of the wound should be performed.

This is a most important aspect of the care of an open fracture. The skin should be sparingly excised but the underlying fascia must be extensively divided to prevent development of tension within muscular compartments, which may jeopardize the blood supply to the limb. In addition, all doubtfully viable or dead muscle must be excised in order to reduce the incidence of anaerobic infections.

After debridement, delayed primary suture is carried out, not later than 10 days from the time of injury. Internal fixation should, if possible, be avoided in this type of fracture.

At the time of admission, prophylactic measures should be taken to avoid both tetanus and gas gangrene (see Vol. 1, Ch. 8).

7. Common complications of fractures

The complications of fractures may be divided into *early* and *late*, *local* and *general*. In some cases the effects of the fracture will be enhanced by the presence of a dislocation.

EARLY LOCAL COMPLICATIONS

Injury to the skin overlying a fracture

1. *Friction burns.* Such burns should be thoroughly cleansed of particles of dirt ground into the dermis otherwise an ugly tatoo mark will result.
2. *Compromised skin circulation.* This is most commonly the result of a gradual increase in internal tension rather than a direct injury to blood vessels (see below).
3. *Plaster sores.* Badly applied or unpadded plasters may lead to plaster sores as a result of direct pressure over a bony prominence. A complaint of unremitting localized pain suggests that this complication is occurring, and it should be investigated by cutting a window and if necessary replacing the plaster. A window cut in a plaster should never be left open.

Vascular complications

Arterial

The classic symptoms and signs of impending vascular problems are the five P's: Pain, Paralysis, Paraesthesia, loss of Pulses and Pallor. Of these symptoms, the most important are the complaint of pain which is deep, unremitting and poorly localized, and paraesthesia. The presence of neurological signs may occur within 30 minutes if the vascular occlusion is complete and acute whereas functional changes

91

occur in the muscles within 2-4 hours; total ischaemia of longer than 12 hours is always followed by contractures.

Some fractures are more liable to cause vascular compromise than others, e.g. fractures or fracture-dislocations of the head of the humerus may cause damage to the axillary artery; supracondylar fractures of the humerus are notorious for the damage which may occur to the brachial artery and fractures or fracture dislocations around the knee may damage the popliteal artery.

Closed, extensively comminuted fractures may compromise the blood supply to the injured limb in the following ways:

1. By causing contusion of the artery which may lead to:
   a. Spasm.
   b. Thrombosis, caused either by intramural haemorrhage or detachment of the intima accompanied by prolapse into the lumen.

2. By causing a puncture wound in the vessel wall by a spicule of bone. In the presence of signs indicating that arterial obstruction has occurred immediately following the injury an arteriogram followed by exploration of the artery is indicated. If an area of contusion is found and the spasm cannot be relieved by medical means the affected segment of the artery should be excised and an end-to-end anastomosis performed using either 4/0 or 6/0 arterial sutures. If excision results in the loss of more than 2 cm of the artery it may be necessary to bridge the gap using a reversed autogenous venous graft. In all cases the overall prognosis is worse if there is concomitant injury to the venous side of the circulation.

3. By venous engorgement and/or oedema within a tight fascial compartment.

The latter is known as the compartment syndrome, which is defined as a condition in which the circulation and hence the function of the tissues within a closed space are compromised by an increased pressure within that space. It is most commonly seen after fractures of the leg and forearm.

Thus the syndrome may result from:

1. A decrease in the size of the compartment within which the fracture has occurred due to premature closure of fascial defects, tight dressings or localized external pressure.

2. An increase in the contents of a particular compartment as a result of haemorrhage into the compartment or increased capillary permeability. A significant physical sign in this condition is increasing pain on passive movement of the toes or fingers. In some centres

direct intracompartmental pressure measurements are available and are used to indicate the correct treatment.

The treatment of choice of this syndrome – if simple measures such as removal of the dressings or cast do nothing to relieve the problem – is immediate and extensive fasciotomy.

Failure to treat arterial injuries in a satisfactory manner, or delay in diagnosis, leads to a Volkmann's ischaemic contracture, in which the muscle mass is replaced by fibrous tissue or, worse, the necessity to amputate the limb.

Venous

Any fracture requiring immobilization may be complicated by deep venous thrombosis, which may be followed by a pulmonary embolus. Prophylactic measures such as the subcutaneous injection of heparin or intravenous dextran are used, particularly in elderly patients who are likely to be subjected to prolonged immobilization.

Neurological complications

Bony injury, especially if associated with dislocation in the following sites, may lead to nerve damage. Excluding spinal fractures the commonest nerve injury is, however, a neuropraxia from which a rapid recovery will occur. Occasionally an axonotmesis occurs, particularly when the fracture is complicated by a dislocation which causes traction on the nerve. Such cases should recover and can be followed by serial electromyograms allowing a lag phase of 1 month and thereafter a recovery rate of 2.5 cm per month. If distal innervation has not occurred by the expected time the affected nerve should be explored.

Fractures and fracture-dislocations of the spine

Skeletal disruptions at the level of T10 and above, if of sufficient severity, may cause cord damage and as a result no recovery is possible. However, the spinal cord terminates at the level of the intervertebral disc between L1 and L2; caudal to this level the only neural contents of the spinal canal are the roots of the cauda equina. Because the average dimensions of the vertebral canal in an adult are 23.4 mm in width and 17.4 mm in the anteroposterior axis the lumbar region has relatively greater space within it than other regions of the vertebral column, and therefore fractures and fracture-dislocations in the lumbar region require more displacement than in their counterparts in the thoracic spine to produce neurological damage.

In lesions of the cauda equina that part of the deficit due to damage to the motor fibres may recover so long as the fibrous perineurium of the fasciculi remains intact. This is not, however, true of the sensory component if the lesion has occurred proximal to the peripheral nerve cell of origin, i.e. the dorsal root ganglion cell.

Posterior dislocation or fracture-dislocation of the hip

The perineal part of the sciatic nerve is frequently contused in dislocations or fracture-dislocations of the hip joint. Such injuries should be recognized early as the nerve trunk does not tolerate pressure and ischaemic changes soon occur. Thus a posterior dislocation should be reduced as a surgical emergency, and if a posterior fragment remains persistently displaced in the presence of neurological signs an open reduction should be undertaken with internal fixation of the acetabular fragment.

Fractures and fracture-dislocations around the knee joint

These may cause injury to both the medial and lateral popliteal nerves.

Fractures of the shaft of the humerus

Between 5-10% of fractures of the humerus are complicated by an injury to the radial nerve, which is particularly likely if the fracture involves the distal third of the shaft. The diagnosis is easily made because of the concomitant wrist drop. The fingers should be fixed in a dynamic splint and, since the most common injury is a stretching or bruising of the nerve, complete recovery of function can be anticipated within days or months. When a complete injury has occurred delayed repair is said to be followed by as good results as primary repair.

Fracture of the medial epicondyle

This fracture is usually due to avulsion forces with the result that the fracture line is not necessarily limited to the area of the original ossification centre. Such injuries may be associated with damage to the ulnar nerve.

Supracondylar fractures of the humerus

Damage to the brachial artery and the median nerve occur, especially in extension injuries of this area; the sharp fractured end of the proximal fragment projecting forwards into the antecubital fossa may contuse or impale the nerve.

Dislocations of the elbow

These may cause both median and ulnar nerve injuries.

LATE LOCAL COMPLICATIONS

Involving bone

Avascular necrosis (aseptic necrosis)

This condition nearly always affects some fragments of a comminuted fracture, particularly when these are completely separated from all the surrounding tissues. It is also a specific complication of fractures at certain sites which include subcapital fractures of the femur, fractures of the scaphoid, fracture-dislocation of the head of the humerus and less commonly fractures of the radial head, lunate bone and talus. The fundamental cause of avascular necrosis is the loss of the blood supply to the affected bone. Therefore although most commonly associated with fractures aseptic necrosis may also occur following:

1. Too extensive a stripping of the periosteum during surgery.
2. Caisson's disease.
3. As a long term complication of irradiation.

Despite the immediate organic changes during which the lacunae become empty and the marrow contains a formless debris the mechanical properties of the bone are not necessarily immediately affected and the dead bone may continue to function for months or indeed years. The bone adjacent to the fracture line becomes hyperaemic in preparation for the replacement of the dead tissue, causing resorption and thus demineralization and trabecular thinning of the living bone adjacent to the fracture. Since the necrotic bone lacks a blood supply it cannot undergo resorption immediately and so retains its original density and architecture. Thus the ischaemic bone, although of normal density, appears denser than the proximal long bone which has undergone the changes described.

In due course granulation tissue invades the marrow and the Haversian system of the dead bone, phagocytes remove the debris, and osteoclasts absorb the dead bone, thinning the trabeculae and widening the Haversian canals. Osteoblasts then begin to lay down osteoid seams, the trabeculae being replaced by new bone, a process commonly referred to as 'creeping substitution'.

The articular cartilage overlying dead bone does not itself become necrotic because it derives its nutrition from the synovial fluid; thus the joint space may be preserved for a considerable period until subchondral fractures occur in the necrotic trabeculae as a result of weightbearing pressures.

In the case of intracapsular fractures of the neck of the femur the incidence of segmental collapse of the head due to this complication varies considerably depending on the series examined. In Garden stage III/IV fractures, defined as complete fractures with partial displacement (III) and complete fracture with full displacement (IV), the incidence of segmental collapse according to a series published by Barnes and his colleagues in 1976 increased over time from 3–10% at 12 months to 18–28% at 36 months, the lower figure being related to males, in whom this type of fracture is much less common.

Factors affecting the incidence of collapse over which the surgeon has no control are: old age, sex, decreased mobility prior to the accident, and level of the fracture.

Factors over which the surgeon does have control include: acceptance of extreme valgus or varus deformity; extensive retroversion or anteversion following reduction; position of the fixation device; and postoperative ambulation.

Infection

Infection may follow a compound fracture or open reduction of a closed fracture. The infecting organism may be either Gram-positive or Gram-negative, more commonly the former, e.g. staphylococcus. If infection is not eradicated delayed or non-union may follow.

Delayed union and non-union

Delayed union may be defined as a failure of the bone to unite within the usual time space. To estimate the time taken for union and consolidation to occur reference is frequently make to Perkins' formula which provides a rough guide, although both clinical and radiological evidence of union should be present before whatever splintage has been used in a particular fracture is abandoned.

a. Spiral fractures of the upper limb unite in 3 weeks and consolidate in 6 weeks.
b. Transverse fractures of the upper limb unite in 6 weeks and consolidate in 12.
c. Spiral fractures of the lower limb unite in 12 weeks and consolidate in 24 weeks.
d. Transverse fractures of the lower limb unite in 24 weeks and consolidate in 48 weeks.

In children these figures may be halved.

The common reasons for non-union, assuming that the fracture is not pathogical, are as follows:

1. Infection.

2. Avascular necrosis, which may be the result of extreme comminution or too extensive a stripping of the soft tissues surrounding the fracture when performing internal fixation.

3. Distraction, either due to excessive traction or faulty internal fixation

4. The interposition of soft tissues, e.g. a flap of periosteum may become interposed between the shaft of the tibia and the medial malleolus, muscle may become interposed between the fractured ends of the femoral shaft; in fractures of the lateral condyle of the humerus rotation of the fragment may occur so that the cartilaginous articular surface faces the shaft.

5. Inadequate immobilization.

Specifically, fractures occurring in areas in which there is a poor blood supply may undergo delayed union, such areas being the lower third of the tibia and the neck of the femur.

Once there has been failure to unite the bone fragments usually become linked with fibrous tissue. However, consolidation is still possible, even in the presence of infection, if the bone fragments are immobilized. When the bone ends are sclerotic, cancellous or cortical autogenous bone grafts may be necessary to promote union as well as fixation together with compression. If non-union is due to inadequate fixation a pseudoarthrosis forms, which again makes union impossible without the use of bone grafts.

6. *Mal-union.* This is a complication of treatment rather than of the fracture itself. It may be treated conservatively if the deformity is acceptable both cosmetically and functionally or require osteotomy.

7. *Post-traumatic osteoporosis.* There is considerable variation in the individual response to immobilization, from little or no change to severe changes. Bone pain is frequently marked in demineralized bone and patients suffering from rarefaction after a fracture frequently exhibit marked bone tenderness. The condition is usually accompanied by muscle atrophy and its onset is accelerated when the bone is not subjected to functional stress. It is preventable by early mobilization and by activity within the splint or plaster. Osteoporosis takes longer to recover from than it does to develop and all methods other than the restoration of normal bone loading have proved ineffective.

8. *Sudeck's atrophy.* This condition is now referred to by a number of synonyms including reflex sympathetic dystrophy. It is fortunately rare and most commonly seen following a Colles' fracture of the lower radius or a fractured scaphoid. The precise aetiology is unknown but it is presumed that the sympathetic nervous system plays some part in its development. The symptoms of this condition are pain, which is variously described as excruciating or burning in character. The pain is not restricted to specific dermatomes and is characteristically out of all proportion to the initiating injury and often accentuated by emotional factors. In addition to pain there is associated joint stiffness; in the early stages the skin is red and the skin temperature raised, whereas in the later stages, when the pain may extend to involve the whole limb, the skin may appear pale, cool and atrophic.

Muscular complications – myositis ossificans (traumatic subperiosteal ossification)

This condition is characterized pathologically by fibrous, cartilaginous and osseous proliferation which may be situated in an extraosseous, periosteal or paraosteal position. The commonest site is in the brachialis following a fracture of the lower end of the shaft of the humerus but it also occurs in the absence of a fracture in the adductor region of the thigh in riders. The factors which have been implicated are:

1. Delayed treatment of a fracture leading to the need for excessive force when manipulation is finally undertaken.

2. Extensive soft tissue injury.
3. Too brief a period of immobilization.
4. Passive stretching to promote mobilization.

The pathogenesis of this condition is incompletely understood. An essential prerequisite is the formation of a haematoma in the damaged soft tissues, after which it is thought that an alteration in the ground substance of the connective tissue occurs followed by a proliferation of undifferentiated mesenchymal cells which then assume the morphological characteristics of osteoblasts. Mineralization follows and bone is formed. The changes appear first in the least damaged tissues and then spread centrally to involve the more damaged tissues.

Clinically the affected area becomes swollen and painful with loss of movement. As the pain subsides a circumscribed indurated palpable swelling is found. In the arm active extension is obstructed by the inelasticity of the muscle and flexion by the mass itself.

Treatment

Under no circumstances should the affected limb be manipulated. If the elbow region is involved the elbow joint should be immobilized in the position of maximum function, i.e. in 45° of flexion. Occasionally, when the process appears to have settled, excision of the residual swelling may be worthwhile but often this is followed by unsatisfactory results.

Tendon rupture

This complication is seen after Colles' fracture at the wrist or following crush fractures of the lower end of the radius. The tendon of extensor pollicis longus ruptures as it crosses the tubercle on the dorsal surface of the bone. The tendon usually ruptures between 4–8 weeks after the fracture and indeed at the time this event occurs the wrist may still be in plaster. Examination shows that whilst there is a passive range of movements of the thumb joints active extension at the interphalangeal joint is impossible and active extension at the meta-carpophalangeal joint is restricted.

Treatment

The most reliable operation is to transfer the tendon of extensor indicis to activate the distal stump of the extensor pollicis longus.

Joint stiffness

Joint stiffness may result from:

1. *Adhesions*. Adhesions may develop in joints after fractures have occurred in proximity to joints particularly when the injury has been followed by a haemarthrosis. The majority of blood is either aspirated or absorbed but that which remains may form filmy adhesions which later after organization become stronger. Joints such as the knee, elbow and fingers stiffen easily and often suffer permanent impairment of movement whereas the hip and wrist usually regain their full mobility.

2. *Periarticular changes*. Periarticular changes are a much more common cause of joint stiffness and cause loss of resilience in the periarticular tissues.

Joint stiffness complicating fractures should be prevented from developing by the early mobilization of adjacent joints by the use of functional bracing if this is possible. Following immobilization active exercises are required, sometimes over a long period. If manipulation is indicated, especially of the knee, it should be performed gently since the patella is easily fractured if more than moderate force is used. Repeated gentle manipulation is more appropriate to the situation.

Osteoarthritis

Any irregularity of a joint surface as a result of a fracture involving a joint may precipitate osteoarthritis. Even a slight step between the opposed fragments may lead to subsequent disability, particularly in a weightbearing joint. For example, ankle fractures in which a posterior tibial fragment has occurred are followed by degenerative arthritis in some 30% of patients. Even in fractures not directly involving the joint incorrect alignment may cause malalignment of the joint surfaces and thus excessive stress on one part of a joint leading eventually to degeneration.

EARLY GENERAL COMPLICATIONS

1. *Shock* – see Volume 1, Chapter 9.
2. *Fat embolus* – see Volume 1, Chapter 13.
3. *Pulmonary embolus* – see Volume 1, Chapter 13.
4. *Anaerobic infections* – see Volume 1, Chapter 8.

LATE GENERAL COMPLICATIONS

1. *Renal failure* – see Volume 1, Chapter 14.
2. *Renal calculi*. These may form due to a variety of factors, the most important of which are recumbency and infection. The former, particularly when associated with immobilization, leads to hypercalciuria, the latter to the deposition of triple phosphate. The stones of recumbency typically develop in the inferior major calyces which are the most dependent in the supine position.
3. *Accident neurosis*. Following a major injury a certain degree of neuroticism often develops. This usually resolves once full function has returned but in some patients if may persist even beyond the settlement of all legal claims.

8. Fractures of the cervical spine

FREQUENCY AND CAUSATION

Severe injuries to the cervical spine, i.e. those complicated by spinal cord injury, are relatively rare. In contrast, lesser injuries known to the community as the 'whiplash' injury are commonplace. The two commonest causes of severe injury are road traffic accidents and sporting injuries. Among the latter are diving, trampolining, and body contact sports such as rugby although, in the latter, efforts have been made to reduce the frequency of these injuries by tighter controls of the ruck. In some patients in whom a bony injury occurs cord damage could have been avoided by careful movement of the injured person at the scene of the accident, i.e. turning the patient with the head fixed in relation to the trunk, a manœuvre which may require as many as five persons co-operating or, alternatively, in a motor accident not attempting to move the injured person at all unless there is a danger of fire, until paramedical or medical help is available. Then the normal procedure is to stabilize the neck prior to moving the victim by means of a semi-rigid cervical collar extending from the occiput to the level of the nipple line anteriorly.

Mechanisms of injury

Great forces are required to produce damage to the normal cervical spine and the mechanism of injury is frequently complex, involving rotational forces as well as simple flexion or extension. In addition, particularly in diving accidents or potential suicides, axial compression is exerted on the spine producing the typical 'bursting' injury of the vertebral body or bodies.

The major factors modifying the effects of cervical injury are: the age of the patient since this affects the 'strength' of the vertebrae and the surrounding ligaments; the presence of degenerative disease; and whether the muscles surrounding the cervical spine are 'on guard' at the time of the injury.

Causes of death

A fracture of the upper cervical spine may result in sudden death from damage to the brain stem; indeed survival after complete occipito-atlantal dislocation is exceptional. Later deaths were commonly due to urinary tract infection leading to secondary renal damage or respiratory complications. The frequency of both these complications has been much reduced in recent years; indeed the life expectancy of the healthy young tetraplegic patient has now been extended to some thirty years.

Pathology of the spinal cord

When the bony injury is so severe that damage to the spinal cord occurs a spreading haemorrhagic necrosis occurs, the white fibres being secondarily involved with spreading oedema, so that not only does a transverse but also a longitudinal lesion occur healing with gliosis and cyst formation.

INJURIES DUE TO FLEXION AND HYPERFLEXION

When forcible flexion of the head on the neck occurs, the first effect is to produce compression of the anterior part of the vertebral body, causing the typical wedge-shaped appearance. The common area in which this type of injury occurs is in the lower three cervical vertebrae. As the force producing hyperflexion continues, particularly if a rotational element is added, so the posterior longitudinal ligament may be ruptured and one or both facets subluxated or dislocated. When a bilateral facet dislocation has occurred only the anterior longitudinal ligament remains intact. Whilst a partial subluxation is usually associated with minimal neurological impairment, bilateral facet dislocation is normally accompanied by a tetraplegia although prompt reduction may result in a minimal neurological defect.

Radiology of flexion–rotation injuries

The correct interpretation of lateral and oblique X-rays of the spine is of great importance and full depression of the shoulders, 'the swimmer's view' and a 45° supine oblique view usually demonstrate injuries at the cervico-thoracic junction. CAT, if available, is of course an additional aid to the correct diagnosis.

If forward displacement of one vertebral body on another is less than half a diameter it indicates that there has been a unilateral facet dislocation, whereas greater displacement indicates a bilateral dislocation. Nevertheless when there is more than 3.5 mm of horizontal displacement of one vertebra in relation to another it indicates that the spine is potentially unstable.

When no bony injury is seen on the lateral and oblique radiographs it must be assumed that there has been momentary subluxation followed by spontaneous reduction. Such an injury may only become obvious when the neck is X-rayed in flexion although careful scrutiny of a routine lateral film may show that the outer articular facets are not parallel.

INJURIES DUE TO HYPEREXTENSION (HYPERDEFLEXION OR RETROFLEXION INJURIES)

Whereas in a flexion injury the neck is buttressed by the approximation of the head onto the chest, no such natural barrier exists when the head is forced into hyperextension. As a result the anterior longitudinal ligament is ruptured causing a compressive force on the facet joints with the result that a fracture of the articular facets may occur. The radiographic appearances may be minimal or there may be an enlarged prevertebral shadow, anterior widening of the disc space or an anterior marginal fracture. In young patients fractures of the bases of the spinous processes may occur. In very severe injuries of this type they may be mistaken for flexion injuries because of anterior displacement of the vertebral body. However, a careful examination of the head for bruising over the forehead or severe facial lacerations or injuries accompanied by a lateral X-ray demonstrating fractures of the laminae, pedicles or bases of the adjacent spinous process all point to the correct diagnosis.

The accompanying neurological deficit following this type of injury is extremely variable. Skull traction is not required for the majority of these injuries, the neck being immobilized in a collar. A lower motor neurone paralysis of the upper limbs occurs, accompanied by a spastic paralysis of the legs, the legs recovering better than the arms but with the prehensile function of the hands permanently impaired.

Grossly displaced fractures of this type require reduction and bone grafting.

COMPRESSION FRACTURES

These are extremely rare and are usually caused by falling from a height onto the head. At the level of the atlanto-axial joint such an injury may produce severe damage to the ring of the atlas, because the force of the blow is transmitted through the two lateral masses and the ring of bone then breaks at its weaker points.

Should the atlas be displaced in a forward direction, instantaneous death may follow if the transverse ligament bracing the odontoid process is torn. If, however, this ligament remains intact, it holds the odontoid to the arch, which minimizes cord damage. Thus these fractures are not necessarily associated with a cord lesion and there may therefore be a complete absence of neurological signs; alternatively there may be a complete tetraplegia.

To demonstrate this type of fracture the patient should be X-rayed through the open mouth.

Wedging or comminution of the vertebral bodies may occur whether the neck is flexed or extended at the time of injury. If a large anteroinferior fragment is produced, the remainder of the vertebral body and the disc material is pushed backwards into the spinal canal. In other cases severe compression may burst the vertebral bodies and damage the discs, with the result that the bony fragments are thrust into the anterior aspect of the cord.

CLINICAL FEATURES OF CERVICAL INJURIES

Any conscious patient admitted following an accident that might have given rise to a cervical injury should be regarded as suspect if a complaint of neck pain is made, particularly if, following the injury, the patient complains of tingling or weakness of the feet or hands. Some conscious patients may walk into the accident and emergency department holding their head supported by their hands. Incomplete cord injuries may be associated with stiffness rather than paralysis of the limbs. The diagnosis of tetraplegia should not be difficult to make but on two occasions in the author's clinical experience such 'paralysis' has been caused by hysteria.

General examination

The aim of the general examination is to determine the severity and distribution of associated injuries and in addition carefully examine the head and face to ascertain the position of bruising, lacerations, or areas of tenderness, which may give a clue as to the mechanism of the spinal injury.

Neurological examination

The aims of a thorough clinical neurological examination are to:

- Establish the presence of absence of a cord lesion.
- Establish whether this is complete or incomplete.
- Establish the nature and extent of any root involvement.

These features are established by an examination of:

1. The sensory system.
2. Movement.
3. The presence or absence of reflexes, superficial or deep.

Sensation

This is assessed by reference to the response to light touch, pinprick, vibration, and joint position sense.

Sensation should be tested by proceeding from innervated to denervated areas, marking the denervated areas with a skin pencil to indicate the level of the cord lesion or an involved nerve root.

The following points of reference are useful to remember:

a. The occipital area of the scalp is supplied by C2.
b. The front of the neck by C3.
c. The shoulders C5.
d. The outer aspect of the forearm, thumb, index and middle finger C6.
e. The fourth and fifth finger C7.
f. The ulnar border of the hand and forearm C8.

When examining the remainder of the body, of particular importance are the anal skin reflex, the 'anal wink' and the bulbocavernosus reflex, the latter being elicited by squeezing the glans penis or clitoris whilst noting the contraction of the anal sphincter on the gloved finger. Both these reflexes are cord mediated and are absent in the stage of spinal shock, which normally lasts for 48 hours. If both these reflexes return in the absence of any sensation, the cord lesion can be judged complete.

Motor examination

The following are key movements indicating the level of the lesion:

a. Deltoid and biceps C5.
b. Extensors of the wrist C6.
c. Triceps, pronator teres and flexor carpi radialis C7.
d. Finger flexors C8.
e. Intrinsic muscles of the hand T1.

Reflex examination

In the stage of spinal shock deep tendon, superficial and the cremasteric reflexes are seldom present but their early return after 24–48 hours is a hopeful sign.

Five main neurological lesions associated with cervical injuries have been identified:

1. *Incomplete lesions*, in which partial preservation of motor and sensory function is present. Should a rapid improvement occur in the first week, near normal function may return.

2. *Anterior cord syndrome*, which presents a similar clinical picture to that produced by thrombosis of the anterior spinal artery. In this syndrome there is complete paralysis below the level of the lesion with loss of pain and temperature sensation but sparing of deep pressure sensation, two-point discrimination, joint position and vibration sense.

3. *Posterior cord syndrome*. This syndrome is most frequently associated with hyperextension injuries and fractures of the posterior elements of the spinal column. There is no loss of muscle power but there is loss of deep pressure sensation, deep pain and proprioception.

4. *Brown–Séquard syndrome*. This syndrome may follow a stab wound of the neck or more commonly a fracture of the lateral mass. Motor loss, impairment of joint position sense, two-point discrimination and vibration sense occur on the side of the injury accompanied by loss of pain and temperature sensation on the opposite side. These sensory losses are accompanied by minimal motor loss.

5. *Central cord syndrome*. This is the commonest of incomplete cord lesions and although it may occur following any cervical fracture it is more usual after hyperextension injuries involving the spondylitic spines of older patients. It is caused by haemorrhage into the central grey matter with varying degrees of involvement of the

white matter. Classically a flaccid paralysis of the upper limbs occurs accompanied by a spastic paralysis or paresis of the lower limbs.

Radiological diagnosis

The following views of the cervical spine are required: anteroposterior, oblique and lateral.

Special types of injury

1. Fractures of the atlas or odontoid – anteroposterior views through the open mouth.
2. Fractures in the C5/6/7 region – to obtain a clear radiological view it may be necessary to depress the shoulders.
3. Suspected posterior spinal ligament injury – X-ray in slight flexion in order to demonstrate the flexion-induced displacement.
4. Suspected extension injury – radiographs in extension may be necessary.

TREATMENT OF CERVICAL INJURIES

The treatment of cervical fractures remains very much a matter of opinion. Some surgeons adopt a conservative approach; the most conservative of all would never operate. Others adopt a radical approach, fusing the spine in all cases and performing an open reduction, if this is necessary.

Between these two extremes is the area in which most orthopaedic surgeons operate, adopting a conservative approach for some patients and a more radical approach for others. Few surgeons, for example, fuse or reduce the spine by operative techniques in the presence of neurological signs within the first 24 hours of injury, for no one has yet proved that early operation promotes recovery. Furthermore, when there is no improvement in the neurological defect within 24 hours it is highly probable that the spinal cord injury is permanent.

The great improvement in survival of those patients who sustain severe spinal cord injury is due more to improved medical care in the general sense than to advances in surgical technique.

Treatment of complete cord lesion

When the cord lesion is complete, management of the patient is dominated by a desire to avoid complications. These include:

1. *Pressure sores*, avoided by 2-hourly turning and careful attention to the skin.
2. *Pulmonary complications*, avoided by frequent chest physiotherapy.
3. *Contractures*, avoided by regular passive movements through a full range of all joints in the paralysed limb.
4. *urinary tract infection.*

The proper management of the bladder is of great importance. In the past, urinary tract infection associated with pyelonephritis was the commonest cause of death following cervical injuries.

The management of the bladder and the place of urethral catheterization are extremely controversial. If a catheter is used in the stage of spinal shock, should it be passed intermittently or should it be permanent?

An alternative is to use a small suprapubic plastic catheter; a paediatric peritoneal dialysing catheter has been found adequate. This is inserted and the bladder allowed to drain at night, but in the daytime the catheter is clipped and released at 2-hourly intervals. The suprapubic catheter can be removed when the residual urine has fallen to less than 100 ml, which is usually within 3 weeks, by which time a true automatic bladder has been established. No antibiotics need be given unless the patient develops signs and symptoms of infection.

Specific fractures

Compression fractures

In the absence of a cord lesion, compression fractures may be treated by continuous skeletal traction for 6 weeks followed by a polythene collar until interbody fusion takes place. If the cord has been damaged, the patient is put on traction and the spine slowly distracted so that the damaged intervertebral space is widened to a limit of not more than twice the width of the normal. Persistent neurological symptoms and signs are an indication in some quarters, especially in the United States, for surgical decompression of the disc space.

Technique of decompression. The spine is approached through an anterolateral cervical incision. The damaged area is located and the disc is removed from between the shattered vertebrae; the posterior vertebral ligament is then divided so that the epidural space can be explored and any prolapsed disc tissue removed.

If the cartilaginous end-plates are intact they are removed and a graft is inserted. The neck is completely immobilized for 6 weeks, after which a protective collar must be worn.

Fracture-dislocations

Fracture-dislocations of the cervical spine are unstable and, therefore, are frequently associated with cord damage.

The immediate treatment of such an injury is to institute skull traction. The leather sling which gained purchase from the jaw and occiput, originally used for this purpose, has now been replaced by a variety of metal devices for procuring skeletal traction. These include the Halo device, Crutchfield tongs, the Blackburn caliper and many others. Once the device is in situ, in the adult, traction should begin with weights of 15–20 lb (6.8–9 kg). This is gradually increased, and when radiographs show the articular processes are in accurate apposition, the weight is reduced to 10–12 lb (4.5–5.5 kg).

If the X-ray has shown a unilateral dislocation of a facet, gentle manipulation without an anaesthetic may be tried, tilting the neck away from the affected side. When there has been bilateral dislocation of the articular facets a straight pull of 20 lb (9 kg) is used at first. At intervals, the X-rays are repeated and, if necessary, traction is increased. Once reduced, the traction force is reduced to 10 lb (4.5 kg) and the neck is kept in slight extension.

If reduction cannot be achieved solely by traction, gentle manipulation under anaesthesia may be tried, and if this also fails an open reduction and fusion is required.

The surgical literature suggests that reduction of facet dislocation is of great importance in producing a pain-free patient. Among those patients in whom healing is allowed to occur in the displaced position, the majority suffer pain.

When there has been a severe flexion injury the posterior spinal ligament is destroyed, leaving the neck unstable, liable to cause persistent pain, and to undergo early degeneration. Because of this, fusion is nearly always required.

If an early operation is performed for 'locked' facets, a posterior fusion is nearly always carried out. However, if the operation is delayed, an anterior fusion is probably the method of choice.

Extension injuries

These do not require traction and are usually treated by immobilization in slight flexion for 3 months in a collar.

Psychological problems

Since many of the victims of cervical injuries are young adults, such an injury produces grave psychological problems which must be dealt with if possible before they arise. There can be little doubt that the life of a tetraplegic patient, whilst not to be compared with that of a normal individual, has altered for the better in recent years even though the physical defect remains the same as in yesteryears.

9. Lumbar disc lesions

DEVELOPMENTAL ANATOMY

The intervertebral discs are formed from the axial notochord. By the time of birth the annulus fibrosus has differentiated from the primitive tissues and the nucleus pulposus has been formed, by the rapid proliferation of notochordal cells followed by the liquefaction of the surrounding fibrocartilage and the elaboration of a mucoid matrix. The nucleus pulposus of the infant is predominantly notochordal but cells of this nature disappear within the first decade of life, to be replaced by a sparse population of fibroblasts and cartilage cells within a soft matrix which is rich in randomly orientated collagen bundles.

Anatomy of the adult disc

The adult intervertebral disc is composed of several elements:

1. A thin layer of hyaline cartilage lying directly on the end plate of the vertebral body.
2. The annulus fibrosus, which is divided into a peripheral laminated layer in which the fibres are most numerous anteriorly and are attached to the vertebral body deep to the epiphysial ring, an intermediate layer passing from one vertebral body to the epiphysial ring of the vertebral body below, and an inner group of fibres which run between the cartilaginous plates. The anteriorly placed outer fibres are strongly reinforced by the anterior longitudinal ligament, whereas the posterior fibres are considerably weaker.
3. The nucleus pulposus, which is contained within the annulus and acts as a ball-bearing upon which the vertebral bodies can roll on extension and flexion of the spine.

AGING AND DISC DEGENERATION

In youth, the nucleus is composed of a three-dimensional collagen lattice in which is enmeshed a mucoprotein gel, and the efficient functioning of the discs is entirely dependent on the elasticity of the nucleus. This, in turn, is dependent on the water-binding properties of the mucopolysaccharide complex which is lost with advancing years, a change associated with a progressive decrease in the degree of hydration.

Cells derived from the annulus invade the nucleus, which slowly alters in colour and texture. There is still doubt as to whether the disc forms an osmotic system or whether it imbibes water. Degeneration of the nucleus leads to increasing stresses on the annulus which may split in a radial fashion allowing the escape of nuclear material.

Effects of disc degeneration

As the disc degenerates the movement between adjacent vertebrae becomes uneven or excessive. At this point the spine is vulnerable to trauma causing acute attacks of backache. As repeated trauma occurs, secondary degenerative changes develop in the capsule and the zygapophysial joints. When the anterior fibres of the annulus are weakened the involved segments may hyperextend, and as the disc loses height the posterior joints subluxate, so that again minor trauma may cause severe pain. Such changes in the spine may give rise to backache together with referred pain which, passing from the lower back, may be referred down the back of the thigh as far as (but usually no further than) the knee.

Should degeneration of the disc proceed, a protrusion may develop which results in sciatic pain of variable distribution according to the level affected. The effect of the disc protrusion may be made worse by the bony changes which accompany the osteoarthritis of the facet joints.

LUMBAR DISC PROTRUSION

Classification (after MacNab)

1. *Contained disc protrusion.* This type of protrusion is a localized bulging of the disc with the annulus remaining intact.
2. *Non-contained disc protrusion.*
   a. Subligamentous, i.e. the herniation remains contained within the posterior longitudinal ligament.

b. *Transligamentous disc,* i.e. the herniated material of the intervertebral disc has extruded through the posterior longitudinal ligament.
c. *Sequestered disc,* in which the disc tissue has not only penetrated the annulus and the posterior longitudinal ligament but has completely separated so that the fragment lies free in the spinal canal. Such fragments tend to migrate upwards to lie behind the cephalad vertebra but can also migrate caudally.

In addition to the anatomical effects of protrusion, which causes compression of the nerve root, an inflammatory response also occurs between the extruded disc material and the nerve root. It is probably this inflammatory response which is responsible for the 'sciatica' since simple physical pressure on a peripheral nerve does not produce pain but parasthesia.

Symptomatology of disc protrusion

Symptoms of disc degeneration most commonly occur in the fourth decade, males being much more commonly affected than females. The most significant complaint is of pain, which may arise with extreme suddenness, or develop gradually over a period of days. In many patients a long history of intermittent backache (lumbago) precedes the development of sciatica. The pain of a disc protrusion has three components:

1. Aching in the back, exacerbated by spinal movements.
2. Deep pain in the buttocks and thighs, aching in character, influenced by posture.
3. Radiating pain extending a variable distance down the thigh, leg and foot, exacerbated by coughing, sneezing or evacuation of the bowels.

Physical signs associated with disc protrusion

Postural deformity

During an acute attack postural deformities and extremely limited spinal movements are experienced due to protective spasm of the erector spinae muscles. The lumbar lordosis is often flattened and the trunk may be tilted on the pelvis. The tilt may be either towards or away from the affected side and may sometimes be observed only on bending forwards. The direction of the tilt is in large measure determined by the relation of the nerve root to the protrusion. When the nerve is displaced laterally the tilt is usually to the side of the lesion, but when the nerve is displaced medially the tilt is in the opposite direction. Reversal of the normal spinal rhythm on attempting to regain the erect position after forward flexion is characteristic of a posterior joint lesion, the patient bringing the pelvis under the spine when trying to regain the erect posture.

Sensation

When nerve roots are irritated muscle tenderness is frequently present; an L4 lesion produces tenderness in the quadriceps; L5, tenderness in the anterior tibial muscles; and S1, tenderness in the calf.

Pinprick sensation is reduced over the skin in the anteromedial aspect of the thigh in L4 lesions, over the dorsum of the foot and anterior part of the leg when L5 is involved, and over the outer part of the foot and the sole in S1 lesions.

Muscle weakness, reflexes, and straight leg raising

Lesions of the 4th lumbar root cause weakness of the quadriceps, tested by resting the limb on the examiner's arm and asking the patient to extend the knee against resistance. Lesions of L5 cause weakness of extensor hallucis longus and later weakness of the dorsiflexors of the foot. Lesions of S1 cause weakness of flexor hallucis longus and later weakness of the gastrocnemius, which can be discerned by asking the patient to repeatedly stand on tip toe.

Reflexes. L4 lesions cause loss of the knee jerk, L5 lesions weakness of the ankle jerk, and S1 weakness or absence of the ankle jerk.

Straight leg raising is a test of root tension. The leg should be raised slowly; pain evoked by forced dorsiflexion of the foot is highly suggestive of root tension, as is relief from pain by flexing the knee. If straight leg raising of the opposite leg produces pain in the affected limb it suggests that the protruding disc is lying medial to the affected root.

INVESTIGATIONS

Screening investigations in patients suffering from low back pain

1. *ESR.* The most important is the erythrocyte sedimentation rate (ESR) or plasma viscosity, a raised ESR suggesting an inflammatory

or neoplastic cause, whereas a normal result suggests a structural problem. Occasionally this investigation is misleading, for example, in early ankylosing spondylitis and brucellosis the result may be within normal limits.

2. *Serum calcium.* Hypercalcaemia suggests hyperparathyroidism or secondary carcinomatosis with osseous involvement.

3. *Serum acid phosphatase.* This is a valuable screening investigation in older men in whom back pain may be the first overt sign of carcinoma of the prostate.

Methods of investigation

Plain X-rays of the spine

Standard anteroposterior views are taken of the patient supine, centring on L3, with lateral views centred on L3 and L5 with the patient lying on his side. These views are then supplemented by erect lateral films looking for alterations of posture, and oblique views useful in looking for abnormalities of the vertebral arches as in spondylolisthesis. In view of recent diagnostic developments, however, the major value of the plain X-ray is to exclude other causes of backache, including infection, ankylosing spondylitis and neoplasia.

Myelography

This is another investigation which has largely been overtaken by events. This examination was first applied to the diagnosis of spinal tumours by Sicard and Forestier in 1921 but it was not until the development in the 1970s of water-soluble contrast agents which could be introduced into the arachnoid space that myelography came to be regarded as a safe procedure. Nevertheless it is still followed by occasional neurological complications, chief among which is headache usually beginning within 4–8 hours, resolving within 48 hours. Both anaphylactoid and renal toxicity are also occasionally seen.

The myelographic changes indicating a herniated disc include:

1. *Defects in the sac alone.* Simple smooth midline defects are not to be interpreted as herniations. They are more commonly caused by annular bulging as part of degenerative disease. Indicative of a disc herniation is a double density defect.

2. *Defects in the root sleeves.* Because of the low viscosity of water-soluble contrast materials the root sleeves (radiculogram) fill with ease if they are not obstructed.

3. *Computerized axial tomography (CAT)*. Whilst myelography is often capable of showing the level of the pathology it does not necessarily show the nature of the lesion or its precise location. CAT was introduced into clinical medicine in 1972. Normally the spine is scanned at cuts of 2–5 mm. The chief evidence of an abnormal scan is: focal protrusion of the disc distorting the normal configuration of the margin of the annulus; obliteration of the epidural fat; deformity of the dural sac; displacement of a nerve root; or swelling of the nerve root.

4. *Magnetic resonance imaging (MRI)*. Introduced by Damadian in 1981, this technique is of greater value than CAT in that it produces excellent soft tissue detail. It will show intradural lesions such as tumours and arachnoiditis but it has one disadvantage – it takes longer than CAT and is therefore difficult for the patient in pain to endure.

TREATMENT

1. *Conservative.* The majority of patients suffering from an acute disc prolapse will settle on conservative therapy. This takes the form of:
   a. Complete bed rest.
   b. Muscle relaxants.
   c. Non-steroidal anti-inflammatory agents.
   d. Exercises.
2. *Operative.* The indications for intervention are:
   a. Recurrent attacks of sciatica.
   b. An increasing neurological defect associated with increasing pain and marked reduction of straight leg raising.
   c. Bladder and bowel involvement, a situation which indicates a sequestrated disc.
   d. Failure of conservative treatment as measured by failure to relieve pain or produce improvement in leg raising ability.

INTERVENTIONAL PROCEDURES

Chemonucleolysis

In 1960 the first enzymic dissolution of the nucleus pulposus in the human was reported using the enzyme, chymopapain. After a somewhat chequered career in the United States the drug was once more licensed in 1982 and has been used with increasing frequency since that date. The beneficial action of this enzyme is exerted by its action on glycosaminoglycan side chains of the non-nuclear matrix of the disc. By splitting these it interferes with the ability of the proteoglycan to hold water, thus deflating the nuclear bulge. Because an extruded/sequestrated disc lying free within the spinal canal is chiefly made up of collagen it is unaffected by the enzyme and therefore in this situation useless. Other contraindications to the use of chymopapain according to MacNab are:

1. Degenerative disc disease associated with mechanical instability due to degeneration of the facet joints.
2. Patients suffering from spondylolisthesis.
3. Previous surgery with recurrent symptoms on the same side and at the same level.
4. Patients sensitive to the enzyme.

Complications

a. *Anaphylaxis.* All patients should be tested for sensitivity to avoid this complication.
b. *Neurological complications.* These are normally due to injecting the enzyme into the subarachnoid space but may also be due to penetration of a nerve root at the time of needle insertion.

Postoperative care

In some patients severe spasm and back pain may occur which requires the use of narcotic analgesics, muscle relaxants and corticosteroids for its control.

Results

About 70% of patients benefit from this type of treatment, which is said not to make surgical intervention more difficult if the method fails.

Surgical intervention

The original surgical treatment of 'prolapsed' intervertebral disc was introduced by Barr and Mixter in 1941. The original optimism that followed was tempered by two factors: the realization that the majority of patients respond to conservative therapy, and the reports of indifferent results as the operation became more widely used.

The original approach was via a formal laminectomy and through the dura. This has now been modified to an extradural approach. The majority of surgeons do not perform a laminectomy but, instead, approach the cord and its coverings by excising the ligamentum flavum from adjacent laminae and then, if necessary, removing small portions of the laminae themselves. It is necessary to find the lateral border of the nerve root and to do this the medial edge of the superior facet of the anatomical segment below may require to be removed. 95% of the exposures will be of the L4/L5 and L5/S1 levels. How much of the disc apart from the protrusion itself needs to be removed is a matter of opinion.

Complications

Apart from the complications common to all surgical procedures the specific complications of disc surgery are:

a. The operation is performed at the wrong level.
b. Dural tears.
c. Increased neural deficit due to nerve injury.

Results

When patients are carefully selected approximately 90% will have an excellent result as defined by a total absence of residual symptoms or the presence of minimal residual symptoms with relief from backache and sciatica.

Complete failure may occur due to one or more of the following causes:

1. Too long a delay between the onset of symptoms and operative intervention.
2. Neuroticism or accident neurosis.
3. Degenerative changes in the spine leading to bony encroachment which goes unrelieved.
4. Removal of the wrong disc.
5. Incorrect diagnosis, e.g. a tumour of the spinal cord or spinal metastases.

However, Hakelius in 1970 reported a retrospective study of 583 patients suffering from unilateral L5/S1 sciatica and found that surgically treated patients initially had a better result but that 6 months after operation there was no difference between those patients treated surgically and those treated conservatively, although at 7 years the conservatively treated group had more sciatic discomfort, more recurrences, and had lost more time off work. Similarly Weber in 1983 found that the early results of surgery were appreciably better than those patients conservatively treated, but at 4 and 10 years there was no statistically significant difference between the two groups of patients.

SPINAL STENOSIS

No essay on the organic causes of back pain would be complete without reference to the condition of spinal stenosis. Although acquired types of this condition had been recognized and subjected to decompression laminectomy as early as 1911, it was the Dutch surgeon Verbiest in 1950 who established that developmental spinal stenosis could also occur.

The condition, whether developmental or acquired, produces a classic syndrome of low back pain and widespread pain in the legs on walking. The condition therefore symptomatically resembles intermitten claudication but all the peripheral pulses are present, even in the presence of pain. A further feature of the condition is that, whilst the symptoms may be present on walking, the lumbar spine being in extension, activity in flexion, e.g. cycling, does not lead to the onset of pain.

Spengler in 1985 suggested that the space available to the cauda equina should be measured as an area rather than as a diameter. An area less than 100 mm^2 is indicative of spinal stenosis at the L5/S1 level. The great majority of cases are secondary and are caused by narrowing of the spinal canal due to:

1. Severe kyphosis with secondary lordosis.
2. Severe degenerative spondylosis.
3. Degenerative spondylolisthesis.
4. Bone pathology.
5. Trauma.

The diagnosis can be made by the investigations already described. When the condition is disabling, operative relief of the leg pain may be gained by laminectomy and removal of the articular facets on the side of the lesion, the latter manoeuvre removing the pressure on the lateral recess through which the spinal roots pass to the exterior. However, if the facets are interfered with fusion is required to stabilize the spine.

10. Principles involved in the treatment of tendon and nerve injuries, with special reference to the hand

Factors influencing the results of tendon repair in general include:

1. The site of the injury.
2. The tendon involved.
3. The presence of associated injury which may involve:
   a. Soft tissues covering the tendon.
   b. Nerves.
   c. Joints.
4. The extent of damage to the tendon itself; the type of injury, whether partially divided, wholly divided, crushed; whether the injury is clean or contaminated.
5. The length of time between injury and treatment.
6. The age, attitude and occupation of the patient.
7. The skill and experience of the surgeon.

INJURIES TO THE FLEXOR MECHANISM OF THE HAND

Even without the long flexor tendons, the sublimis and profundus, the fingers can be flexed to 90° at the metacarpophalangeal joint due to the action of the interossei and lumbricals. The goal of extrinsic tendon repair is to re-establish interphalangeal joint flexion, and a simple formula for assessing the results of such efforts is provided by the following formula, which establishes the percentage of the total active motion (TAM), normally equal to 260°. The formula used is:

$$\frac{\text{PIP} + \text{DIP flexion} - \text{extension lag} \times 100}{175}$$

= percentage of normal proximal and distal interphalangeal motion

The measurement of flexion should be made whilst making a fist.

Using this formula the results of treatment can be graded as: poor, 0-24; fair, 25-49; good, 50-74; and excellent, 75-100.

Anatomy

In 1967 Verdan designated five zones in the hand in which tendon lacerations correlated with prognosis, the zones corresponding to the site of the tendon injury rather than the actual laceration in the skin which led to the injury.

The five zones are:

- *Zone I*, extending from the insertion of flexor digitorum profundus on the distal phalanx to the insertion of flexor digitorum sublimis on either side of the mid-shaft of the middle phalanx.
- *Zone II*, extending from Zone I to the opening of the proximal pulley at the head of the corresponding metacarpal or, in the thumb, extending proximally to the metacarpophalangeal joint.
- *Zone III*, extending from Zone II proximally to the distal edge of the carpal tunnel.
- *Zone IV*, within the carpal tunnel.
- *Zone V*, proximal to the carpal tunnel.

Zone II, located between the distal palmar crease and the distal interphalangeal flexion crease, represents the portion of the tendon within the fibro-osseous canal, once known as 'no man's land'; it was in this area that there was until recently great controversy as to the manner in which repair of divided tendons should be approached and whether or not both the sublimis and profundus should be repaired at the time of the injury. This controversy has now been resolved with the great majority of surgeons favouring repair of both tendons.

Principles

Exposure

When exploring the fingers or palm, longitudinal incisions should *not* be made over the midline of the fingers or palms. Instead, incisions in the fingers should be made in the mid-lateral position; if extensive exposure is required this should be achieved by Z-plasties and, in the palm incisions, should follow the skin creases. Thus the local circulation should be preserved, incisions must not be made on surfaces which will be subjected to trauma, and flexion creases must be crossed at an angle of less than 90° in order to avoid scar-related flexion contractures.

Repair

Tendons are relatively avascular structures in which few cells are found. The blood supply upon which repair is dependent comes chiefly via the vincula longi and brevia. Mishandling may produce delayed healing and, more importantly, adhesions between the tendons themselves, or adjacent structures may result in limitation of movement.

Sutures and suture material

The most commonly used material for tendon suture is 4/0 nylon. Originally the Bunnel pull-out stitch was most commonly used but this has now been superseded by the core suture described by Kessler. In addition to this stitch, whose chief function is to anchor the two ends of the tendon together, great emphasis is now placed on the repair of the epitendinous tissue using a running suture of 8/0 nylon.

Immobilization

Views on the duration of immobilization have also been a source of controversy. In the recent past complete immobilization was recommended after the repair of the flexor tendons in the fingers or wrist, followed by a 3-week period of supervised active movements. This regime has now been modified so that although no *active* flexion is permitted for 3 weeks, movement of the tendon or tendons is encouraged in the following manner. At the termination of reconstructive surgery two rubber bands are sown to the fingernail of each involved digit. A circumferential short arm plaster is applied maintaining the wrist in 30° of flexion and the metacarpophalangeal joints at 45°, this position causing relaxation of the flexor mechanism. A safety pin is inserted into the plaster at the level of the scaphoid. After 3 days an ellipse is cut from the palmar surface of the plaster and the rubber bands are attached to the safety pin, thus drawing the finger or fingers into flexion. The patient is now encouraged to extend the fingers within the plaster cast, the rubber band bringing the fingers once more into flexion. This exercise is repeated many times several times daily. After 3–4 weeks the plaster is removed and active flexion encouraged although power gripping is restrained for a further month.

Repair within specific zones

Zone I

If an adequate length of the distal stump of the flexor digitorum profundus is available a Kessler stitch is used to approximate the two ends of the tendon. If, however, the tendon has been sheared off the distal phalanx leaving no tendinous material, a pull-through technique can be employed, drilling a hole through the base of the distal phalanx, inserting one half of the Kessler stitch, pulling the tendon through the canal thus formed, and then bringing the stitch to the surface, anchoring it to a button.

Zone II

Whereas in the past, in this 'no man's land', it was considered that only the profundus tendon should be repaired, it is now generally agreed that both sublimis and profundus should be repaired.

It is, however, important to remember that the proximal ends of tendons divided in this zone may retract upwards to the level of the distal transverse skin crease and counter incisions may therefore have to be made at this level. The original laceration is extended as above and the entry wound in the sheath enlarged by what is known as the 'flag' type of incision. The palmar incision is then made and having located the proximal end of the tendon a small catheter is passed proximally through the tendon sheath until it exists in the palmar wound. At this point the core stitch is inserted into the tendon and attached to the catheter, which is then used to draw the tendon distally through the sheath. Prior to the repair of the profundus tendon the slips of the sublimis are attached to the sides of the intermediate phalanx with 5/0 nylon. The advantage of repairing both the sublimis and profundus tendons is that the vincular blood supply is preserved and a smooth gliding bed for the profundus tendon is retained. The profundus repair follows, after which the sheath itself is repaired. The flexor digitorum sublimis, which flexes the proximal interphalangeal joint, is especially important in labourers because it contributes to power grip.

Zone III

The mid-palmar area. In this area retraction of the profundus tendon is limited by the lumbrical muscle which tethers the tendon. Assuming that the lumbrical is intact the tendon can always be found by following the belly of the muscle proximally. On the other hand the flexor digitorum sublimis tendon frequently retracts as far proximally as the carpal tunnel and therefore counter incisions at this level may need to be made, followed by catheter retrieval in the manner previously described. If the excursion of the repaired tendon is impaired by the first annular pulley this can be sectioned without loss of function.

Zone IV

Repair of the flexor tendons at the level of the carpal tunnel should not be attempted without formal, complete carpal tunnel release. A mid-palmar incision is made parallel to the thenar crease but to the ulnar side so as to avoid damage to the palmar cutaneous branch of the median nerve.

When tendons are divided within the carpal tunnel all the tendons should be tagged. The tendons of profundus lie side by side along the floor and the sublimis flexors, lying superficial to these, are arranged in two layers, the tendons to the middle and ring fingers (3 and 4) being superficial to the tendons of the index and little fingers (2 and 5). Repair should naturally proceed from deep to superficial.

EXTENSOR TENDON INJURIES

Injuries to the extensor tendons over the dorsum of the hand and fingers have a favourable prognosis because of the location of the tendons within the loose areolar tissue, which means that there is rarely any restriction of function due to adhesions. This is not the case on the dorsum of the wrist at which point tendons may adhere to the extensor retinaculum. Injuries at this site are best treated by repositioning the repaired tendon within the superficial tissue and closing the retinaculum deep to the repaired tendon.

Specific injuries

'Mallet finger'

This deformity is due to disruption of the extensor tendon from its insertion into the base of the distal phalanx. This causes the distal interphalangeal joint to be held in the flexed position although it can be straightened passively. Seen early the condition may be treated by splinting the finger with the proximal joint held in flexion and the distal joint in hyperextension. If seen late, or no improvement occurs after a period of splintage, open operation with attachment of the tendon or the small fragment of bone that is commonly avulsed at the time of injury may improve the situation.

A similar condition, known as the 'Mallet thumb', occurs if the extensor pollicis longus is divided. Direct repair is indicated in simple lacerations, but in other situations such as rupture due to fractures at the lower end of the radius, or in rheumatoid arthritis, the ends of the tendon are so frayed that direct repair is frequently impossible. Reconstruction is then best performed by transposition of the extensor indicis or the extensor carpi radialis longus.

Boutonnière deformity

This deformity results from disruption of the central slip of the extensor tendon from its insertion into the base of the middle phalanx. Initially the condition may be unrecognized, but in due course the lateral bands of the extensor tendon slowly assume a more volar position anterior to the axis of rotation of the joint. When this state of affairs develops the lateral bands flex the proximal interphalangeal joint and extend the distal interphalangeal joint.

The condition is treated by open operation. A variety of techniques have been described, one of which is to suture the lateral slips of the extensor tendon together over the proximal interphalangeal joint via a posterior incision.

NERVE INJURIES

Seddon classified the severity of peripheral nerve injuries as follows:

1. *Neuropraxia.* This is often caused by ischaemia, compression, or a blow. The axons remain in continuity and recovery is spontaneous and complete.
2. *Axonotmesis.* Most commonly this is caused by crushing. The axons are disrupted within the intact sheaths but the nerve trunk remains in continuity, and therefore each axon grows down its own tunnel and recovery is eventually complete.
3. *Neurotmesis.* This implies total disruption of the nerve. There can be no recovery without repair and some axonal confusion is inevitable; recovery is slow and may be incomplete.

While this classification is useful it is somewhat artificial since in practice there is often a mixture, particularly of neuropraxia and axonotmesis. Lacerated nerves should be repaired by primary suture; delayed primary suture carried out within 4–10 days do as well, but repair delayed beyond 2–3 weeks is not so satisfactory. If delayed repair is contemplated, both ends of the severed nerve should be tagged with non-absorbable sutures to make their later identification easier. In the following conditions primary repair may be expected to yield a good result:

1. The wound is fresh and expected to heal promptly.
2. The skin defect, if any, is easily closed.
3. The nerve is sharply cut across.
4. The nerve ends can be easily brought together. This is the single most important factor.
5. The ends are lying in healthy tissue.

The technical difficulties are considerable since the epineurium is tenuous and does not easily hold suture material; should a gap be present after dividing the ragged ends of a nerve with a single clean transverse cut, the gap may be closed by flexion of the joints above and below the lesion. Neither catgut nor silk should be used, but four stitches of 9/0 nylon should be used for a digital nerve. Care should be taken to handle the nerve carefully, using non-toothed forceps and holding the nerve by the epineurium. When repairing high lesions such as the median nerve it should be remembered that the blood supply to the nerve arises from a vessel on the volar aspect.

Nerve repair produces satisfactory functional sensation but this is never entirely normal. The recovery of motor function and muscle bulk, particularly in the small muscles of the hand, is much less predictable, and it is for this reason that the ulnar nerve lesion is particularly serious.

Tests of functional recovery of nervous continuity

1. *Tinel's sign*. Percussion over the advancing edge of the regrowing nerve fibres produces a characteristic tingling sensation. The rate of advance approximates to 1 mm per day after a lag of 10 days which follows the injury.
2. *Sweat test*. The presence of sweating can be demonstrated by a hand print on ninhydrin-impregnated paper. Sweat is absent in denervated skin but recovery is unpredictable and correlates poorly with the quality of sensory recovery.
3. *When light touch returns*, it is called protective sensation, but more precise testing, using two-point discrimination or distinguishing

between differing materials can be used to expose incomplete recovery.

4. *Electromyography*. This indicates that the nerve is recovering function some weeks before clinical tests become positive; action potentials can be demonstrated in a recovering nerve before any increased muscle strength can be detected.

SECTION THREE

11. Benign prostatic hypertrophy

Benign prostatic hypertrophy is the most common neoplastic growth in the male. Normally the prostate slowly increases in size from birth to puberty, after which it undergoes a rapid increase in size until the third decade. It then remains stable until the middle of the fifth decade, when it either commences to atrophy or becomes the seat of benign hypertrophy and continues to increase in size. Although the majority of men over 50 will have histological evidence of benign prostatic hypertrophy, many of whom may suffer minor symptoms, the number requiring prostatectomy is relatively small. Bell reviewed over 100 patients in whom minimal symptoms were present and prostatectomy was not indicated. He found that after 10 years only 10% had required surgery and only 2% had suffered acute retention.

AETIOLOGY

The cause of the disease remains unknown although several facts support the hypothesis that benign hypertrophy is an endocrine induced condition. Firstly, it does not occur in males castrated before puberty; secondly, regression occurs following castration; and thirdly, the disease can be reproduced in animals by the administration of hormones.

ANATOMY

The apex of the normal prostate rests upon the external sphincter, its posterior surface is separated from the rectum by two layers of rectovesical fascia and has a depression towards its upper extremity through which the ejaculatory ducts enter the gland to open into the prostatic urethra on either side of the utriculus masculinus which itself lies on the crista urethralis. The plane of the ejaculatory ducts divides the gland into a number of lobes. Below the level of the ejaculatory ducts in the midline is the posterior lobe, above this level is the middle lobe. On each side of the middle and the much larger posterior lobe is situated the major portion of the gland, i.e. the lateral lobes, which weigh 6-7 g. The lateral lobes are joined anteriorly by the anterior lobe, which contains few, if any, glands.

Two sets of glands are present in the normal prostate: an inner group, which lie in the inner zone and directly surround the urethra, and an outer group, which lie in an outer zone separated from the true capsule of the prostate by a plexus of veins.

PATHOLOGY

It must be appreciated that prostatic symptoms may develop in the absence of gross enlargement of the prostate and conversely a grossly enlarged prostate may be associated with minimal symptoms. The hyperplastic gland may be large and soft, or small and hard, depending on the relative contribution made by the glandular elements and the fibromuscular ground substance.

When the gland is large and soft histological examination shows that the number of glands in the stroma has increased, 'adenosis' and that the number of cells forming these new glands has also multiplied, 'epitheliosis', although there may be little or no increase in the stromal elements. Approximately 25% of all large adenomatous glands show evidence of secondary change such as infarction and in about 10% an unsuspected carcinoma will be found. In addition if secretions are retained within the new glands cyst formation will occur. Such changes most commonly occur in the lateral lobes so that rectal examination readily reveals the enlargement. If they occur only in the middle lobe the prostate may feel normal in size even though middle lobe enlargement can produce severe obstructive symptoms. A further pertinent point is that prostatic hypertrophy begins in the inner zone of the prostate producing compression of the outer zone which then forms the false capsule from which the 'adenomatous gland' is enucleated.

When the gland is small and hard a minimal degree of epithelial proliferation is present accompanied by a considerable overgrowth of the fibromuscular components of the gland. Such a gland may feel almost normal on rectal examination but cystourethrography may reveal a so-called median bar seen best with a fore-oblique lens with the urethroscope situated just proximal to the veru so that the prostatic urethra above this level can be viewed as a whole. Normally the bladder neck forms a circle but in the presence of a median bar the circle is interrupted inferiorly by a ridge which appears to stretch across and interrupt the inferior boundary of the circle.

If outflow obstruction occurs hypertrophy of the bladder musculature follows, causing trabeculation of the bladder wall, which can be readily seen on cystoscopy because the muscle fibres of the detrusor muscle are reticulate. Later, if nothing is done to correct the condition, saccules and diverticula develop between the hypertrophied muscle fibres. Continuing obstruction may finally progress to atrophy, producing an atonic bladder. In the presence of residual urine, infection may develop leading to the formation of bladder calculi; renal failure may result as a consequence of obstruction to the intramural parts of the ureters and partly to vesico-ureteric reflux.

CLINICAL PRESENTATION

Normally, benign prostatic hypertrophy presents with a constellation of symptoms which include:

- Diminution of the calibre and force of the urinary stream.
- Hesitancy in initiating voiding.
- Inability to terminate micturition abruptly, with post-voiding dribbling.
- Recurrent attacks of infection.
- Nocturnal wakening.
- Haematuria, which is somewhat commoner in benign hypertrophy than in malignant disease.
- Chronic retention with overflow incontinence.
- Acute retention. This may occur following a long history of increasing difficulty or may occur without any prior symptoms should infarction, infection or congestion of the prostrate occur. A common cause of congestion is haemorrhoidectomy or the recent administration of diuretics.

Such obstructive symptoms must be distinguished from the irritative symptoms such as dysuria, frequency and urgency.

Clinical examination

Little may be found, but the presence of longstanding obstruction leading to renal failure may cause loss of weight, a secondary anaemia, or tenderness in the renal angles.

In chronic obstruction the bladder wall may be so thin and the bladder muscle so atonic that the grossly enlarged bladder may be impalpable. In acute retention the bladder is extremely tender to palpation and can be felt above the level of the pubis.

Rectal examination may reveal an apparently normal-sized prostate, especially if only the median lobe is enlarged; alternatively, if the lateral lobes are hypertrophied, a mass will be felt bulging backwards into the rectum with the lateral sulci and the median sulcus clearly palpable. This examination is also valuable in establishing the tone and contractility of the anal sphincters, which if normal indicates that the nerve supply to the bladder is intact.

INVESTIGATIONS

1. *Residual urine.* Catheterization to determine the volume of the residual urine is now never employed, since this volume can be estimated with accuracy by means of ultrasonic scanning of the bladder or by intravenous pyelography.
2. *Microscopy of the urine.* Microscopy of the urine would be regarded as essential if the presenting symptom consisted of haematuria.
3. *Blood urea.* This investigation is simple to perform and valuable in that a much raised value indicates that there is no purpose in performing an intravenous pyelogram.
4. *Intravenous pyelography.* This investigation may show a variety of physical changes in the urinary tract, including:
    a. Non-function of the kidneys.
    b. Dilatation of the pelvi-calyceal system.
    c. Hydroureter.
    d. Bladder trabeculation and diverticula formation.
    e. Filling defect at the bladder base
    f. Measurable quantities of residual urine.
5. *Acid phosphatase.* (see p. 147)
6. *Bacteriological examination of a midstream specimen of urine.* In the majority of patients suffering from prostatism the urine will be sterile, but in the presence of longstanding obstructive symptoms and a large residual urine infection is commonplace – a feature of great importance since one of the commonest causes of shock after a urological procedure is bacteraemic shock.
7. *Measurement of peak flow.* This is a simple measurement to perform. If the peak flow rate is greater than 15 ml/second after loading the patient with 2 litres of fluid, this indicates that there is no infravesical obstruction. When the peak flow rate falls to below 10 ml/second, not only does this indicate that an operation

is required – it also indicates that if surgery is not undertaken in the relatively near future acute or acute-on-chronic retention is almost bound to occur sooner rather than later.

8. *Cystourethroscopy.* This examination establishes:
   a. Prostatic size.
   b. The degree of bladder trabeculation, which is an anatomical indication of the physiological difficulty.
   c. The presence or absence of bladder diverticuli.
   d. Whether the urinary obstruction is due to prostatic hypertrophy or some other cause such as urethral stricture, hypertrophy of the bladder neck or carcinoma of the bladder.

MEDICAL MANAGEMENT OF PROSTATISM

Two recent medical trials have recently been reported:

1. The use of a pollen extract, Cernilton. Given over a 6-month period this drug produced subjective improvement in 69% of a treated group as compared to a comparable group receiving a placebo, in which only 30% improved. There was a significant decrease in the volume of the residual urine and in the anteroposterior diameter of the prostate as measured by ultrasonography, but the flow rate and voiding volume were not significantly altered.

2. The use of a pumpkin seed extract, Curbicin. In a series of 53 patients treated over a period of 3 months, symptomatic improvement occurred.

In addition to the above, two mechanical aids have recently been subjected to trial:

1. The use of balloon dilatation of the prostrate, first introduced in 1987, dilating the prostatic urethra up to a diameter of 35 mm. This method has no role in the treatment of acute retention, but may be of value in younger patients wishing to avoid prostatectomy and the risk of retrograde ejaculation.

2. The insertion of a permanently implanted urethral stent made from woven stainless steel in the form of a tubular mesh. Such a stent is implanted using both ultrasound and endoscopic control. Within 6 weeks the stent can be easily removed and can therefore be resited but after some 6–8 months it becomes covered with epithelium.

Regardless of the above the 'gold standard' against which all other methods of treatment must be compared is the operation of prostatectomy, either by the transurethral route or by open retropubic surgery.

Indications for prostatectomy

The most frequent indications for prostatectomy are:

1. To relieve the various symptoms of urinary obstruction.
2. To eradicate an infected area, e.g. chronic prostatic abscess.
3. To correct the physiological imbalance associated with a neurogenic bladder.

However, when considering surgical treatment for obstructive symptoms, the age and general condition of the patient, as well as the severity of the symptoms, must be taken into account. This is important because:

a. If the effects of back pressure are limited to the bladder there may be long asymptomatic intervals.
b. The introduction of stents makes a viable alternative for the elderly patient.

PROSTATECTOMY

The operation may be performed by closed techniques, i.e. by transurethral resection, or by open methods.

In general a prostate weighing 60 g or less is always treated by resection, and above that weight by retropubic prostatectomy, although there are no hard and fast rules since the choice of operation depends to a great extent on the experience of the operator, especially when considering transurethral resection. Recorded experience indicates that approximately 80% of patients are now treated by transurethral resection using the 'hot' loop.

The most frequent causes of death following prostatic surgery are cardiovascular, respiratory and renal.

Retropubic prostatectomy

Although the technique was described as long ago as 1908 by van Stocken, this method of removing the prostate, which involves enucleation of the 'adenoma' from the false capsule which it creates, did not come into general use until its reintroduction in 1945 by the Irish surgeon Terence Millin.

Complications

Immediate.

1. *Clot retention.* This can usually be dealt with by per-urethral means, using one of the many forms of evacuator followed by continuous bladder irrigation by means of a three-way Foley catheter. Occasionally, however, the wound must be reopened together with the capsule, and the bleeding vessel dealt with under direct vision; or, if no specific bleeding point can be identified, the prostatic cavity can be packed and both a urethral and a suprapubic catheter inserted for some days.

This complication is avoided by:
   a. Careful control of bleeding prior to closure of the capsule.
   b. The use of diuretics to flush out the bloody urine in the early postoperative period.
   c. Continuous bladder irrigation using a three-way Foley catheter if this is felt necessary at the time of the operation.

Many series have been published performing the operation without introducing a catheter at the termination of the operation, but examination of the data shows that in nearly half such patients catheterization is necessary within 24 hours.

2. *Shock.* This is due to excessive blood loss after enucleating the adenoma and should not occur if the blood loss is corrected by immediate transfusion.

Intermediate.

1. *Fistula formation.* This complication usually arises when the capsule has been difficult to close or excessive coagulation has led to extensive necrosis. Such a fistula normally closes if continuous catheter drainage is instituted.

2. *Epididymitis.* It was once considered that this complication could be avoided by ligation and division of the vas and this was originally a routine procedure, now abandoned.

3. *Secondary harmorrhage.* This is fortunately rare. It is more common if the bladder is infected at the time of the operation.

Late.

1. *Incontinence.* This is nearly always temporary and usually improves within 3 months.

2. *Osteitis pubis.* This should be suspected when a patient complains within a few weeks of operation of pain in the pubic area and down the inner side of the thigh. Typically the patient walks with a

shuffling gait, taking small steps due to spasm of the adductor muscles. The condition normally improves spontaneously, but very occasionally pus formation occurs, which may track for long distances through tissue planes.

3. *Stricture formation.* Strictures can develop at the external meatus, in the urethra or at the bladder neck. The latter tend to develop when there has been too limited a resection of the bladder neck. Strictures of the urethra and the external meatus are normally due to irritation by the indwelling catheter, which should be as small as possible and removed as soon as possible.

4. Retrograde ejaculation leading to sterility.

Complications of transurethral resection

Peroperative.

1. *Perforation of the prostatic capsule*, which if unrecognized results in the extravasation of the irrigating fluid into the periprostatic and perivesical space, elongating the prostatic urethra and elevating and compressing the lateral borders of the bladder. The earliest symptoms of this mishap are restlessness, nausea, vomiting and abdominal pain despite spinal anaesthesia, together with a rise in the pulse rate and a fall in blood pressure.

2. *Haemorrhage.* This may occur at the time of resection from small arteries or from the venous sinuses. The former is usually easily recognized since the blood emerges from the point of resection in a pulsating manner and can be easily controlled by electrocoagulation, whereas bleeding from venous sinuses due to too deep a resection is non-pulsatile and cannot be so easily controlled, requiring the use of three-way Foley catheter drainage with careful positioning of the balloon for a longer period than is normal. Because the pressure in the venous sinuses is below that of the pressure of the irrigation fluid used during resection, the irrigation fluid may intravasate, causing hypovolaemia, hyponatraemia and haemoglobinuria – hence the use of 1.5% gylcine as the irrigating fluid.

Intermediate.

1. *Stricture formation.* Normally a 26F sheath is used; care must be taken that the external meatus and the urethra will easily accept this diameter of instrument, otherwise instrumental trauma will lead to stricture formation at the external meatus, the proximal end of the fossa navicularis or just distal to the bladder neck. If it is considered

that the urethra is too narrow, an extensive meatotomy should be performed prior to commencing the operation, or even an internal urethrotomy.

2. *Incontinence.* Incontinence following transurethral resection is nearly always permanent and is due to damage to the external sphincter. It can be avoided by restricting the lower limit of the prostatic resection to the level of the verumontanum.

Late. The principal late complication is continued prostatism, indicating that the initial resection was too conservative.

12. Prostatic cancer

Prevalence

The true prevalence of prostatic cancer is unknown but, if the incidental cancers found at prostatectomy and at autopsy are counted, it is believed that prostatic cancer is the most prevalent of all malignancies in the male, ranking third as a cause of cancer death after bronchial and colorectal tumours.

AETOLOGY

The aetiology of the disease is unknown but, since it does not occur in eunuchs, it is thought that the changing hormonal patterns of advancing age must be of some significance. Further validating the importance of the hormonal activity is the fact that a considerable percentage of prostatic cancers can be controlled, at least temporarily, by hormonal manipulation and that the tumour tends to develop in the outer subcapsular glands, which appear to be more sensitive to androgens than the inner group from which benign hypertrophy arises. Other subsidiary factors may be genetic, the incidence of the disease being several times higher in northern Europeans and North Americans than it is in the Japanese.

PATHOLOGY

Gross appearance

Unless the tumour has penetrated the capsule of the gland and invaded the surrounding structures, there are no gross features characteristic of prostatic cancer. Since nodular hyperplasia is commonly present, the areas of the gland affected by neoplastic change may only be recognized by the slight butter-yellow colour of a nodule, by the grittier feel on cutting, and by the ill-defined manner in which malignant nodules infiltrate the surrounding tissues.

Microscopic appearance

The majority (95%) of prostatic cancers are adenocarcinomas in which acinar formation is well marked. The tumour arises from the epithelial cells of the ducts or acini of the glands in the outer zone of the gland and may have a multifocal origin. This, together with the production of mucous by the tissue, indicates a well differentiated tumour. In some tumours the degree of de-differentiation is so great that the tumour cells are arranged in compact groups or solid columns. The surrounding stroma may be densely collagenous, producing a scirrhous cancer, or scanty, so that the growth is encephaloid.

The degree of differentiation is considered to be of prognostic importance but prostatic cancers tend to vary in their histological pattern from area to area. This may correlate with the clinical observation that some metastases may respond to hormonal therapy whilst metastases in other parts of the skeleton continue to progress.

Dissemination

Direct spread

This normally results in infiltration of the base of the bladder, the seminal vesicles and the urethra. Posterior spread is usually halted by the rectovesical fascia of Denonvilliers, which acts as a very effective barrier to involvement of the rectum. However, occasionally this fascia is breached and the rectum is then involved. This is of clinical importance since the tumour may then present with rectal symptoms and be mistaken for a primary rectal growth.

Lymphatic spread

This takes place to the internal and external iliac, to the lumbar, para-aortic, thoracic and supraclavicular nodes.

Perineural spread

This is not uncommon, tumour cells being frequently found in the perineural spaces.

Haematogenous spread

This most commonly results in metastases in the pelvis, lumbosacral vertebrae, femora, thoracic spine, and ribs, in descending order of frequency. The lungs are involved in about 20% of patients dying of the disease. Some osseous metastases are osteolytic in which case the alkaline phosphatase is elevated because of bone destruction, but the majority are osteosclerotic appearing denser than normal bone on a plain X-ray. All may be associated with a pathological fracture.

CLINICAL PRESENTATION

Many tumours are now being diagnosed at routine 'health checks' in completely symptomless males but, when symptoms are present, approximately two-thirds of patients will have problems relating to the lower urinary tract and one-third symptoms due to disseminated disease. Lower urinary tract symptoms include frequency, difficulty, passing urine, haematuria or retention. There may be diffuse perineal pain and, eventually, as the tumour spreads across the pelvis, sciatic pain develops together with bilateral venous oedema due to obstruction of the external iliac veins. Bloodstream dissemination may be associated with severe bone pain, pathological fractures or leucoerythroblastic anaemia.

In the majority of patients in whom symptoms are present the diagnosis can be made by digital examination of the prostate, although an infarct of the gland or, occasionally, a prostatic calculus may simulate a solitary nodule. When the tumour is more advanced the normal sharp palpable outline of the gland and the median sulcus are lost; once this stage has been reached the only real differential diagnosis is chronic prostatitis.

Natural history

The natural history of prostatic cancer is variable and unpredictable. Some have a malignant potential so great that metastases occur before there are any local symptoms, whereas others are so indolent that the life of the afflicted individual remains unaltered. As with the response to all malignancy, the natural history is dependent on the interaction between the host and his tumour.

STAGING

As with any tumour, to stage carcinoma of the prostate there must be cytological or histological verification of the diagnosis. If this cannot be met the symbol T_x, N_x or M_x must be used.

The following T categories are recognized, adding the suffix m if multiple tumours are present:

T_x – Minimum requirements not met.
T_{IS} – Pre-invasive carcinoma, carcinoma-in-situ.
T_0 – No tumour palpable, incidental finding in an operative or biopsy specimen.
T_1 – Intracapsular tumour surrounded by palpably normal gland.
T_2 – Tumour confined to gland, a smooth nodule deforming the contour of the gland leaving the lateral sulci and seminal vesicles uninvolved.
T_3 – Tumour extending beyond the capsule, with or without involvement of lateral sulci or seminal vescicles.
T_4 – Tumour fixed and invading neighbouring structures.

Methods of diagnosis and staging

Physical examination

Although a small percentage of carcinomas of the prostate are first recognized only because of the effect of distant metastases, e.g. backache from skeletal metastases, the majority of patients present with obstructive urinary symptoms and rectal examination reveals a small hard nodule in the prostate – or, in the case of a more advanced tumour (T_3), a hard, fixed, irregular mass encroaching on the lateral sulci. Indeed, 70–80% of all prostatic carcinomas have extended beyond the organ's boundaries at the time of diagnosis and are therefore easily diagnosed as unsuitable for any form of radical surgery. Local signs are best established in the fully anaesthetized patient by bimanual examination. However, investigation by sophisticated methods has shown that 40% of all prostatic tumours are understaged using digital examination alone. Assuming that rectal examination suggests the presence of a carcinoma of the prostate the following investigations can be used to verify the diagnosis, the stage the tumour has reached and the possible outcome.

Non-invasive investigations

Tumour markers. The commonest marker used for the identification of cancer of the prostate is acid phosphatase, which is produced by the acinar cells and secreted into the seminal fluid in the prostatic ductal system. In prostatic cancer the acid phosphatase level may be raised, either because acid phosphatase produced by the cancerous cells which have lost their connection with the prostatic ducts is absorbed directly into the bloodstream, or because compression of the ductal system has caused back-diffusion into the circulation. Acid phosphatase is also derived from the erythrocytes although the phosphatase derived from this source is inactivated by 0.5% formaldehyde. The upper limit of normal is 3.5 KA units and this level is not usually exceeded unless the tumour has extended beyond the capsule of the gland. A level of 10 units indicates that metastases are definitely present, but in as many as 40% of patients suffering from skeletal metastases the acid phosphatase is normal. When skeletal metastases are present the alkaline phosphatase is also raised. However, when a prostatic neoplasm responds favourably to orchidectomy or oestrogens, the level falls. Other markers recently recognized and investigated, some of which may also be used to indicate prognosis, are:

1. *Prostatic specific antigen (PGA)*. Isolated by Wang in 1979, PGA is a glycoprotein found in prostatic tissue and seminal plasma. Its normal concentration is 0–4 µg/l. Its exact physiological role is unknown. It is distinct from acid phosphatase both enzymatically and immunologically.
2. *Neopterin*, a protein derived from and secreted by activated T-lymphocytes. It represents the immunological response to tumours associated with antigens; unfortunately, however, it does not signal an increased ability of the immune system to defeat the tumour, but merely an increased outflow of tumour analogues foreign to the species.
3. *Thymidine kinase*.
4. *C-reactive protein*. Both thymidine kinase and C-reactive protein levels are elevated when DNA proliferation is increased.
5. *Osteocalcin*. This is a GLa protein indicating osteoblastic activity; its presence indicates a more aggressive tumour type.
6. *Tissue polypeptide antigen*, a non-specific marker.

Using multivariant analysis it has been found that the concentration of thymidine kinase provides the best indicator of prognosis, although unchanging values of PGA indicate that the disease is stable.

Ultrasonography. First applied by Wantake in 1974; advances in technique and the development of high frequency transducers allow the identification of the internal zonal anatomy of the gland, and high resolution now permits the recognition of tumours 4 mm in diameter, the involvement of the seminal vesicles and bladder base, and the discontinuity of the anterolateral part of the capsule before this is evident on digital examination. Ultrasonography can also be used to indicate the presence of ureteral obstruction and the development of hydronephrosis, and in many centres is used in place of intravenous pyelography to assess the upper urinary tract.

CAT and NMR. Both these methods have been used in the investigation of prostatic cancer. Both CAT and NMR appear to be less effective than ultrasound in identifying carcinoma of the prostate. However, NMR allows the detection of lymphadenopathy and bony metastases in the pelvis and lumbosacral region, although neither method will satisfactorily identify microscopic malignancy.

Plain X-rays of the pelvis, spine and chest. These may reveal the presence of soft tissue or bony metastases. So far as bony metastases are concerned it should be noted that at least 50% of the bone must be replaced by tumour before changes can be detected on plain X-rays.

HISTOLOGICAL CONFIRMATION

This histological structure of malignant disease of the prostate is graded in the following manner:

G_x – Grade cannot be assessed.
G_0 – No evidence of anaplasia.
G_1 – Low grade malignancy.
G_2 – Medium grade malignancy.
G_3 – High grade malignancy.

Tissue for histological identification of the tumour is usually obtained at the same time as bimanual examination of the prostate under anaesthesia, in which situation a transurethral resection of the prostate is performed. However, transurethral biopsy may not confirm the diagnosis in early prostatic cancer since it tends to arise in the periphery of the gland. Histological confirmation of the diagnosis in the absence of any obstructive symptoms is most commonly made by the use of a needle biopsy using a Tru-cut biopsy needle (Travenol). This may be performed via the perineum or per rectum, the former method obviating the danger of infection. The original technique of transrectal biopsy was described by Astradi in 1937 and the technique has been much improved by the use of a per rectal ultrasonic probe, which allows the operator to guide the needle into a solitary nodule. The biopsy is performed with the patient in the left lateral position. In a series of 150 patients in whom this technique was used by Eaton, a positive blood culture followed in 85% of patients within 10 minutes of the biopsy due to a transient bacteraemia, and in 20% of patients an overt urinary tract infection occurred. It is therefore now common practice to administer, prior to perineal biopsy, a wide-spectrum antibiotic such as gentamycin 2 mg/kg in patients in whom renal function is normal. Needle biopsy has an approximately 10% false negative rate.

Aspiration cytology

Fine needle aspiration biopsy has been extensively used in Scandinavia, where the accuracy of their results is comparable to those obtained by core biopsy. However, in other centres the diagnostic accuracy using this method has not been so high; errors up to 30% being reported, false negative results being commonest when the tumour is well differentiated.

Lymphangiography

This investigation is now rarely used since the results are often flawed. This is due to the fact that the hypogastric and presacral nodes are not consistently visualized by bipedal lymphangiography and because the sensitivity of the method is low, nodal metastases being detected in only approximately 50% of patients in whom they are present. Staging pelvic lymphadenectomy has been advocated by some workers in this field but has never gained general acceptance because of the considerable morbidity of the procedure. In particular, extensive nodal dissection followed later by X-ray therapy may lead to extremely disabling oedema of the genital area or lower limbs. Modified lymphadenectomy, although associated with a lower morbidity, gives a very high false negative rate as a consequence of the limited dissection.

Bone scanning

Bony secondaries appear on bone scans before their appearance on plain X-rays, false negative scans occurring in less than 2% of patients. The most commonly used agent is 99m Tc methylene diphosphonate, which has a high bone:soft tissue ratio and allows imaging 2 hours after injection of the isotope. Since bone isotopes are taken up in any area of increased bone turnover they are relatively non-specific hence the need for plain radiographs to rule out the presence of degenerative, traumatic, infective, or metabolic bone disease. The bone-seeking nuclide is taken up in areas in which new bone is being laid down in an attempt to repair the destruction caused by tumour invasion, so the area is depicted as a zone of increased uptake. The scan may not only be used to diagnose the presence of secondaries but also to assess progress after treatment.

TREATMENT

In general terms the majority of patients suffering from prostatic cancer are treated by palliative means. Ferguson rightly pointed out that the overall merits of any particular form of treatment should be judged more by the relief of symptoms than by survival time since in most patients the latter is in any case limited. It has indeed been estimated that the overall life expectancy of untreated cases from the onset of symptoms is 31 months, although 7% may survive for 5 years. This demonstrates the great variability in biological activity of these tumours. If metastases are present when the patient is first seen two-thirds of the patients are dead within 9 months.

Methods

Surgery

Theoretically, prostatic cancer should be as radically treated as any other neoplasm by surgical means. However, in less than 5% of patients is radical prostatectomy possible and, in the UK, the operation of radical prostatectomy, which involves the removal of the fascia of Denonvilliers, the prostate and the prostatic capsule, the vesical neck and trigone, the seminal vesicles and the ampullae of the vas deferens, has gained few adherents. The operation carries a relatively high mortality rate of 1–5% according to the series examined, an incontinence rate of 2–57% again according to the series examined, and impotence follows in nearly every patient.

Although retropubic and transvesical prostatectomy can be performed, this results only in a limited excision of malignant tissue; such operations are usually carried out when the correct preoperative diagnosis has not been made since the preferred method of dealing with obstructive symptoms is by transurethral resection.

Radiation therapy

Radiation therapy was first used in the treatment of prostatic cancer at the beginning of this century but poor results led to its use being abandoned. However, with the development of megavoltage external beam radiation generated by cobalt units and linear acceleration, interest in this modality of treatment has revived. In patients in whom distant metastases are not already present a 5-year tumour-free survival of approximately 50% has been reported by some centres. Local tumour control correlates with tumour grade, occurring more commonly in low-grade than in high-grade tumours.

However, external beam therapy is not without its complications. Acute gastrointestinal side-effects, commonly diarrhoea, rectal discomfort and tenesmus occur in 30–40% of patients, usually within the fourth week of therapy. Chronic symptoms due to radiation proctitis, which may later result in strictures or fistulae, occur in 1% of patients. Urinary side-effects also occur, consisting of frequency, dysuria and haematuria, and chronic urinary symptoms have been reported in as many as 5% of patients.

Hormonal therapy

Prostatic cells are dependent upon androgen to carry out their normal metabolic functions, the androgens being converted to dihydrotestosterone (DHT) within the prostatic cells. The major androgen is testosterone, 90% of which is produced in the testes, after which most is bound to sex steroid-binding globulin and albumin, some 3% remains free, which is the functionally active form of the hormone.

In the absence of androgens the prostate undergoes atrophy. Unfortunately, however, prostatic cancers are composed of a heterogenous population of cells that differ in their androgenic requirements. Some require near physiological levels of androgens to survive whilst others may thrive in the virtual absence of androgen. Thus a variable response to hormone deprivation can be expected.

Androgen production by the testes and adrenals is regulated by the hypothalamic–pituitary axis through two separate negative feedback mechanisms. Testosterone secretion by the testes is stimulated by luteinizing hormone (LH) released from the anterior pituitary upon stimulation by the LH-releasing hormone (LHRH) from the anterior hypothalamus. Androgen secretion by the adrenal is stimulated by adrenocorticotrophic hormone (ACTH) released from the anterior pituitary by corticotropic releasing factor (CRF) from the hypothalamus.

The seminal work on the hormonal control of prostatic cancer was performed by Huggins and his co-workers in Chicago in the 1940s and early 1950s and, following their work, it became a routine procedure in all cases of prostatic cancer to remove the testicular endocrine secretion by orchidectomy or subcapsular enucleation or, alternatively, to inhibit the secretion of androgens by the administration of high doses of stilboestrol.

Bilateral orchidectomy reduces the circulating testosterone levels from approximately 500 ng/dl to some 50 ng/dl, a reduction effectively arresting the metabolism of the androgen-dependent population of prostatic cancer cells, thereby inducing a high proportion of clinical remission. A similar result been also obtained by means of subcapsular orchidectomy.

Medical orchidectomy

The oestrogens have many influences on androgen metabolism: suppression of pituitary LH secretion; increasing the level of sex steroid-binding globulin; reducing testosterone production in the testes; and decreasing DNA synthesis in prostatic cancer cells. The principal effect appears to be the suppression of pituitary LH secretion. It may also be that the oestrogens have a direct cytotoxic action on the cancer cells.

The early uncritical use of high-dose oestrogen therapy has now been superseded by a more cautious approach, chiefly as a result of the Veterans Administration Co-operative Urological Research Group, who published a series of papers between 1964 and 1967 that indicated that treatment with high doses of oestrogens could be harmful, causing premature deaths from such causes as myocardial infarction, congestive heart failure and pulmonary embolus. More recently it has, however, been shown that, by reducing the dose of diethylstilboestrol to 2 mg daily, the death rate from these complications is reduced to that anticipated in patients of matched age.

Medical orchidectomy is not superior to surgical orchidectomy.

Signs of relapse may be subjective, and may include loss of weight, onset of pain either in the perineum from local extension or from the development of bony secondaries and loss of performance. Objective signs of recurrence may be gained from repeated ultrasound studies of the prostate itself or from repeated bone scans showing an increase in the number of 'hot spots' or new 'hot spots' developing in previously clear areas.

In general the prognosis appears to be extremely poor in patients with poorly-differentiated tumours subjected to orchidectomy as compared to the results obtained by the use of oestrogens. More recently, newer agents have been developed, including:

Cyproterone acetate, which was first isolated in 1971. This drug acts in two ways:

a. It acts as an antiandrogen by binding with receptor protein for DHT.
b. It controls the release of pituitary LH and LSH.

Clinical trials with this drug have shown that over 60 percent of patients respond as shown by radiological regression of skeletal metastases and regression of metastatic lymphadenopathy on CT scans. However the median duration of response is a mere 25 months.

LHRH analogue. Acting by suppressing luteinizing hormone and testosterone, this drug has also been shown to produce a response in about half the sufferers from prostatic cancer, with a median duration of response similar to that of cyproterone acetate.

Megestrol. In patients who have failed to respond to hormonal therapy, the drug megestrol may stabilize the disease, although a recently reported trial by Patel el al in 1990 showed that objective responses to this drug are rare.

13. Cryptorchidism

This term means 'hidden testis' and is applicable to any testis which has failed to descend into its normal postnatal anatomical position. Since the testes develop in the abdomen their descent may be inhibited anywhere along their normal pathway or they may be diverted from their route into the scrotum into an ectopic position.

Incidence

This incidence of undescended testis varies somewhat according to the series examined, but in general terms the average incidence of the condition is approximately 3% in the fullterm infant, falling to less than 1% at the end of the 1st year.

Why descent?

The reason for descent is the necessity for the testes to find a cooler environment. Situated in the abdomen, in which the temperature may be as much as 2°C higher than in the scrotum, spermatogenesis is impossible. However, in some animals the testes are situated within the abdomen during hibernation, descending only during the breeding season.

EMBRYOLOGY

By the 6th week of gestation the primordial germ cells have migrated from the wall of the embryonic yolk sac along the dorsal mesentery of the hindgut to invade the genital ridges; at this stage the gubernaculum appears as a ridge of mesenchymal tissue extending from the genital ridge through a gap in the anterior abdominal wall, which is the future inguinal canal to the genital swellings, the future scrotum. By the 7th week the indifferent gonads differentiate into the fetal testes and by the 8th week the fetal Leydig cells begin to secrete testosterone under the influence of the maternal chorionic gonadotrophin, which induces the Wolffian ducts to form the vasa deferentia and the epididymis. At the same time the fetal Sertoli cells begin to secrete a hormone known as the Müllerian inhibiting factor, which causes regression of the Müllerian ducts – leaving only the appendices testis (hydatids of Morgagni). At the same time the processus vaginalis appears ventral to the gubernaculum, alongside which are the fibres that will form the cremaster. Between the 8th and the 16th week the external genitalia develop. Testosterone secreted by the embryonic testes is converted to DHT by 5-α-reductase in the tissues of the genitalia, and this induces this differentiation. The testes now lie on top of the gubernaculum awaiting descent, the gubernaculum running from the lower pole of the epididymis through the inguinal canal to the genital swellings, which are slowly transformed into the scrotum proper. The process of descent remains dormant between the 12th week and the 7th month of gestation, during which the processus vaginalis slowly extends into the scrotum. At about the 7th month, just prior to descent, the vasa deferentia and the testicular vessels increase in size. The gubernaculum begins to swell and the processus extends rapidly into the scrotum. As the testes begin their descent they are preceded by the epididymis and, with descent completed, the scrotal part of the processus persists as the tunica whilst the upper part is normally obliterated.

Mechanism of descent

There are four chief theories regarding the actual mechanism of descent, all of which have their protagonists and detractors:

1. That traction on the testes by the gubernaculum is responsible.
2. That increasing intra-abdominal pressure pushes the testes through the inguinal canal, which has been dilated by the swelling of the gubernaculum.
3. That differential growth of the body wall in relation to a relatively immobile gubernaculum is responsible.
4. That the development and maturation of the epididymis is responsible.

Regardless of the actual mechanism, an important aspect appears to be the endocrine influence since both gonadotrophins and testosterone itself will induce premature testicular descent in experimental animals. Nevertheless the exact mechanism by which androgens act to promote testicular descent is unknown.

Most testes are situated within the scrotum at 3 months of age, except in premature infants when descent may be delayed until 6 months of age. If the testes are not found in the scrotum at the end of the first year, spontaneous descent is unlikely. Once in the scrotum, testicular development takes place in three phases:

1. From birth to the 4th year is the resting phase, during which the seminal tubules remain small and there is no evidence of cellular differentiation in the seminiferous tubules.
2. From the 5th to the 9th years is the growth phase, during which the seminal tubules elongate to become tortuous and the tubular diameter increases, although there is still no differentiation of the lining cells.
3. From the 9th to the 15th years maturation takes place, in which the seminiferous tubules become increasingly tortuous, their diameter increases and cellular differentiation occurs into the various spermatogenic layers.

Should the testes remain in the undescended position, positive histological changes from normal appear beginning at about 2.5 years of age, by which time it can be recognized that the seminiferous tubules are smaller than normal, with fewer spermatogonia and an increase in the peritubular tissues.

CLASSIFICATION

Based on their location, undescended testes can be classified as:

- *Abdominal*, situated within the internal ring. This accounts for 25%.
- *Within the inguinal canal*, situated between the internal and the external ring. This accounts for 70%.

The remaining 5% are *ectopic*; having traversed the inguinal canal in the normal way they come to rest in an abnormal site. Commonly the maldescended testis lies in the superficial inguinal pouch, less commonly in the suprapubic region, and rarely in the perineum or the femoral canal; each of these sites represents one of the many divisions of the gubernaculum.

Retractile testes

In addition to the above fixed, abnormal positions is the retractile testis, which is due to the development of the cremasteric reflex at between 5–6 years of age, resulting in a testis which can be elevated as high as the external ring. After the age of 13 years the testis is usually no longer retractile.

Hinman also described the dysgenetic testis. This is a testis which is grossly and histologically abnormal and, in all, some 20% of all undescended testes belong to this group, its importance lies in the fact that in such males 30–60% of the contralateral testes – even though occupying a normal position – will also be abnormal. Neither the abdominal testis nor one situated in the canal are palpable, although when the inguinal region is explored in a child suffering from an intra-abdominal testis it is commonly found that gentle abdominal pressure will lead to the extrusion of the testis into the canal – although normally the cord will be so short that no further descent is possible without a radical dissection.

ASSOCIATED CONDITIONS

Inguinal hernia

Following normal descent, the processus vaginalis closes between the 8th month of fetal life and within 1 month of birth. However, when the testis fails to descend the processus remains patent, leading to either a hydrocele or a congenital inguinal hernia. If the hernia is clinically evident at the first examination of the child, this is an indication for immediate operation to prevent the potential danger of strangulation. All that need be done is division and ligation of the processus at the level of the internal ring, which in the infant lies almost immediately posterior to the external ring.

Trauma

Whereas an ectopic testis is definitely at increased risk of injury, an inguinal testis resting in the canal is only a little more in danger than its scrotal counterpart.

Torsion

This is an important association because if urgent operation is not performed the affected testis will be lost due to infarction.

Malignancy

The incidence of non-descent in cases of testicular tumour has been found in retrospective studies to be between 5.9 and 14.3%. The risk of tumour development is put at 30–50 times that of a testis in the normal scrotal position, and the risk associated with an abdominal testis is four times greater than that of a testis lying in the inguinal canal. The bilateral cryptorchid is particularly at risk because if a tumour develops on one side the chance of malignancy in the opposite testis is one in four. Because testicular tumours have occurred in patients who have undergone orchidectomy as early as 5 years, the majority of paediatric surgeons recommend surgical correction at or before 2 years of age.

An important point from the surgeon's viewpoint is that orchidopexy does not appear to lessen the risk of malignant change in the testis that is brought into the normal position. Furthermore, almost 20% of testes which become malignant are the contralateral, normally placed testes. This fact suggests that the abnormal position is not in itself the carcinogenic agent, but rather that there is a primary testicular defect responsible for both non-descent and the increased risk of malignancy. The only value of orchidopexy is that a tumour developing in a scrotal testis is more easily diagnosed and, therefore, theoretically at least can be treated at an earlier date.

However, the incidence of testicular tumour in the male population is only 2.1 per million, so the problem posed by undescended testes is relatively insignificant.

Absence of lower segments of the recti

The 'prune belly syndrome'. In this condition the lower abdominal muscles are absent, leading to a typical deformity in the lower abdomen. The syndrome is commonly associated with bilateral cryptorchidism, together with abnormalities of the urinary tract, especially dilatation of the bladder.

Psychological effects

The importance of this is open to doubt. Various authors have quoted differing opinions, some considering that the child becomes increasingly disturbed between 3 and 6 years of age by the absence of a testis or testes. Such an argument can be used in favour of surgical treatment between these ages.

Infertility

Since tubular maldescent retards the production of spermatozoa, it is hardly surprising that males suffering from bilateral undescended testes are normally infertile. The higher and longer the testes reside away from the bottom of the scrotum the greater is the likelihood of permanent damage to the seminiferous tubules, and the earlier the testis is brought down the greater is the potential for the recovery of spermatogenic activity. In addition to defects in spermatogenesis there is also clinical and experimental evidence to suggest that cryptorchidism may also affect the interstitial compartment of the testes, although this does not appear to be of clinical importance since sufferers from bilateral maldescent develop the normal secondary sexual characteristics common to all males.

TREATMENT OF THE UNDESCENDED TESTIS

Hormonal treatment

This form of therapy was introduced in 1931, using human chorionic gonadotrophin (HCG), a hormone that is produced in the placenta and found in both the blood and urine of pregnant women. In the female, its action is predominantly that of the pituitary luteinizing hormone, and in the male it stimulates the interstitial cells of the testes and consequently the secretion of androgens. Various courses have been suggested, 500–1500 units once or twice daily for 4–8 weeks, 500 units twice weekly for 6 weeks and, latterly, a short course of 3300 units on alternate days for 6 days. At first, extravagant claims were made for the efficacy of hormonal treatment and even as late as 1938 it was being reported as successful in 65% of bilateral and 47% of unilateral cases of cryptorchidism. Only later was it appreciated that many of these apparently satisfactory results had been obtained in patients suffering from retractile testes.

It is now the general opinion that hormonal treatment is only worthy of trial in cases of bilateral cryptorchidism. The optimum age for starting treatment appears to be between 2 and 5 years, and a success rate of only about a third can be expected. It has been pointed out by some observers that the fertility in those patients with bilateral cryptorchidism who respond to HCG is greater than those who require surgery, but this is not unexpected since a proportion of those children not responding to hormone therapy will possess dysgenetic testes, the function of which is unlikely to be improved by surgery.

Surgical treatment

At present, orchidopexy is usually performed before the child enters schools at the age of 5 years. The essential operative features of orchidopexy are:

1. *Dissection of the spermatic cord from its surroundings,* so that the cord as a whole may be lengthened sufficiently to allow the testis to lie without tension within the scrotum. A hernial sac, if present, is divided above the testis, dissected from the cord and ligated at the level of the deep inguinal ring. Difficulty encountered in removing the sac from the cord can be minimized by infiltrating the cord with saline, thus separating its various parts.

2. *Cord lengthening.* If, after careful dissection of the cord, the testis cannot be brought into the scrotum, several techniques may be attempted:
   a. Division of the suspensory ligament of Browne. This is composed of a group of fibres, which radiate upwards and laterally from the cord at the level of the deep inguinal ring, and are best seen when the cord is drawn downwards and medially.
   b. Further lengthening can also be achieved by incising the medial edge of the internal ring and so taking the 'kink' out of the cord. There is no indication to divide the inferior epigastric artery which can usually be displaced medially.
   c. A further technique that may lengthen the cord is division of the spermatic artery itself which leaves the viability of the testis dependent upon the vasal vessels. This method is theoretically possible if the former can be divided at a sufficiently high level to preserve an anastomosis between the two systems.

Prior to such action the spermatic artery should be temporarily occluded in order to be certain that the testis remains viable. Since the length of the artery rather than the vas forms the limiting factor in 'cord length', microvascular techniques have recently been described in which the origin of the spermatic vessels is brought lower down the aorta.

3. *Fixation of the testis.* The older operations such as that described by Torek, in which the testis is temporarily fixed by implantation into a subcutaneous tunnel in the thigh, have now been generally abandoned because the tension created normally led to a high incidence of testicular atrophy. It is now more common to fix the testes within a subcutaneous pouch by dividing the prepubic fascia, which is identified by a finger from within the scrotum (Denis Brown's technique) or, alternatively, by placing the mobilized testicle through the scrotal septum into the opposite side of the scrotum (Ombrédanne's operation).

If the testis, despite the manoeuvres described previously, cannot be satisfactorily brought into the scrotum, it has been suggested that it should be fixed at the lowest point attainable without undue tension and then re-explored some time in the future when cord lengthening according to the advocates of this procedure will have occurred. However, the author has never found this satisfactory; usually at the second operation the testis is merely surrounded by scar tissue.

Results of orchidopexy

Testicular atrophy. The incidence of testicular atrophy following orchidopexy has been variously reported at between 2 and 50%. However, many of the results from which these figures were obtained were from older series in which undue strain had been placed on the testicle by placing it in the thigh.

Fertility studies. Fertility studies, although difficult to perform, show a variation in results between 30 and 70%.

Percentage paternity ratios. This is defined as the percentage of married patients who have become fathers. In a recent study in which 112 patients who had undergone orchidopexy were traced (with a response rate of 54%) it was found that the paternity rate for patients in whom a unilateral orchidopexy had been performed was equal to that of a normal individual, whereas when bilateral orchidectomy had been performed the percentage was considerably less.

Orchidectomy

Assuming that the opposite testis is normally placed in the scrotum, orchidectomy becomes an acceptable method of treatment of the undescended or maldescended testis if it cannot be brought into the scrotum. However, in cases of bilateral non-descent it is as well to bury the testis deep to the external oblique until the position on the opposite side has been properly established. This, at least, ensures that testosterone formation will occur, which will result in the development of the normal secondary sexual characteristics.

14. Swellings of the scrotum and testicular tumours

Swellings of the scrotum may be divided into cystic and solid.

CYSTIC SWELLINGS

Unilateral

Hydrocele

A hydrocele is a collection of fluid within the tunica vaginalis. Seen in childhood, it may be either congenital – when the communication between the tunica and the abdomen remains open via the processus vaginalis; or infantile – when this communication has already been cut off. Rarely hydroceles of the cord occur when fluid accumulates in a portion of the processus which has not been completely obliterated.

The obvious differential diagnosis is from a congenital hernia, and it is therefore contraindicated to attempt to aspirate such a swelling. If the baby is in no discomfort time should be allowed to observe whether the communication will close spontaneously or, alternatively, whether the fluid will be absorbed from the tunica. If neither of these events occur operation is required – the processus divided or, if the hydrocele is of the infantile type, the sac can be everted.

Adult hydroceles are primary or idiopathic, in which case there appears to be no underlying disease of the testis itself, or secondary to testicular disease, usually trauma, infection or malignancy.

Idiopathic hydroceles may be treated by intermittent aspiration, which is accompanied by the danger of infection, or by open operation, e.g. Jaboulay's operation.

Other unilateral cystic swellings

1. *Spermatoceles.* These are cystic collections of turbid fluid in the ducts of the vasa efferentia, the turbidity being due to the spermatozoa present.

2. *Cystic collections in embryonic remnants.* Neither of these two conditions require active treatment unless they have become an irritation to the patient.

Bilateral

Epididymal cysts

These are normally multiple cystic swellings, frequently bilateral, which develop in the epididymis. Unlike spermatoceles they contain clear fluid. Excision can be performed if they recur following aspiration.

SOLID SWELLINGS

Swellings of the epididymis

Inflammatory conditions

Acute epididymitis normally occurs during an acute urinary tract infection.

Chronic tuberculous epididymitis, always a secondary manifestation of genitourinary tuberculosis. The testis becomes craggy and hard and may break down to produce a chronic discharging sinus in the scrotum. In a previous era the treatment consisted of excision of the epididymis but at the present day the condition, now rare in the western world, responds to antituberculous drug therapy.

Swellings of the testes

Inflammatory conditions

Mumps. Viral orchitis occurs in 25% of post-adolescent cases of mumps. It is associated with severe pain and swelling of the body of the testis. The treatment consists of corticosteroids.

Gumma. Gummatous orchitis is a manifestation of tertiary syphilis, causing a painless enlargement of the testis to develop.

Granulomatous orchitis A relatively rare condition, which may follow a traumatic episode. It is considered to be due to a reaction of the interstitial tissues of the testis to the presence of spermatozoa, the responsible agent being an acid-fast lipid which chemically resembles the mycolic acid of *Mycobacterium tuberculosis*.

Neoplastic swellings (see below)

Swellings of the tunica vaginalis

Haematocele. Caused by severe trauma to the body of the testis, blood slowly organizes to produce a solid swelling in the scrotum, which may in the course of time liquify.

TESTICULAR TUMOURS

Testicular tumours are relatively uncommon. Their incidence is about 3 per 100 000 of the population, or 1% of all male tumours. They represent an interesting group of tumours, however, in view of the altered management and prognosis in recent years.

Clinical presentation

The majority of testicular tumours are brought to the attention of the patient by observing that one testis has become larger or heavier than the opposite member. Because the tumour is contained within the tunica albuginea the overall shape of the testis is retained. Pain is seldom a feature but insensitiveness of the testis to pressure is commonplace once the normal testicular tissue has been destroyed.

Very occasionally metastatic deposits, either in the retroperitoneal lymph nodes or in the lungs, draw attention to a hitherto unsuspected testicular swelling. Rarely, a tumour may produce hormonal side-effects: a choriocarcinoma, a rare form of teratoma, may produce sufficient gonadotrophins to cause gynaecomastia; Sertoli cell tumours and Leydig cell tumours may both secrete sufficient oestrogen to cause gynaecomastia; and Leydig tumours may also secrete sufficient androgen to produce sexual precocity in affected children.

In looking at a male with an enlarged solid swelling of the testes it is as well to remember that there are only three other important causes of swelling of the body of the testis: mumps, in which a typical history of severe pain is always obtained; gumma, a rare condition in the West, which normally occurs in a much older age group; and granulomatous orchitis, which is also rare. Whereas teratomas are found at all ages, seminomas are most common in the fifth decade.

Pathology

90% of all testicular tumours are either derived from epithelial tissue (seminoma), or are tumours of embryonic origin (teratoma), although both seminoma and teratoma elements are to be found in many. A further group of tumours principally occurring in infancy has also been recognized: the yolk sac tumour, formerly referred to as the orchioblastoma.

The classification of these tumours has always presented a considerable problem since so many factors may be taken into consideration, including the microscopic appearance of the tumour, and its histogenesis, morphology, and immunological and biochemical characteristics.

So far as testicular tumours are concerned, consideration of these various factors has led to an increasing subdivision of the various tumour types. The recognized World Health Organization (WHO) classification of testicular germ cell tumours drawn up in 1977 is given below, and contrasts with the slightly earlier classification of the British Testicular Tumour Panel (BTTP) based on the work of Pugh, 1976 (see Table 14.1).

The proportions of the various types are: seminomas, 40%; teratomas, 32%; mixed tumours in which seminomatous elements are found in teratoma, 14%; and lymphomas, 7%. The remaining tumours are the rarer Leydig, Sertoli cell and yolk sac tumours.

Seminomas are rare in the very young; their peak incidence is in the 30s, after which their incidence falls so that they are comparatively rare after the age of 50. On section they are usually soft and greyish-white in colour although areas of haemorrhage and necrosis can be seen. Enlarged veins may be seen beneath the thickened tunica, and bisection of the tumour shows the normal testicular tissue squashed to one side. Microscopically the tumour is composed of uniform polyhedral cells, which are occasionally arranged in tubular fashion. Direct spread may involve the epididymis and the spermatic cord, and invasion of the lymphatics and bloodstream also occurs. Lymphatic spread carries the tumour to the retroperitoneal lymph nodes, whilst bloodstream spread, which is especially common in MTT tumours, results in deposits developing in the lungs and liver. Two aetiological factors have been described: trauma and maldescent of the testes.

In many cases of established testicular tumour a preceding history of trauma is elicited but it is more probable that the traumatic incident itself draws the patients attention to his scrotum and hence

Table 14.1 Classification of pathology of testicular tumours

WHO	BTTP
Tumours of one histological type	
Seminoma: typical, spermatocytic, anaplastic	Seminoma
Teratoma: mature	Teratoma differentiated (TD) – fully differentiated tissues
immature with malignant transformation	Malignant teratoma intermediate (MTI) – incompletely differentiated tissues with elements having characteristics of malignancy
Embryonal carcinoma	Malignant teratoma undifferentiated (MTU) – mature or organized components lacking
Yolk sac tumour	Malignant trophoblastic teratoma (MTT) containing trophoblastic elements in combination with MTI or MTU
Choriocarcinoma	–
Tumours of more than one histological type e.g. Embryonal carcinoma + seminoma	–

Thus the approximate equivalent for the two systems is as follows:
TD (*BTTP*) = Teratoma, mature and immature (*WHO*)
MTI (*BTTP*) = Teratoma with malignant transformation (*WHO*)
MTU (*BTTP*) = Embryonal carcinoma (*WHO*)
MTT (*BTTP*) = Choriocarcinoma (*WHO*)

to his enlarged testes. So far as maldescent is concerned the weight of evidence leads to the conclusion that there is an increased incidence of seminoma in the maldescended testis, but whether this is due to a direct effect of maldescent, the increased environmental temperature associated with the condition, or some unknown agency remains an enigma. The risk of developing a tumour in an undescended testis is estimated to be 17 times greater than in the normal testis and 30 times greater in an abdominal testis.

Teratomas account for the majority of the remaining neoplastic types. They are derived from all three germ layers but, unlike ovarian teratomas, they are usually extremely active, behaving in the manner of all malignant disease. Less than 1% of teratomas are differentiated to such a degree that a dermoid cyst is produced. On section, teratomas have a varied appearance. The tumour mass is predominantly solid but some cysts are always present, some of which contain mucoid material. Islands of bone and cartilage may be found. In undifferentiated tumours the cut surface is soft and pinkish-white, and areas of necrosis and haemorrhage may be seen.

Tumour markers

Two tumour markers are related to malignant disease of the testis: the glycoprotein, α-fetoprotein, and the β-subunit of human chorionic gonadotrophin. The former is a normal serum protein of the human fetus and is synthesized from the 10th week onwards by fetal liver cells, the cells of the gastrointestinal tract and the yolk sac. The neosynthesis of this protein after the age of 3 months indicates the presence of increased hepatocyte turnover or neoplasia of tissues originally capable of synthesizing this protein in embryonic life. The latter, i.e. HCG, is produced by the syncytial trophoblast and non-gestational trophoblastic elements in gonadal and extragonadal tissues. Not all testicular tumours secrete these markers; only 5–7% of pure seminomas are associated with raised levels of HCG, whereas nearly 90% of teratomas caused raised levels of α-fetoprotein and HCG to appear in the serum.

TREATMENT OF TESTICULAR TUMOURS

Assuming that no obvious metastases are present and a clinical diagnosis of testicular tumour has been made on clinical examination and by the use of ultrasonography, the scrotum is explored by means of an inguinal incision. No biopsy should be attempted through the scrotal skin prior to this, in case seeding occurs. The external oblique aponeurosis is opened and the cord and its vessels clamped, after which the testis is delivered from the scrotum. Assuming that the diagnosis is correct the cord is divided at the level of the internal ring and the wound closed. Following recovery from the operation the tumour is 'staged'.

Unfortunately, many systems of staging have been devised, many of them modifications of the UICC method, which is somewhat complicated. Three examples of the many staging classifications are shown in Tables 14.2–4, including the UICC classification. In addition, the pathologist is consulted in regard to the histological nature of the tumour, where again the classification is anything but simple. However, in an examination of 259 patients suffering from

Table 14.2 The UICC staging classification

T: Primary tumour (In the absence of orchidectomy the symbol T_x must be used)
T_0	No evidence of primary tumour
T_1	Tumour limited to body of testis
T_2	Tumour extending beyond the tunica albuginea
T_3	Tumour involving the testis and epididymis
T_4	Tumour invading the spermatic cord or scrotal wall
T_{4a}	Invasion of spermatic cord
T_{4b}	Invasion of scrotal wall

N: Nodes
N_0	No evidence of regional lymph node involvement
N_1	Involvement of single homolateral lymph node
N_2	Involvement of contralateral nodes, bilateral nodes or multiple regional lymph nodes
N_3	A palpable abdominal mass or fixed inguinal nodes
N_4	Invasion of juxta-regional lymph nodes

M: Distant metastases
M_0	No evidence of distant metastases
M_1	Distant metastases present
M_{1a}	Evidence of distant metastases based on biochemical and/or other tests
M_{1b}	Single metastasis in a single organ
M_{1c}	Multiple metastases in a single organ
M_{1d}	Metastases in multiple organ sites

Table 14.3 Royal Marsden classification, in conjunction with the Medical Research Council (slightly modified from the staging proforma devised by Peckham and his co-workers in 1980)

Stage	Definition
IM	Rising serum markers after orchidectomy

II	Abdominal node metastases
	    A < 2 cm in diameter
	    B 2–5 cm in diameter
	    C > 5 cm in diameter

III	Supradiaphragmatic lymph node metastases
	    0 No abdominal lymph nodes
	    ABC Lymph nodes as defined in II

IV	Extralymphatic metastases
L_1	Less than 3
L_2	More than 3, all less than 2 cm in diameter
L_3	More than 3, at least 1 more than 2 cm in diameter
H	Liver involvement

Table 14.4 A simple staging system

Stage I	Tumour restricted to the testis
Stage II	Small or moderate volume noted on CT scan of para-aortic infradiaphragmatic lymph nodes
Stage III	Nodal involvement above and below the diaphragm
Stage IV	Visceral metastases present

non-seminomatous germ cell tumours Freedman and his co-workers found that four histological features enabled them to predict relapse:

1. Invasion of the testicular veins.
2. Invasion of the testicular lymphatics.
3. An absence of yolk sac elements.
4. The presence of undifferentiated tissue, which they found in the majority of specimens which they examined although their findings did not reflect that tumours categorized as MTU were any more likely to relapse than MTI tumours.

In the past the following investigations were regarded as essential:

a. Tomography of the chest in the presence of a normal radiograph.
b. Intravenous pyelography, which by demonstrating any displacement of the ureters gave some indications of the presence and size of the para-aortic nodes.
c. Bipedal lymphangiography.

CAT is now commonly used to assist staging, where it is available.

Both lymphangiography and CAT do, however, produce a proportion of both false-positive and false-negative results, and in view of this many workers in this field consider that retroperitoneal lymphadenectomy is the only accurate method of staging.

In all patients the tumour markers must be assayed. The HCG level may possibly be elevated in seminoma and, if so, it should return to normal following orchidectomy if no extratesticular tumour tissue is present. The level of α-fetoprotein is not raised in pure seminoma, but is raised when tumours of mixed variety, 14% of the whole, are present.

The treatment of metastatic disease caused by these tumours, either occult or overt, has been greatly influenced in the last two decades by the introduction of chemotherapeutic regimes which have been highly effective in both seminomas and non-seminomatous germ cell tumours (NSGTs) following orchidectomy.

However, so far as seminomas are concerned, occult metastases are present in 10–15% in the abdominal lymph nodes when the patient is first seen, and the first line of treatment of such nodes remains radiotherapy – followed by chemotherapy only in those patients who relapse. Using this regime a relapse rate of only 3–5% can be anticipated, such relapses being controlled by further radiotherapy or by chemotherapy. If nodal disease is already present both above and below the diaphragm when the patient is first seen, chemotherapy alone is the treatment of choice.

Prior to the introduction of vinblastine and bleomycin in 1975, the cure rate for advanced testicular neoplasms was virtually nil. The agents which have played a significant role in improving the outlook in testicular tumours are bleomycin, cisplatin, carboplastin, etoposide and vinblastine. All these drugs are used in combination – never singly.

In 1988 Peckham and others published their results following the treatment of 320 patients suffering from non-seminomatous germ cell tumours. Following orchidectomy and staging, one of the following regimes were used, the combinations altering with time as less toxic ones were developed: VB – vinblastine and bleomycin; PVB – cisplatin, vinblastine and bleomycin; more recently, BEP – bleomycin, etoposide and cisplatin; and even more recently, in an attempt to reduce the myelosuppressive effects, CEB – carboplastin, etoposide and bleomycin.

In all, four to six treatment courses were given, and thereafter localized residual tumour masses were resected in patients in whom the tumour markers had returned to normal levels. The reasons for retroperitoneal para-aortic lymphadenectomy are:

1. Many residual tumour masses contain areas of active but benign teratoma which may continue to grow causing the development of large masses.
2. Despite the presence of normal marker levels, foci of malignancy may be found indicating the need for further courses of chemotherapy. In many centres retroperitoneal lymphadenectomy is not performed if no residual masses are present at the end of the treatment schedule and the tumour markers have reached normal concentrations, since obviously in the absence of tumour tissue the procedure – although allowing very accurate staging in skilled hands – is non-therapeutic. Furthermore it has been shown in some reported series that even if the abdominal lymph nodes are tumour-free, a relapse can occur due to the appearance of intrathoracic nodes. A further problem is that bilateral dissection may cause ejaculation failure.

Using these regimes the actuarial survival at 5 years in a series reported by Peckham and his co-workers was 85% in patients suffering from Stages II, III or IV NSGTs, although survival was short once treatment failure had occurred. In the entire series of 320 patients, 3% died, not of recurrent disease, but due to the complications of chemotherapy. Factors considered to be most important were the tumour volume and a high level of tumour markers, i.e. AFP $>$ 500 ku/l and a serum HCG $>$ 1000 IU/l.

SECTION FOUR

15. Common benign swellings of the breast

DEVELOPMENTAL ANATOMY

In the 6th week of embryonic life a thickened ridge of ectoderm develops, the milk line, extending from the axilla to the groin. Normally in *Homo sapiens* this line regresses, except in the pectoral region where by the 20th week of life, cords develop; after canalization, these cords become confluent at the areola, onto which the ducts open. At birth some 20 channels open at the rudimentary nipple; in the large majority of infants, shortly after birth, the breasts swell and, for about 3 weeks, excrete a cloudy secretion, probably due to increased secretion of prolactin in response to loss of maternal oestrogen. Thereafter the swelling settles and until adolesence the breasts remain undeveloped.

At adolescence either one or both breasts may enlarge in the male, most commonly for only a short period, but in the female great changes occur and indeed continue to occur throughout life until finally atrophy occurs with the onset of menopause.

ANATOMY OF THE BREAST

Gross anatomy

The breast is divisible into three zones:

1. The nipple and areola.
2. The breast disc, which is a thick white fibrous structure containing all the ducts and lobules.
3. The skin and subcutaneous fatty tissue that surrounds the disc.

Microscopic anatomy

Ductal system

The ducts of the breast fan out into the breast disc from the lactiferous sinuses on the undersurface of the nipple. Each duct is lined by pseudostratified columnar epithelium outside which is a thin layer of myoepithelial cells together with a network of loose connective and elastic tissue in which there is a subepithelial lymphatic plexus. External to these is a final layer of rather denser connective tissue. The main ducts are connected by the terminal ducts to the lobules, in which lie the acini embedded in loose intralobular connective tissue. As the terminal duct reaches the acinus it loses the various connective tissue layers and is eventually surrounded only by a thin basement membrane. Throughout active 'hormonal' life the epithelium of the ducts and lobules secretes and absorbs its secretions.

Structure of lobule

Each lobule contains a variable number of acini, from less than 10 to more than 100. Each acinus is lined by a double layer of cells; the cells resting on the basement membrane have a relatively clear cytoplasm whereas the inner layer of cells are more deeply staining. In the active lactating breast, distension of the acini reduces the lining membrane to a one-cell structure.

Involution

Involution is a process caused by lack of hormonal stimulus during which the breast passes into the postmenopausal state. In normal circumstances the growth of the breast disc is controlled by somatotrophic hormone and oestrogen and acinar development by prolactin and progesterone. All four hormones are required to maintain the normal architecture of the breast following development.

During involution, the breast may enlarge because of the deposition of fat, but the glandular tissue, as represented by the number of acini per lobule, decreases and the fibrous tissue becomes increasingly dense and hyalinized.

In about one-third of women at between 30 and 40 years of age the lobules shrink and collapse, only an occasional acinar-like structure persisting, often with cyst-like dilatation. The latter change is possibly brought about by the involuting acini coalescing to form small intralobular cysts which then enlarge.

As involution progresses, the lobular elements continue to disappear and the surrounding stroma increases in density.

The proliferation and deposition of fibrous tissue within the lobules and its fusion with the basement membrane has been named 'lobular sclerosis' by some pathologists. Excessive fibrosis or sclerosis often appears to halt the development of involution so that even in old age small clumps of cells may be seen within a dense stroma. By the mid-50s sclerosis and obliteration of the small ducts has usually taken place, even in a perfectly normal breast.

BENIGN SWELLINGS

The nomenclature and nature of benign swellings of the breast have been bedevilled by the multiplicity of terms and eponyms that have been used to describe similar conditions. Further, the term 'chronic mastitis' applied to certain benign conditions of the breast wrongly suggests that many of these conditions are inflammatory in origin.

Based on physical findings at the bedside, benign breast swellings may be classified as follows:

1. *Discrete with well-circumscribed margins*
   a. Solid – fibroadenoma.
   b. Cystic –   (i) tension cysts
              (ii) lymphatic cysts
              (iii) galactocele.

2. *Diffuse, ill defined swellings*
   a. Irregularities of breast without histological change.
   b. Uneven involution across the breast disc.
   c. Cystic disease leading to –
      (i) excessive fibrosis (lobular sclerosis)
      (ii) cystic lobular sclerosis
      (iii) cystic lobular degeneration.
   d. Duct ectasia.
   e. Fat necrosis.
   f. Breast abscess.

Further consideration will now be given to the aetiology of these various conditions.

Discrete breast swellings

Fibroadenoma

These develop in the breast prior to the menopause, pericanalicular tumours usually being found below the age of 30 and intracanalicular thereafter. Either tumour may be multiple, and successive tumours may develop in the same or contralateral breast. The pericanalicular tumour forms a firm discrete mass, which is freely mobile in the breast tissue, hence the term 'breast mouse'.

The intracanalicular tumour tends to be softer and may grow to such a size that there is necrosis of the overlying skin. To such a condition the terms serocystic disease of Brodie or cystosarcoma phylloides have been given. However, despite the implications of malignancy in the latter term, the tumour is benign.

Pathology. This swelling has been variously regarded as a simple hyperplasia of the epithelial and/or connective tissue elements, or as a composite neoplasm of the breast tissue in which the epithelial and mesenchymal components grow simultaneously.

Treatment. Treatment consists of excision.

Tension cysts

These are relatively common and may be both bilateral and multiple. They form smooth, obviously cystic swellings, usually in the central or middle zones of the breast tissue.

Pathology. Cysts of this type probably arise from obstruction to the ducts of a breast which is already in a state of cystic lobular degeneration. Such cysts are usually surrounded by a dense connective tissue stroma, which may obliterate the lymphatic drainage with the result that, although secretions may form, they cannot be absorbed. Large cysts may be formed from coalescing microcysts rather than by the dilatation of a single acinus.

The lining membrane of a tension cyst is often aprocrine in type and many cells show intense eosinophilic staining due to pink cell metaplasia.

Treatment. Cysts should be treated by simple aspiration. The aspirate is commonly light yellow, green or brown in colour, and is normally acellular.

All should be sent for exfoliative cytology. If suspicious cells are found or a palpable mass remains after aspiration the affected area of the breast should be excised. This is extremely rare.

Lymphatic cysts

These are clinically indistinguishable from the common tension cysts but the diagnosis may be suspected if the aspirating needle meets no resistance as it penetrates the cyst wall.

Galactocele

These are probably formed by obstruction to a duct in the puerperium. The milk retained proximal to the obstruction eventually becomes cheese-like. This condition has become less frequent in the UK and USA as better ante- and postnatal care has become available to the general population. The common complication of this type of swelling is infection.

Diffuse and ill-defined swellings

Routine examination of the breasts, particularly in women who have borne children, often reveals painless irregularities in the breast tissue. In approximately 25%, these irregularities, particularly those situated in the upper and outer quadrant of the breast, are painful and tender, especially in the week preceding menstruation.

The term mastodynia was applied to such a breast by Geschiekter in 1945 but the term is virtually meaningless since nodular breasts are not necessarily painful, and in young women the breast may be painful in the absence of any palpable abnormality. These common irregularities in the breast are often without a radiological or histological basis, but in older women uneven involution may lead to a nodularity that has a true structural basis.

When the breast is painful some relief may be achieved by administration of bromocriptine, which inhibits the secretion of prolactin by the pituitary. Controlled trials in some centres have shown that it is better than a placebo in relieving breast pain but it is only useful in cyclical pain, i.e. pain immediately prior to the onset of menstruation. Constant breast pain remains unaffected. It is recommended that 1.25 mg are administered at bedtime, increasing the dose after 2–3 days to 2.5 mg at bedtime and then after an interval to 2.5 mg twice daily. Various series suggest that 70–80% of women will achieve symptomatic improvement on this medication.

Variants of involution

The variants of involution, regarded by some pathologists as distinct entities, include lobular sclerosis and cystic lobular degeneration. Both conditions present clinically as irregular, ill-defined swellings in the breast which are *not* associated with any of the classic signs of malignancy.

Lobular sclerosis is a condition in which excessive fibrosis is followed by hyalinization within the lobules, in which some acini persist. Once cystic changes take place in the persistent acini the condition may be regarded as cystic lobular degeneration.

In the past, such changes have been variously known as chronic mastitis, adenosis, and cystic hyperplasia.

Treatment. A mammogram is sometimes necessary in this type of breast to eliminate cancer. If the mammogram is negative the decision to excise the affected area depends upon the degree of localization of the pain, tenderness, and swelling. When diffuse, relief can often be obtained by the use of diuretics during the week prior to the period. If the swelling is well localized and extremely tender it can be excised.

Duct ectasia

Clinically, this condition presents as solitary or multiple tender swellings in the sub- or periareolar region of the breast. Palpation reveals a number of cord-like swellings which radiate from the areola, a physical finding which led Bloodgood to apply the term 'varicocele tumour of the breast' to this condition.

The ducts are dilated and contain an inspissated yellow cheesy material that can be expressed like toothpaste from the cut end of a duct. The periductal elastic tissue is destroyed and the surrounding tissues are infiltrated with lymphocytes and plasma cells.

Occasionally, the inflammatory response may be so acute that skin changes occur and the condition may be mistaken for a breast abscess.

Fat necrosis

This is traumatic in origin and is met with only in women with large fatty breasts. Clinically, the patient develops severe bruising after a moderately severe injury. When the bruise settles the woman notices a swelling which it is clinically impossible to distinguish from carcinoma of the breast because the irregular mass is often attached to the skin.

The excised lesion is an infiltrative yellowish white mass. Microscopically a central area of necrotic fat cells are surrounded by a granulomatous reaction consisting of macrophages and mononuclear cells.

Breast abscess

This condition is usually found during lactation. As a rule the infecting organism is *Staphylococcus aureus,* less commonly *Streptococcus pyogenes.* The usual mode of infection is via the nipple, the infection being carried by the suckling infant in the nasopharynx. In maternity wards the condition may occasionally reach epidemic proportions. The infection is at first limited to the segment drained by the lactiferous duct but it may subsequently spread to involve other areas of the breast.

The majority of breast abscesses present clinically as ill-localized areas of painful cellulitis, often associated with redness of the overlying skin and general malaise.

In the early stages the inflammation may respond to antibiotic therapy, but as oedema of the overlying skin develops drainage is required. All loculi must be broken down, and under antibiotic 'cover' the dead space can be closed and the wound sutured without drainage. Alternatively, the abscess can be treated on traditional lines by 'saucerizing' the cavity and allowing it to heal by secondary intention.

16. Breast cancer

Cancer of the breast is the commonest malignant growth in women, and in females aged between 40 and 50 years it is the commonest cause of natural death.

The most important risk factors are:

1. *Sex.* 99% of all breast cancers occur in females. The incidence of breast cancer increases from 20–45 years of age and then falls in the perimenopausal period, presumably due to hormonal influences, only to rise again later in life.

2. *Race.* The annual death rate in Japan is 5/100 000 as compared to 25/100 000 in the Netherlands. This difference in incidence is associated with the finding that Japanese women secrete a wet cerumen in the ears, whereas Western women secrete a dry wax.

3. *Family history.* Daughters of women who have suffered from breast cancer have a two- to three-fold risk of themselves developing breast cancer, the risk increasing if the mother's cancer was diagnosed in the premenopausal period of life.

4. *Genetic factors.* Two genetic syndromes are associated with an increased incidence of breast cancer:
   a. Klinefelter's syndrome, in which the male possesses an extra X chromosome and in consequence suffers from gynaecomastia, small testes and azoospermia.
   b. Bowden's disease, in which soft tissue hamartomas occur, together with an increased risk of cancer of the breast.

5. *Fecundity.* Some protection against breast cancer is conferred by early pergnancy but this protection is lost if the first pregnancy occurs after the age of 35 years.

6. *Previous history of breast cancer.* Patients who have suffered cancer of the breast in one breast are at an increased risk of developing malignancy in the opposite breast, the risk being estimated at 1 percent per year.

PATHOLOGY

The great majority of breast cancers arise from the epithelium of the mammary ducts, only a minority arising from the epithelium of the acini and small intralobular ductules – so-called lobular carcinoma. Invasive ductal carcinomata show a wide spectrum of differentiation.

An attempt to grade breast tumours by examination of their histological features was first made by Greenhough in 1925 followed by Patey and Scarff in 1928. These workers assessed three separate histological characteristics and then combined the results to give a composite histological picture.

The three aspects were as follows:

- The degree of structural differentiation as shown by the presence of tubular arrangement of the cells; tubule formation.
- Variation in size, shape and staining of nuclei; pleomorphism.
- Frequency of hyperchromatic and mitotic figures; mitoses.

This method was further refined by Bloom and Richardson (1957) who used a points system based on each of the above criteria to arrive at an overall estimation of the degree of malignancy.

Tumours were graded from I–III and Bloom found that when no nodal involvement was present 94% of patients classified as suffering from Grade I tumours were alive and well after 5 years, whereas only 16% of those suffering from Grade III tumours survived for this period.

In general, Bloom found that the presence of tubule formation produced a favourable prognosis, that great cellular pleomorphism led to a worse prognosis, and that the more hyperchromatic the nuclei the more gloomy the outlook.

Bloom and Richardson also investigated the possibility that metastatic tumours might develop a different histological grade from the primary growth. Their findings showed that the pattern was identical in 82%, higher than the primary in only 12%, and lower in the remainder. Thus the distant metastases may show remarkably little change even though there may have been an interval of many years between the removal of the primary tumour and the appearance of metastases. Within this group of tumours are the rare colloid or mucoid carcinomas in which the production of a secretion, albeit abnormal, indicates some degree of differentiation.

Other histological types include the medullary carcinomas, comprising 2–5% of all breast tumours. These tumours are well circumscribed on cut section, having a well defined margin as compared to the common invasive ductal carcinomata with their irregular extensions into the surrounding breast tissue. The characteristic feature of this type of tumour is the dense lymphocytic infiltration both within and around the tumour.

Lobular carcinoma

These tumours may be:

1. *In situ.* This lesion is not usually diagnosed clinically but is merely a pathological diagnosis arrived at after removing breast tissue for some other reason. It occurs in premenopausal women, and is multifocal in the majority and bilateral in nearly half the patients in whom it is found. If such a finding is made close surveillance of the patient is required both by clinical and mamographic means.

2. *Invasive.* This tumour is characterized by a homogenous pattern of small cells arranged in strands diffusely infiltrating the lobules. Often multiple, it is frequently bilateral. Clinically it may be associated with breast pain rather than a swelling, and since microcalcification is not present an early lesion may be missed on mammography.

Intraduct carcinoma

This condition usually presents with a clinical lump in which, on mammography, speckled calcification can be seen. Often multifocal, the malignant epithelial cells are confined within the ducts and have by definition not penetrated the basement membrane. Nevertheless even after excision of the lesion, follow-up shows that an invasive carcinoma frequently develops in the same breast at a later date.

CLINICAL PRESENTATION

In the great majority of patients the presenting symptom of breast cancer is a swelling found by the woman herself, by accident or during routine self-examination. This has been widely canvassed as a possible means of reducing the mortality from this disease since in general terms the smaller the swelling when first treated the better the prognosis. In the majority the swelling is painless, unlike many benign conditions of the breast. Nevertheless the absence of confirmatory signs – such as skin attachment, recent nipple retraction, deep attachment to the pectoral fascia, palpable nodes in the axilla, or the presence of pain or tenderness on examination – does not exclude the possibility of malignancy. A further rare physical sign is a crusting eczematous lesion of the nipple which may extend outwards to involve the adjacent skin, the nipple undergoing erosion and destruction. Histologically the dermis of the involved skin shows a non-specific chronic inflammatory response, being invaded by lymphocytes, and the epidermis contains large, undifferentiated pale-staining cells among the epithelial cells – Paget cells, which are now believed to be cancer cells which have spread along ducts and ductal epithelium to infiltrate the skin from an underlying cancer of the breast.

The commonest site of breast cancer is in the upper and outer quadrant, and the least common is the lower and inner quadrant. Occasionally the presence of an intraduct papilloma or carcinoma may be revealed by the presence of a blood-stained discharge from the nipple. Other conditions which may mimic early cancer, all of which are rare, are tuberculosis, fat necrosis and Mondor's disease.

Although breast cancer spreads by the bloodstream, lymphatic extension to the regional lymph nodes also occurs leading to their enlargement. The only accessible palpable nodes are in the axilla and the supraclavicular fossa, both of which should be examined. However, so far as the axilla is concerned, there is a good deal of observer error, up to 40% in some series.

Later tumours present with ulcerating lesions, which are quite obviously malignant. All patients in whom cancer of the breast is suspected should also have a complete physical examination, paying particular attention to the presence or absence of tumours in the opposite breast, pleural effusions, hepatomegaly and ascites.

DIAGNOSTIC CONFIRMATION

Mammography

Mammography has become so refined that clinically undetectable lesions can now be identified. Normal X-ray film can be used or, alternatively, the technique of xeroradiography, which is said to define the lesion more clearly. False-negative and false-positive results are obtained in approximately 10% of patients.

Mammographic appearance of the normal breast

The overall appearance of a mature breast depends on the relative amounts of fat and glandular tissue present. The margins of the glandular tissue are irregular due to the crescentic incursions of fatty tissue. Lactiferous ducts may be identified, although they are never clear-cut unless contrast medium has been injected into them. At the menopause the breast as a whole shrinks and the glandular portion involutes. In a heavy breast the actual amount of fat is increased, thus accentuating the natural contrast between the various tissues and structures in the breast so that even small lesions can be identified. The trabeculae of the breast appear more prominent even though they are thinner, and the lactiferous ducts also stand out against the translucent fatty background. As involution progresses, the glandular portion becomes increasingly dense due to the relative increase in fibrous tissue, thus making small lesions difficult to detect.

Mammographic evidence of malignancy

The two direct signs of malignancy are: the presence of an abnormally dense opacity in the breast, and calcification.

Abnormally dense opacity in the breast. If malignant, such an opacity usually has an irregular outline, leading to the use of such descriptive terms as 'spicules' and 'tentacles'. Even in those rare cases in which a malignant tumour appears to have a smooth outline, at least one part of the circumference usually appears to be ill-defined.

Calcification. Although this may occur in a benign lesion it is usually coarser and smoother, whereas in a malignant lesion it is more commonly fine and irregular, producing the appearance of small dots of calcification in relation to the lesion. However, such calcification occurs in only about 50% of tumours even when they are X-rayed again after section. In cystic disease, scattered discrete opacities may be seen; in duct ectasia, there may be widespread elongated calcific shadows in all four quadrants; and in fibroadenomas, plaque-like deposits may be observed, apparently plastered to the surface of the lesion.

An additional sign of malignancy is known as Leborge's law. A mass which is larger on clinical examination than its apparent size on a mammogram is almost certainly malignant; conversely, the clinical size of a benign lesion is equal to or less than the radiographic size.

Screening mammography

Not only is mammography used as a diagnostic investigation in a female presenting with a swelling of the breast, it is also used in developed countries as a screening tool. Screening is based on the assumption that mammography is more sensitive than clinical examination and will therefore bring to light early breast cancer with a greater chance of cure.

The first results showing that this was indeed the case were the reports by Shapiro in 1977, who demonstrated that 10 years after a screening programme had been set up the breast cancer mortality was 32% lower in women 50–59 years of age and 45% lower in women aged 60–64. This lowering of mortality was considered to be due to the reduction in mean tumour size, from 2.8 cm to 1.3 cm, and fewer women with involved axillary lymph nodes at the time of surgery. Taking the mean doubling time of a breast tumour as 312 days, the time saved by earlier diagnosis may be assumed to be in the region of 3 years.

In the initial studies no apparent benefit was conferred on women below the age of 50, explained by the inability of mammography at that stage in its development to detect lesions in the parenchyma-rich breasts of pre- and perimenopausal women.

However, recent surveys in various European countries have shown that using newer techniques a similar reduction in mortality can be achieved. In the United States it is now recommended that a baseline mammograph should be performed at 35–40 years of age, and thereafter from 40 years onwards an annual mammograph until the age of 50, when the investigation should be repeated at 2-yearly intervals. Various countries throughout the western world are now proceeding with similar protocols, although with slight variations.

Other non-invasive diagnostic methods which have been used to confirm the diagnosis are thermography and sonography, neither of which are in common use.

Invasive diagnostic measures

Fine needle biopsy

This is performed using an 18G needle and a 20 ml syringe attached to a suction device. Normally performed on a palpable swelling under tactile control, it can also be applied to non-palpable swellings by using mammographic stereotactic control. A variety of cells can be found in the aspirate in addition to malignant cells, indicating that a highly competent cytopathologist is required to confidently apply this method. So far as the indications of malignancy are concerned, the cytologist is looking for hyperchromasia, polymorphism, irregular chromatin, clumping, enlarged nuclei, multiple nuclei, and mitoses or atypical mitotic figures.

The incidence of false negatives varies, as would be expected, according to the series examined, but the causes, assuming a competent cytologist is available, are:

a. The needle misses the tumour.
b. The tumour is cell poor, e.g. in a scirrhous carcinoma in which the relative proportion of malignant cells to stroma is small.

Tru-cut needle biopsy

The advantage of this method is that, by removing a core of tissue as opposed to a number of separate cells, the histological characteristics of the tumour can be ascertained, which are now considered of considerable prognostic importance. Citoler, in 1985, reported that the method was superior to fine needle biopsy.

Biopsy

When no physical signs are present but mammography has demonstrated a potentially malignant lesion in the breast, under radiological control a fine hooked wire can be guided down to the area, after which the surgeon can remove the area immediately surrounding the hook.

STAGING METHODS

In order to compare methods of treatment and prognosis in patients suffering from breast cancer, various methods of staging have been designed. One relying only on simple clinical assessment, and which gained almost universal acceptance until the development of the TNM classification of tumours, was the Manchester system, which was simple to use in a clinical setting. In this system the following stages were recognized:

1. *Stage I* Tumour is 5 cm or less in diameter. Skin involvement, if present, is limited to that overlying the tumour.

2. *Stage II* Tumour is 5 cm or less in diameter with skin involvement still limited to the tumour area. The ipsilateral axillary nodes are involved but mobile.
3. *Stage III* Tumour is larger than 5 cm in diameter. It is fixed to the underlying pectoralis major and the ipsilateral lymph nodes are also fixed to the chest wall.
4. *Stage IV* Regardless of the local signs in the breast, there is evidence of generalized dissemination.

This simple classification has now been displaced by the infinitely more complex TNM staging introduced by UICC (see Table 16.1).

Table 16.1 TNM staging of breast cancer

T: Tumour	
T_{is}	Preinvasive carcinoma, carcinoma in situ, non-infiltrating intraductal carcinoma, or Paget's disease of the nipple with no demonstrable tumour
T_o	No demonstrable tumour in the breast
T_1	Tumour of 2 cm or less in its greatest dimension T_{1a} less than 0.5 cm T_{1b} 0.5–1.0 cm T_{1c} 1.0–2.0 cm
T_2	Tumour more than 2 cm but not more than 5 cm in its greatest dimension T_{2a} No fixation to underlying pectoral fascia or muscle T_{2b} With fixation to underlying pectoral fascia and/or muscle
T_3	Tumour more than 5 cm in its greatest dimension T_{3a} With no fixation to underlying pectoral fascia or muscle T_{3b} With fixation to underlying pectoral fascia and/or muscle
T_4	Tumour of any size with direct extension to the chest wall or skin T_{4a} With fixation to the chest wall T_{4b} With oedema, infiltration or ulceration of the skin, including peau d'orange or satellite skin nodules confined to the same breast T_{4c} Both of the above T_{4d} Inflammatory carcinoma
N: Ipisilateral axillary nodes	
N_1	mobile
N_2	fixed
N_3	internal mammary nodes
M: Metastases	
M_o	No metastases
M_1	Distant metastases

If the TNM classification is to be adopted, it is essential that a 'box' chart is used, otherwise the great variety of options will lead to inaccurate recording of the data.

Using the simple Manchester classification, the 5-year survival for the four stages is 85, 45, 20 and 10%, respectively. At 10 years the overall survival for Stage I tumours has fallen to 65% and for Stage II to 26%, and if the follow-up is continued – as was done by Brinkley and Haybrittle – patients even classified as Stage I at presentation continued to die, thus leading to the hypothesis that cancer of the breast is a generalized disease by the time the great majority of patients present themselves for treatment.

Staging is, however, subject to certain difficulties, which include:

1. *Observer variation*, which particularly affects two features:
    a. The estimation of the size of the primary tumour. This is important, since the greater the size of primary tumour the higher the incidence of involved axillary lymph nodes.
    b. The presence or absence of lymph nodes in the axilla – an error of about 40% can be expected in this one aspect alone. This is important since the prognosis can be linked to: the number of nodes involved, since as the number increases so the prognosis worsens; and the site of the involved lymph node, apical lymph node involvement carrying a much worse prognosis than the involvement of a low pectoral node.

2. *Internal mammary lymph node involvement* is particularly liable to occur when the tumour is situated in the medial quadrants of the breast and unless an open biopsy is performed, as was advocated by Handley, such involvement will go undetected.

3. *General dissemination*. Unfortunately the various methods of detecting distant micro-metastases remain crude. They include:
    a. Skeletal survey. Conventional radiographic techniques are notoriously unreliable since the calcium content of the bone must be reduced by half before there is radiological evidence of bone involvement on plain X-ray.
    b. Bone scans. This method of detecting bony metastases is more sensitive, but the available reports suggest that both false-negatives and false-positives occur, and this investigation is now rarely performed.
    c. Biochemical tests. Interest centres on the measurement of the urinary hydroxyproline, an amino acid restricted almost entirely in collagen, of which about one-third is in bone. Thus the hydroxyproline level can be used as a measure of collagen metabolism. Any condition in which increased bone destruction is occurring will raise the hydroxyproline level above normal.

4. *Palpable but uninvolved lymph nodes.* Recent experience in the King's trial, in which enlarged lymph nodes were left untreated, suggests that all enlarged nodes are not involved by tumour – many disappeared within 3 months of treating the primary tumour.

OTHER FACTORS INFLUENCING PROGNOSIS

1. *Characteristics of the tumour.* Reference has already been made to the work of Bloom (see p. 186).

2. *Elastosis.* The amount of elastic tissue as estimated from sections stained by the Van Giesen method has been shown to influence prognosis; increasing amounts of elastic tissue are associated with an overall better prognosis.

3. *Rate of tumour growth.* Gershon-Cohen considered that the rate of tumour growth was all-important in determining prognosis. He considered that survival may not be due to cure or total elimination of the tumour by treatment, but rather an expression of extremely slow tumour growth rates. He considered that the growth rate of tumours is exponential and constant. From an analysis of available data he estimated that the doubling time for breast tumours may vary from 21 to 209 days. Assuming that the parent cell is 10 μm in diameter and the doubling time is 200 days, a tumour of 1 cm in size would develop only after 17 years. However, if the doubling time is as little as 23 days, the tumour could reach a size of 1 cm after 2 years, after 30 doublings. Three more doublings, taking 2 months, would then result in a 2 cm tumour. Gershon-Cohen considered that an important factor governing the development of metastases was the doubling time, probably because the percentage of axillary metastases is low if the primary tumour is small, whereas tumours 2.5 cm in diameter are associated with axillary nodal involvement in 60% of cases. However, as with all solid tumours, the exponential growth pattern must be lost as the tumour increases in size because of the decreased oxygen tension in the interior of the tumour.

The work of Greshon-Cohen has now been expanded by the ability to study the kinetic status of the tumour by measuring the fraction of cells actively synthesizing DNA, which can be determined in vitro by the titrated thymidine labelling index (TLI) of tumour samples; proliferative activity correlates with a poor prognosis, although there is some evidence that highly proliferative tumours respond better to chemotherapy. Another method of providing the clinician with information as to the biological activity of the tumour is by the technique of DNA flow cytometry, which within a day can provide information on ploidy and the S-phase fraction of the tumour. Anaploides show the amount of extra DNA in the tumour cell and the percentage of cells in the S-phase gives information on proliferation.

4. *Cell mediated immunity.* In 1922 MacCarty concluded that the prognosis in breast cancer was determined not only by the degree of cellular anaplasia of the tumour but also by certain stromal features such as fibrosis, hyalinization and lymphocytic infiltration. Although this work aroused considerable criticism, Black and his co-workers found that a well-marked lymphocytic infiltration of the primary tumour together with sinus histiocytosis was associated with high survival regardless of the presence or absence of axillary metastases.

This work has continued to receive attention from many workers, and one of the papers on the subject by Paola and others showed that it was possible to grade the 'cellular host resistance' into three divisions. To achieve this, the degree of lymphocytic infiltration in and around the tumour and the degree of follicular hyperplasia and sinus histiocytosis in the regional lymph nodes was scored from 0-3. The sum of the scores then became the host defence factor (HDF).

Paola found a good correlation between punitive host resistance and long-term survival. If those patients with an extremely good host reaction are discounted because of the smallness of their numbers, there still remained two large groups in which host reaction was either poor or moderately good. In the former the overall 5-year survival was approximately 40% as compared to nearly 70% in the latter.

5. *Vascular permeation.*

6. *Oestrogen receptor status.* It was at one time thought that the sensitivity of the tumour to endocrine therapy was related to the presence and amount of oestrogen receptor (ER), although even when no oestrogen receptor was present it was recognized that about 10% of metastatic tumours still responded to the drug tamoxifen. It is also possible to assess the progesterone receptor level, but this does not appear to have similar importance.

7. *Other biological parameters* that have also been studied, but which appear to have little importance are:
   a. The binding of lectin helix promatia.
   b. Epidermal growth factor.
   c. The take-up of the monoclonal antibody K167.

The Nottingham group, who have been particularly prominent in breast cancer research, have concluded as a result of multivariant analysis that the features in breast cancer that have the most influence on the disease free interval (DFI) and survival are tumour size, node status, menstrual status, and oestrogen receptor status. They have also constructed a prognostic index based on tumour, grade, and the presence of lymph node metastases, linking these features in the following manner:

Tumour size × 0.2 + grade (1–3) + lymph node status

Lymph node status is scored 1–3 according to: no lymph node involvement, low axillary node involvement, or both apical or low and internal mammary involvement present.

TREATMENT OF EARLY BREAST CANCER

Until the latter part of the last century the treatment of carcinoma of the breast was simple mastectomy. Then, appreciating the importance of the axillary lymph nodes Halsted (1894) devised the operation of radical mastectomy, in which the breast was removed together with the pectoralis major and minor and the whole of the axillary contents. With the introduction of this operation the frequency of local recurrences fell from approximately 50% to 5%. Later, when it was appreciated that tumours in the medial quadrants might well spread to involve the internal mammary nodes, these too were removed; similarly, in the so-called supra-radical mastectomy, the supraclavicular nodes were removed. In the period immediately following the First World War, stimulated by Sampson Handley, extensive local surgery was supplemented by irradiation of the skin flaps, the axilla and the mediastinal nodes. Whilst many patients developed some degree of lymphoedema of the arm – and a small percentage were crippled by this complication – this method of treatment continued to be applied in the majority of centres until after the Second World War, when McWhirter of Edinburgh questioned the necessity for radical mastectomy. He based his argument on the contention that if surgeons were prepared to trust radiotherapy to 'sterilize' the lymph nodes of the supraclavicular fossa and the internal mammary chain, it seemed only reasonable that irradiation might be expected to produce the same effect on the axillary nodes. Slowly, McWhirter won his argument, and for many years the standard treatment for carcinoma of the breast was simple mastectomy followed by deep X-ray therapy to the breast area and the axillary, mediastinal, internal mammary and supraclavicular nodes. Over the past two decades the position has shifted once again with the appreciation that in Stage I tumours radiotherapy may well be unnecessary; and furthermore that, if possible, the deformity produced by mastectomy should, if possible, be avoided. Thus at the present time when the tumour is 3 cm or less in diameter many surgeons would perform a local excision of the tumour together with node sampling of the axilla, some surgeons being content to remove a low pectoral node whilst others would also remove an apical node, and yet others remove a number of nodes, since the number of nodes involved is related to prognosis. If further histological examination of the tumour shows that vascular invasion is present, even those surgeons committed to conservation of the breast would re-operate on their patients and remove the remaining breast tissue.

A further argument in favour of total removal of the breast tissue, i.e. what is still regarded by many as a simple mastectomy, is that multifocal invasive malignancy is present in 12% of patients with an apparently solitary palpable tumour, and that the incidence of non-invasive neoplastic change in such a breast may be as high as 30%.

Following local excision of the tumour or mastectomy, if node sampling proves positive, radiotherapy is normally advised by many surgeons to the breast area and the axillary, internal mammary chain and supraclavicular nodes, the patient receiving such treatment in fractions over a 4–6-week period.

Despite the fact that mastectomy is a more mutilating operation than local excision, it is interesting that in many series there appears to be little difference in the psychological impact between the two operations.

Adjuvant therapy

This takes three forms:

1. *Immunotherapy.* The Early Breast Cancer Trialists' Group (EBTG) found no evidence that any benefit derived from agents such as BCG, levamisole and other compounds.

2. *Chemotherapy.* The early protagonists of this form of treatment considered that any benefit, if demonstrated, would be due either to ablation of micro-metastases already present at the time of the operation, or to killing of tumour emboli during surgery. The names which dominated the early history of perioperative chemotherapy are Fisher, Nissen Myer, and Bonnadonna.

3. *Hormonal manipulation.* The principles of hormone manipulation derive from the work of Huggins from Chicago.

Chemotherapy

The various drugs used singly or in combination for the treatment of early breast cancer include adriamycin, cyclophosphamide, 5-fluorouracil, methotrexate, thiotepa and vincristine. These drugs have been administered in various doses, singly, in various combinations, preoperatively, perioperatively and over varying periods of time. A favoured combination is cyclophosphamide, methotrexate and 5-fluorouracil.

Hormonal therapy

The various methods of hormonal manipulation in early breast cancer that have been used include bilateral oophorectomy, irradiation of the ovaries, administration of testosterone and, in elderly patients, oestrogen itself. Latterly the drug tamoxifen has been used, which is a substituted triphenylethylene compound whose anti-oestrogenic properties were first demonstrated by Harper and Walpole in 1966. This drug was first thought to be of use only when the tumour contained large amounts of oestrogen receptor (ER), although it has now been shown that it is effective even when the tumour contains less than 9 fmol of receptor protein per mg of cytosol protein.

The results of the EBCT collaborative group have recently been published in the *Lancet* (January 1992). This group examined the results of 133 randomized trials involving 75 000 women, all of whom had been followed for at least 10 years. Clear evidence emerged that adjuvant therapy enhanced the 10-year survival although the benefit was possibly not as high as had been hoped for.

A highly significant reduction in the annual rate of both recurrence and death was produced by both tamoxifen and ovarian ablation, the latter by either oophorectomy or irradiation, in women below 50 years of age, and by polychemotherapy. But ovarian ablation produced no reduction in older age groups, although it was shown that tamoxifen also reduced the recurrence and mortality in women over 70 years of age – 40% of all breast cancers in British women occur after this age. Indeed, when analysed the findings suggested that tamoxifen was slightly less effective in younger than older women, the cut-off point being 50 years, but even under this age the drug still produced a highly significant difference in the duration of the disease-free interval. Overall it was shown that approximately 12 extra 10-year survivals/100 patients were achieved in females suffering from Stage I disease, and 12 extra 10-year survivals/200 patients in Stage II disease. One-third of this benefit was ascribed to the effects of polychemotherapy and two-thirds to hormonal therapy.

Thus, since 4 out of every 5 females suffering from breast cancer are 50 years of age or over, tamoxifen, which possesses minimal side-effects and little toxicity, appears to be the adjuvant therapy of choice in this age group.

In younger premenopausal patients the effects of tamoxifen were less definite, but were still apparent. However, ovarian ablation by oophorectomy or by irradiation produced a significant increase in the disease-free interval in this age group, especially in those women who were node-positive. For node-negative women under 50 years, the number who had experienced recurrence or died was smaller, but statistical significance was only just reached. Cytotoxic agents were also effective. However, the chief effect of cytotoxic therapy appears to be due to the induction of a chemical castration, since the majority of women receiving this form of treatment become amenorrhoeic temporarily or permanently, and it is in these women that chemotherapy produces its greatest benefit. However, the effect cannot be entirely hormonal since in postmenopausal females a smaller but still significant effect of polychemotherapy is also apparent.

DISSEMINATED OR RECURRENT DISEASE

When recurrent or overt disseminated disease has developed, all methods of treatment must be regarded as palliative. The methods required to deal with this situation depend to some degree on the site involved.

1. *Radiotherapy.* This can be used to control recurrent disease in areas that have not previously been irradiated, and it is most effective in controlling the pain from osseous metastases. Excellent and rapid relief can be obtained in spinal secondaries using fractionated doses of 60 Gy.

2. *Pleural effusions*, which commonly occur, can be controlled by the installation of bleomycin into the pleural cavity, although there is equally good evidence that talc insufflated into a dry pleural cavity is as effective.

So far as systemic treatment is concerned, two options are available: hormonal treatment or chemotherapy.

Hormonal treatment

In the early years of this century, two Scottish surgeons showed that some women suffering from advanced cancer of the breast responded to oophorectomy, which was then of course a highly dangerous procedure. Further progress awaited the work of Huggins, and for a period of some 20 years the standard treatment of disseminated breast cancer was oophorectomy and adrenalectomy, the latter operation becoming commonplace once cortisone became freely available. This method has now been overtaken by the better radiotherapeutic control of ovarian secretion and the development of the drug, aminogluthemide, which blocks the conversion of cholesterol to pregnenolone and thus inhibits the production of adrenal steroids and in addition inhibits the aromatization of androstenedione to oestrone in the peripheral tissues. If the patient has not received tamoxifen, however, the latter remains the first line of treatment because of its lack of side-effects. Treatment with aminogluthemide is associated with some toxicity, including lethargy and a morbilliform rash. In addition, if aminoglutethemide is used the patient must be given either hydrocortisone or dexamethasone, otherwise adrenal insufficiency develops.

In general terms, patients who have had a long DFI between their primary treatment and their recurrence tend to respond better than those with a short DFI, and patients in whom visceral metastases are present do not tend to respond as well as patients with local recurrence or osseous metastases. Approximately one-third of all tumours respond to hormonal manipulation and in the case of postmenopausal women some will respond favourably to the administration of oestrogens themselves, although side-effects such as nausea, vomiting and oedema may develop.

Chemotherapy

Both single and combination regimes have been subjected to intensive trials. One of the problems is that there is as yet no universally accepted definition of a 'favourable' response. The drugs that have been shown to have a beneficial effect in patients suffering from disseminated breast cancer are those which have been used for adjuvant therapy, i.e. cyclophosphamide, 5-flurouracil, methotrexate, doxorubin and vincristine. Of these, cyclophosphamide and vincristine combined with doxorubicin appear to be the most potent.

Unfortunately, generalized toxicity may occur, including bone marrow suppression, alopecia, nausea, vomiting, diarrhoea and malaise, although stopping the administration of the drugs results in relief from these effects. However, vincristine is neurotoxic, an effect again usually reversed on stopping the drug, and doxorubicin may cause a cardiomyopathy, which may be permanent.

Figures in the literature quoted for total response to chemotherapy vary from 5–50% and figures for a partial response from 20–80%. However, no permanent relief is afforded.

17. Malignant tumours of the skin

BASAL CELL CARCINOMA

These tumours most commonly occur on the face, typically above a line drawn from the corner of the mouth to the ear although they may occur elsewhere except on the palms of the hands.

Although locally invasive, so that underlying tissues including bone may be involved, they rarely metastasize – with the exception of the rare anal basal cell tumours of the anal canal, which may spread to distant sites.

The tumour is believed to arise from the basal cells of the epidermis or hair follicle cells, and may be single or multiple. The tumour consists of islets of malignant cells which invade the dermis. The constituent cells markedly resemble the basal cells, with those at the periphery of the islet being oval or columnar, forming a palisade around the islet. Basal cell carcinomas ulcerate early and possess a classic pearly edge, with the lesion frequently appearing to be healing at one edge whilst it is extending at another.

Treatment

Smaller lesions can be treated by cryotherapy. Larger lesions may be excised but may require local flaps to close the resulting defect or skin grafts, or even more specialized plastic techniques. Irradiation using 40–60 Gy (4–6000 rads) is also followed by excellent results, but is contraindicated for lesions near to the eye or over the cartilage of the nose and ear.

SQUAMOUS CARCINOMA

A squamous carcinoma may be invasive ab initio; occasionally, however, dysplastic changes occur in skin epidermal cells, which later progress and present all the features of malignancy with the exception of invasion. This latter condition may involve any squamous epithelium, but is particularly common in the larynx and cervix, and is called carcinoma 'in situ', intraepidermal carcinoma or Bowen's disease. When it involves the squamous epithelium of the penis or vulva it is called erythroplasia of Queyrat.

'In situ' carcinoma of the skin may result from excessive exposure of fair-skinned people to the sun producing the condition of solar keratosis. Similar changes occur in skin exposed to tar or irradiation and, in the past, in patients intensively treated with arsenical preparations such as Fowler's solution for psoriasis. The latent period to the development of invasive cancer in such patients appears to be of the order of 10–20 years. Invasive carcinoma 'in situ' or solar keratosis is much less malignant than that arising in Bowen's disease, chronic ulcers or sinuses (Marjolin's ulcer). However, in approximately 20% of patients in whom there is no predisposing cause a primary systemic cancer will be found within about 5 years.

In all the above conditions, the in situ changes consist of hyperkeratosis and pleomorphism of the prickle cells accompanied by increased mitotic activity. Individual cells might show keratinous degeneration (dyskeratosis) before reaching the surface. Invasion is not evident but the epidermis may be thicker than normal (acanthotic). The underlying dermis usually shows a chronic inflammatory cell infiltrate. The gross appearance of 'in situ' carcinoma is not very pathognomonic. There may be thickening of the epidermis to produce plaques and the surface is usually white and scaly due to hyperkeratosis. In Queyrat's erythroplasia, the lesions are warty or velvet-like and red.

In invasive squamous carcinoma, ulceration of the skin is evident in the later stages, the ulcer having an elevated hard edge. Histological appearances include cell nests with epithelial pearls composed of keratin infiltrating the dermis.

Treatment

Such tumours may be treated by surgical excision, radiotherapy or local destruction by cryotherapy depending on the site and size of the lesion. If local lymph node metastases are present a block dissection must be performed, although an interval of several weeks should follow the treatment of the primary since the nodes may be reactive rather than involved in malignant disease; if the nodes are reactive they will shrink after healing of the primary tumour.

PIGMENTED NAEVI (OTHERWISE KNOWN AS MOLES, NAEVUS CELL MOLES OR MELANOCYTIC NAEVI)

These are benign tumours composed of melanocytes – pigment containing cells which, although most numerous in the basal layer of the epidermis, also occur in the dermis. These tumours, which are all benign, are commonly classified according to their site of origin into junctional, compound or intradermal. This classification is purely descriptive and has no pathological significance.

In the junctional naevus the melanocytes appear to proliferate at the epidermodermal junction. All pigmented lesions on the palms, soles and genitalia are of this type. The lesion, clinically, is usually flat and deeply pigmented and should be removed if it develops in an area liable to irritation.

When the cells appear to 'drop' into the dermis a compound naevus is produced; 98% of moles in children and 12% in adults are of this type. In this position the cells may disappear, producing a zone of depigmentation, the Sutton's naevus.

Naevi arising from the dermal melanocytes are rare and produce the clinical lesion known as the Mongolian spot, usually found in Mongolian and Negro infants and only occasionally in Caucasians. Such naevi commonly occur in the sacral area and commonly disappear at about 4 years of age. Arising in other sites such as the face and forearms they may persist throughout life.

When pigmented lesions develop from melanocytes in the epidermis they produce lesions such as the common freckle, lentigo senilis and the café au lait spots found in association with neurofibromatosis.

Macroscopically moles vary from flat to warty and may even be pedunculated; some are associated with excessive hair, producing the 'hairy naevus'. Microscopically there is a considerable variation in the amount of melanin in pigmented naevi and occasionally special stains such as the Masson–Fontana may be necessary to demonstrate its presence.

MALIGNANT MELANOMA

This is a rare form of malignancy accounting for approximately 3% of all skin tumours. They arise from the melanocytes previously described in connection with naevus cell moles, either de novo or within a pre-existing lesion. The chances of malignancy developing in a pre-existing benign lesion are unknown but modern opinion suggests that it is very small, whereas it was once thought that as many as 40% of malignant lesions arose in this manner.

As well as occurring in the skin, malignant melanoma may occur in the uveal tract of the eye, which comprises the choroid, ciliary body and iris. In addition they are also found in the mouth, vagina and upper respiratory tract.

There are two types of malignant melanoma in situ in which the melanoma cells remain confined to the epidermis.

1. *Lentigo maligna (Hutchinson's freckle)*. This lesion forms an unevenly pigmented macule extending over several centimetres in diameter from which an invasive lesion may take between 10 and 20 years to develop. Indicative of this change is an increasingly rapid rate of spread and the development of superficial nodularity. This type of tumour occurs most commonly in the elderly and rarely metastasizes.

2. *Pagetoid malignant melanoma in situ*. This is a macular lesion developing usually on unexposed skin areas. It is smaller than lentigo maligna and becomes overtly malignant at an earlier stage.

When either of the above lesions become malignant they are known respectively as lentigo maligna melanoma and pagetoid malignant melanoma.

Invasive malignant melanoma

The clinical signs of malignant change in a pre-existing lesion are:

- Increasing pigmentation in a pre-existing lesion.
- Ulceration accompanied by bleeding and crusting.
- The development of satellite tumours in the surrounding skin.
- Overt evidence of metastases.

The clinical signs of malignancy arising de novo are the appearance of a dark area in previously normal skin, which ulcerates and bleeds shortly after its appearance.

Predisposing factors and especially vulnerable situations include:

1. Exposure to ultraviolet light. Malignant melanomas are more common in Australia and the southern states of the US. The death rate from this condition trebles between Hobart and Brisbane.
2. Ectopic pigmentation on the soles of palms of Negroes.
3. Commonest sites include the face, genitalia and feet.

Pathology

The growth of all malignant melanomas starts at the epidermodermal junction, with the exception of the rare melanomas arising from the dermal melanocytes. Histologically, junctional changes are seen, i.e. proliferation of nests of melanocytes in the basal layer of the epidermis. These cells tend to be more pleomorphic than the naevus cells of the benign moles, and mitotic figures are normally present. In some melanomas the tumour cells are spindle-shaped and many resemble the cells of a sarcoma, but normally they are round or polygonal. Malignant melanomas are more cellular than simple moles and the cells show no signs of becoming effete as collagen develops in the underlying dermis, as occurs with a benign mole.

The quantity of pigment produced varies from case to case and between the primary and the secondary tumour. Some tumours produce no melanin or so little that special staining is required to demonstrate it, the amelanotic melanomata. Any pigment produced may be excreted in the urine unchanged or, alternatively, a colourless melanogen is excreted which darkens on exposure of the urine to air or an oxidizing agent. One peculiar characteristic of malignant melanoma is the occasional tendency for highly invasive metastases to appear many years after the apparently adequate excision of the primary, another is the tendency for such tumours to regress in pregnancy.

Prognostic indicators

Bodeham divided melanomas into two large groups, the 'good' and the 'bad'.

The 'good' tumours, that is to say those which remain localized and rarely metastasize, are tumours arising in an area of lentigo. They are slowly growing tumours producing little mass in relation to their surface area, and include the very rare ring melanoma. Included perhaps in this group should also be tumours arising on the extremities, which always carry a better prognosis than tumours arising on the trunk.

The 'bad' tumours metastasize early. In this group Bodeham included tumours which ulcerate rapidly, those whose bulk is out of proportion to their surface area and, lastly, diffuse tumours with satellite formation. Also included in this group are tumours of the trunk.

Ulceration. Australian studies have confirmed Bodeham's view that ulcerating tumours carry a worse prognosis than non-ulcerated. Only 42% of patients presenting with an ulcerating lesion are alive and well after 5 years compared to 77% at the same interval when no ulceration is present. In general, however, the ulcerating lesions are also the thicker.

Invasion. Recently Bodeham's somewhat empirical classification has been refined by pathologists in two different ways. First, Clark and his colleagues related the prognosis to the level of invasion, classifying the latter in the following manner:

a. Level 1: tumour confined to the epidermis.
b. Level 2: tumour involving the papillary dermis.
c. Level 3: tumour fills the papillary dermis but does not invade the reticular dermis.
d. Level 4: tumour invades the reticular dermis.
e. Level 5: tumour invades the subcutaneous fat.

Alternatively Breslow classified the tumour in terms of the depth of invasion, a method difficult to apply in ulcerating tumours. Breslow recognized three stages:

1. Tumour thickness <0.76 mm.
2. Tumour thickness 0.76–3 mm.
3. Tumour thickness >3 mm.

Breslow's classification has proved remarkably accurate as a prognostic indicator. Reports from large series of cases suggest that the chances of metastases being present or developing following the excision of a thin melanoma – as long as this is adequately excised in the first place – are virtually nil. In keeping with this suggestion, 98 out of 100 patients treated will be alive and well after 5 years. With tumours of intermediate thickness there is an increasing risk, up to 80%, of regional and/or distant metastases being present even though these may be micro-metastases when the patient is first seen. In this group only 65 patients out of every 100 will be alive and well after 5 years. When the tumour exceeds 4 mm in thickness the risk of micro-metastases being present when the patient is first seen is 80% or above, and in keeping with this the vast proportion of these patients are dead within 2 years of the diagnosis being made, the remainder dying within the next 3 years. If the tumour proves to be less than 0.75 mm in thickness the outlook is remarkably good, whereas if the tumour is more than 3 mm thick only about 50% will survive.

In disseminated disease, the amount of melanin produced may be such that the whole body becomes pigmented.

Position of the tumour. Survival of patients presenting with melanoma on the trunk is much worse than for those patients presenting with melanoma on the limbs.

Pigmentation. Amelanotic melanomas appear to have a much worse prognosis than pigmented lesions.

Treatment

At various times the following modes of treatment have been applied to malignant melanoma.

1. Removal of the primary tumour and the surrounding skin, the actual area to be excised being a matter of considerable debate. This treatment must be followed by frequent observation of the regional lymph nodes; enlargement indicates that they should be removed.
2. Removal of the primary tumour and after some weeks the regional lymph nodes.
3. Removal of the tumour, the skin and underlying deep fascia and the nodes in one piece at the same operation, an operation pioneered by Sampson Handley.
4. Amputation.
5. Isolated limb perfusion with drugs such as melphalan.

It would now appear from the pathological data presented above that the treatment of malignant melanoma, particularly when occurring in the limbs, can be placed on a more rational level.

With 'thin' lesions the risk of lymph node metastases is so rare that nothing is required other than radical local excision, i.e. a 5 cm margin of normal healthy skin should be removed around a tumour on a limb, possibly 15 cm on the trunk; but on the face only 1 cm because of the cosmetic disability if more is removed.

When the lesion is of intermediate thickness there is a definite case for removing the regional lymph nodes, particularly when the tumour is between 1.50 and 3.99 mm in thickness, because in this group in particular the actuarial incidence of subsequent lymph node involvement within 3 years is almost 60%.

When the lesion is greater than 4 mm in thickness the benefits of regional node excision are much less apparent because of the high risk of distant blood-borne metastases at the time of the initial diagnosis.

Wide excision implies the use of grafts to close the defect. Regional lymph node dissection, particularly when concerned with the inguinal nodes, is associated with considerable morbidity. Necrosis of the skin flaps is common however they are constructed, a lymph fistula may develop and lymphoedema is commonplace. In the upper limb the same morbidity is not encountered and so far as the trunk is concerned lymph node dissection is impossible because the site of potential involvement is difficult to predict.

SECTION FIVE

18. Enlargement of the parotid gland

Enlargement of the parotid gland may be either local or general. When localized enlargement is found in the parotid region it is nearly always due to a tumour within the gland itself, but a number of common and also rare conditions should be kept in mind, including sebaceous cyst, swelling of the pre-auricular lymph node, dental or branchial cysts, hypertrophy or myoxoma of the masseter, lymphangioma, haemangioma, or neuroma of the facial nerve.

GENERALIZED PAROTID ENLARGEMENT

Viral parotitis

The commonest cause of a generalized enlargement of the parotid glands is mumps, caused by a paramyxovirus. This same virus may also cause mild abdominal pain due to pancreatitis, severe testicular pain due to orchitis and, occasionally, encephalitis. Clinically the condition presents as a rapidly enlarging, painful swelling of one or both parotid glands, following an incubation period of 12–20 days. After 2–3 days the swelling begins to diminish in size and the pain gradually decreases.

Pathologically, acinar cell necrosis occurs accompanied by lymphocytic infiltration of the interstitial tissues.

Acute suppurative parotitis

Once commonplace on surgical wards following major surgery, this condition is now rarely seen because of the overall improvement in dental hygiene in the UK and the importance attached to adequate hydration in the postoperative period. It may, however, still be seen occasionally and is particularly liable to occur in patients receiving radiotherapy to the face.

Clinically the disease is most commonly unilateral, the affected gland becoming enlarged, painful and tender on palpation. Pressure over the duct causes pus to discharge into the mouth from the opening of Stenson's duct. As the condition deteriorates the temperature rises and trismus develops making oral rehydration difficult. Should the condition go unrecognized an abscess forms.

Pathologically the appearances are typical of an acute pyogenic infection.

Treatment

This consists of the appropriate antibiotics, e.g. cloxacillin and metronidazole. In postoperative patients, in whom the condition is normally recognized at an early stage, irradiation and rehydration will often produce resolution. Once an abscess has formed, incision and drainage are required.

Sialectasis

This causes an intermittent painful swelling of the parotid glands, due to recurrent infections of the dilated acini. The condition is commonly associated with trumpet players and, in the past, with glass blowers. If such patients are asked to exhale with the lips tightly pursed and the nose obstructed, the glands inflate like balloons. In advanced cases a plain X-ray shows the ducts and acini outlined by air, and sialography shows the ducts and acini to be grossly dilated.

Treatment

If possible the patient should refrain from the activity that predisposes to the ascending infection. Any dental condition should be treated to diminish oral infection, and minor degrees of infection can be treated by the intermittent administration of the appropriate antibiotic. If the gland is grossly disorganized and both recurrent swelling and pain are causing much inconvenience, a superficial parotidectomy is required.

Parotid calculi

In comparison to calculi in the submandibular gland, calculi of the parotid are rare, because the secretion of the parotid is serous. Parotid calculi are largely composed of calcium phosphate with lesser amounts of calcium carbonate.

The typical history is one of sudden swelling and pain in the affected gland, accompanied by a cessation of salivation. If the obstruction is accompanied by infection a suppurative parotitis may develop. If the condition is not accompanied by infection a sudden spurt of saliva into the mouth may herald the relief of symptoms and the sudden regression of the swelling. A sialogram may demonstrate a calculus although in the author's clinical experience this is exceedingly rare. However, a stricture may be present, which will respond to dilatation.

Sjögren's syndrome

This condition, which may be classified as a non-organ-specific autoimmune disease, may affect one or both glands and occasionally the submandibular glands. As with the majority of autoimmune conditions Sjögren's syndrome is more common in women than in men. Recurrent or persistent enlargement of the glands occurs, accompanied by dryness of the mouth (xerostomia), which makes chewing and swallowing difficult. In some patients keratoconjunctivitis sicca develops, due to similar changes in the lacrimal glands and causes soreness of the eyes and occasionally corneal ulceration. In over 50% of those affected there is evidence of overt collagen disease, notably rheumatoid arthritis, polymyositis, scleroderma or systemic lupus erythematosus. In 45%, antibodies to the thyroid are found; in 89%, antibodies to the gastric mucosa; and in approximately 50%, antibodies reacting specifically against the salivary duct epithelium.

Pathology

The affected salivary glands are swollen, and on section are found to be densely infiltrated with lymphocytes and plasma cells, the glandular acini becoming atrophic and tending to disappear. In the ducts the epithelium proliferates and deposits of homogenous eosinophilic material occurs within the cell masses. The diagnosis is made on the basis of finding antibodies to the salivary duct cells and biopsy of a labial salivary gland may show similar histological changes. Previously the condition known as Mikulicz disease was believed to be a separate condition, but it is now recognized that this is a variant of Sjögren's syndrome in which the lacrimal glands also become grossly enlarged.

Treatment

There is no specific treatment of this condition. Dryness of the eyes must be treated by the frequent installation of methylcellulose drops and the wearing of glasses. If this fails to relieve the patient a tarsorrhaphy may be necessary. The dryness of the mouth, which produces difficulty in swallowing, can be overcome only by taking frequent drinks at meal times. Xerostomia predisposes to tooth decay, which in turn predisposes to ascending parotitis; hence it is essential that dental caries should be treated. Only when gross enlargement of the gland causes severe deformity should the gland or glands be excised.

TUMOURS OF THE SALIVARY GLANDS

Tumours of the salivary glands occur most commonly in the major glands, the parotid and submandibular, but they may also involve the lesser glands such as the sublingual, or microscopic glands found in the buccal mucosa of the lips, cheeks, nasopharynx, oropharynx, larynx and trachea. All are uncommon and the great majority of salivary tumours occur in the parotid itself. The cell of origin, i.e. the histogenesis, of many salivary tumours remains a matter for debate, and furthermore, a precise classification of these tumours into benign and malignant is difficult since many tend to grow slowly and their behaviour is unpredictable on histological grounds.

Non-epithelial tumours such as haemangiomas and neurofibromas comprise half of all tumours in the salivary glands of children, but less than 5% in adults. Metastases from primary tumours elsewhere rarely involve the major salivary glands but the gland may be directly invaded by adjacent malignant lymph nodes. Epithelial tumours of the salivary glands are classified by WHO into four groups but, since certain benign and malignant tumours cannot be placed into any of these classes a fifth group, the 'unclassified', has been added.

In terms of their clinical behaviour salivary tumours can also be classified into those of an intermediate nature, those that are benign, and those that are frankly malignant.

Salivary gland tumours of intermediate nature

The intermediate group is in fact the commonest tumour of the salivary glands; 90% occur in the parotid and only 10% elsewhere, chiefly in the submandibular gland.

Pleomorphic adenoma

This tumour is also known as the 'mixed cell tumour'. They are composed of epithelial, myoepithelial and connective tissue cells. Macroscopically they appear to be encapsulated and multilobular, grey, white or yellow in appearance, with patches of translucency corresponding to the 'cartilage-like' areas. Histologically the most arresting feature is the mucous stroma and the pleomorphic nature of the cellular component.

The ultrastructure of the epithelial cells found in the tumour indicates that they are of both duct and myoepithelial origin, but some cells have features of both types of cells and some are indeterminate, being insufficiently differentiated.

If the capsule of such a tumour is inadvertently split or divided during surgery the contents ooze out as pressure is put on the surrounding tissues. Although benign, these tumours have a high recurrence rate due to the following:

1. The tumour may be multifocal.
2. As stated above, the tumour may be fragmented leading to local implantation if the capsule is breached during removal.
3. Tumour cells may have involved the false capsule which is formed by compression of the normal glandular tissue.

Mucoepidermoid tumours

All these tumours are malignant, although the low grade of malignancy of the majority (approximately 80%), puts them into the intermediate category of salivary tumour, their rate of growth being extremely variable. This type of tumour constitutes 5–10% of all salivary tumours, 90% occurring in the parotid. Macroscopically the tumour is either uncapsulated or poorly encapsulated. They are greyish red in colour and may diffusely infiltrate the gland. They arise from the epithelial cells of the ducts of the gland which proliferate and develop chiefly into squamous and mucous secreting columnar cells, although intermediate type cells are also found, as are basal cells, clear cells and oncocytes.

Histologically the tumour consists of small epithelioid cells of variable size, which in some areas may exhibit keratin formation. Admixed with these cells are goblet and clear mucin-producing cells with occasional sebaceous cells. All these different cell types form islets or strands within a connective tissue stroma. Mucin production results in the formation of small glandular structures or cysts containing mucin, the amount of which is an indication of malignancy.

Acinic cell tumours

These tumours constitute only 1% of all salivary tumours and, although always malignant, the aggressive nature of the tumour varies from patient to patient. They form hard nodules in the affected gland and may be encapsulated or show evidence of a pseudocapsule due to compression of the surrounding normal gland. Histologically they are highly cellular with the cells arranged in a solid adenocarcinomatous pattern. The majority of the cells have the appearance of the normal serous acinar cells of the salivary gland, i.e. they have a finely granular cytoplasm. Some cells, however, are clear due to the presence of glycogen in the cytoplasm. Normally they grow slowly and only about 20% metastasize.

Benign tumours

Adenolymphoma (Warthin's tumour)

This is the commonest benign tumour of the parotid, accounting for about 5% of all salivary tumours. It is more common with advancing age and more common in the male than the female; in a small percentage of patients the tumour is bilateral. Macroscopically these tumours are well encapsulated, partly cystic, and often exude an opaque brownish fluid if the capsule is injured in the course of their removal. Microscopically the tumour is composed of delicate fronds of double- or triple-layered epithelium separated by lymphoid tissue containing germinal centres.

Malignant tumours

Adenoid cystic carcinoma

Formerly known as a cylindroma, this is a highly malignant tumour. Macroscopically they are firm, pinkish-grey tumours which are incompletely encapsulated. Histologically they have a typical appearance due to the presence of small cystic spaces within collections of small dark cells with darkly staining nuclei. These tumours are more common in the minor salivary glands than in the parotid, but those arising in the parotid tend to spread along nerve sheaths rather than by lymphatic channels, and bloodstream invasion also results in distant metastases to the lungs.

Other malignant tumours

Adenocarcinoma. These tumours possess a tubular, papillary or undifferentiated pattern.

Squamous carcinoma. This is a rare tumour confined to the parotid gland itself, possessing the same histological structure as squamous carcinoma elsewhere in the body.

Undifferentiated carcinoma. This is a rare tumour so poorly differentiated that it cannot be classified.

Malignant pleomorphic adenoma. Carcinoma arising in a previously benign pleomorphic adenoma represents not more than 10% of lesions of mixed cell category.

Clinical presentation of parotid tumours

The majority of parotid tumours, whether benign or malignant, present as painless discrete swellings that frequently have been present for many years before the patient seeks advice – even when the tumour is frankly malignant, such as the adenoid cystic carcinoma.

However, four other presenting symptoms and signs may be present if the tumour is frankly malignant:

1. *Facial nerve palsy.* As pointed out above, this is particularly common in association with adenoid cystic carcinoma (which specifically tends to spread along the nerve sheaths) and with truly undifferentiated carcinomata.
2. *Lymphatic metastases.* These are particularly common in association with the very rare squamous carcinoma of the parotid.
3. *Distant blood-borne metastases* are observed, particularly with adenoid cystic carcinoma and acinic cell tumours.
4. *Ulceration of the overlying skin*, although this is occasionally seen with large, wholly benign tumours such as giant pleomorphic adenoma.

Investigation

Radiology is of little assistance in determining the nature of the majority of parotid swellings. However, CAT is of use in determining the extent of deep penetration by a tumour.

Treatment

Fortunately the majority of parotid tumours present as localized small swellings varying in size from 1–4 cm in diameter, and occupy the superficial portion of the gland. The treatment of such tumours is superficial parotidectomy, thus avoiding the danger of rupture of the capsule or incomplete removal of the tumour. The statement seen in some surgical textbooks that the aim should be excision of the tumour together with a generous cuff of surrounding normal gland is a contradiction, since generous excision without first identifying the facial nerve is unquestionably going to limit the excision for fear of injury to this all-important structure.

Therefore it is reasonable to advocate total superficial parotidectomy for all localized masses within the parotid. Unfortunately this operation means that the facial nerve must be identified prior to proceeding with the resection and, although simple in theory, it is extremely difficult in practice even with the assistance of nerve stimulators. The nerve can be identified with practice as it leaves the stylomastoid foramen and, since no branches leave its posterior aspect, the main trunk can be traced distally with safety. By performing a superficial parotidectomy the danger of recurrence which follows simple enucleation – which is as high as 40% in some series with long follow-up – is avoided.

As an alternative, local excision followed by irradiation has been proposed but this method has not found favour particularly because secondary operations on the parotid region carry a high risk of facial nerve damage.

Nevertheless superfical parotidectomy is not without its complications. These include:

1. A small number of cases of partial facial nerve palsy.
2. Dryness of the mouth.
3. Salivary fistula.
4. Auriculotemporal syndrome (Frey's syndrome). This consists of gustatory sweating and redness in the cutaneous distribution of the auriculotemporal nerve. One explanation for this syndrome is that divided parasympathetic secretory fibres grow into the sheath of the auriculotemporal nerve so that stimuli which would normally provoke secretion produce sweating. If the symptom is distressing it may be relieved by division of the tympanic branch of the glossopharyngeal nerve in the middle ear.

If the tumour is frankly malignant on clinical grounds, preoperative deep radiotherapy followed by radical parotidectomy is probably the best option open to both the patient and the surgeon.

19. Dysphagia

Definition

The term 'dysphagia' implies difficulty, but not pain, on swallowing. The difficulty may be intermittent or progressive, and may involve the swallowing of solids rather than liquids, or both. The causes may be classified as follows:

AETIOLOGY

Congenital causes

1. Atresia.
2. Stenosis.
3. Dysphagia lusoria.

Acquired causes

Disease of the wall of the oesophagus

1. *Benign tumours:*
   a. Lipoma.
   b. Leiomyoma.
2. *Malignant tumours:*
   a. Adenocarcinoma.
   b. Squamous carcinoma.
3. *Strictures:*
   a. Due to corrosives.
   b. Due to acid/pepsin reflux.
4. *Neurological causes – infective:*
   a. Diphtheria.
   b. Poliomyelitis.
   c. Syphilitic pachymeningitis.
   d. Bulbar paralysis.

e. Polyneuritis.
5. *Neurological causes – non-infective:*
   a. Myasthenia gravis.
   b. Thrombosis or bleeding in the brain stem.
6. *Neuromuscular causes:*
   a. Pharnygeal pouch.
   b. Plummer–Vinson syndrome.
   c. Diffuse spasm.
7. *Connective tissue disease: scleroderma.*
8. *Intraluminal obstruction:*
   a. Foreign body.
   b. Bolus obstruction.
9. *Extrinsic pressure:*
   a. Pressure by enlarged lymph nodes from any cause.
   b. Dysphagia lusoria, where abnormal vessels become dilated due to atherosclerosis.
10. *Psychosomatic: globus hystericus.* This condition presents with dysphagia associated with a lump in the throat. Although the majority of sufferers have no organic abnormality they should be investigated, since in a minority of patients an organic lesion, most commonly a hiatus hernia, will be found.

Discussion in this section will be restricted to the diagnosis and treatment of pharyngeal pouch, Plummer–Vinson syndrome, carcinoma of the oesophagus, benign stricture associated with reflux oesophagitis, and achalasia of the cardia.

PHARYNGEAL POUCH (ZENKER'S PHARYNGEAL DIVERTICULUM)

Pathology

A pharyngeal pouch is a pulsion diverticulum, although there remains considerable disagreement over the causal factor. The following theories have been proposed:

1. Failure of the horizontal fibres of the cricopharyngeus to relax during the act of swallowing.
2. Premature closure of the cricopharyngeal sphincter during the act of swallowing.
3. Hypertonicity of the cricopharyngeal sphincter due to reflex stimulation, possibly because of associated excessive gastro-oesophageal reflux.

Whatever the underlying cause the pouch is formed by an outpouching of the pharyngeal mucosa and submucosa through the weak area which normally exists between the oblique and horizontal fibres of the cricopharyngeus, otherwise known as Killian's dehiscence.

Symptomatology

This condition is commoner in males than females and classically is more frequently seen in the elderly. In some patients severe dysphagia may occur even though the pouch itself is small and in others small pouches may be incidentally found during the course of a barium swallow in the absence of any symptoms whatsoever. As the pouch enlarges it is displaced sideways, usually protruding to the left side of the neck and a swelling may be observed, particularly after eating. The presence of such a high obstruction leads to the spillage of retained fluid or food into the larynx with the result that the patient may develop an irritating cough, paticularly at night. As the dysphagia increases in severity so weight loss and cachexia follow and in longstanding cases actual pneumonitis develops so that the patient may present with the symptoms and signs of a pulmonary infection.

When the patient suffers from an exceedingly large sac he may be aware of the sac filling during eating or drinking. Apart from dysphagia the main symptoms associated with this condition are regurgitation of food and severe halitosis.

Investigation

The only investigation required for the diagnosis of a pharyngeal pouch is a barium swallow, when the pouch can be seen in nearly every view. If the pouch is large the fundus descends into the superior mediastinum.

Treatment

The treatment usually advised for large diverticula is excision of the pouch together with myotomy of the transverse fibres of the cricopharyngeus; otherwise the patient is faced with progressive deterioration and possibly severe pulmonary complications.

The pharnyx is approached through a collar incision in the neck at the level of the cricoid cartilage or by an incision along the anterior border of the left sternomastoid.

Following division of the deep fascia, the left lateral lobe of the thyroid is mobilized by division of the middle thyroid veins, if present, after which the pouch is gradually dissected free. The essential part of the operation is to divide the sac at the neck and close the defect in two layers, after which a myotomy of the horizontal fibres of the cricopharyngeus is performed. Pharyngeal narrowing can be avoided during the reconstruction by passing a large-bore oesophageal tube through the pharynx.

Some surgeons would advise merely a myotomy for this condition, particularly if the diverticulum is small, but since the neck of the diverticulum has to be exposed in order to perform this operation it seems only reasonable that the pouch, however small, should be excised at the same time.

The operation is accompanied by a small mortality, which is hardly surprising since most of the patients are elderly. Specifically, the occasional complication of oesophago-cutaneous fistula may follow excision, and since this is the result of removing the pouch it forms the basis for arguing that, with small pouches, one should be content to perform a careful myotomy only; or, if the pouch is large, some authors have suggested accompanying the myotomy with displacement of the fundus of the sac upwards.

PLUMMER–VINSON SYNDROME

This is often termed the Plummer–Vinson–Paterson syndrome because Paterson and Kelly were the first to describe it.

Pathology

The cause of the dysphagia is, at first, spasm of the circular muscle fibres of the upper end of the oesophagus, which is later associated with the formation of webs arising from the anterior wall of the cervical oesophagus. The mucosa overlying this area of the oesophagus may be hyperkeratotic, or desquamated and friable. The condition is precancerous being associated wih the subsequent development of a postcricoid carcinoma. This condition is always associated with a low serum iron (normal value, 80–160 µg/dl; males 13–31 mmol/l, females 11–29 mmol/l) and a hypochromic microcytic anaemia.

Symptomatology

The main features of this condition are a longstanding dysphagia associated with a sideropenic anaemia and the symptoms thereof.

The syndrome is confined almost exclusively to middle-aged women between 35 and 60 years of age. Glossitis, angular stomatitis, and koilonychia are almost invariably present. The patient complains of progressive dysphagia due to muscular incoordination at the level of the larynx.

Investigations

1. Blood examination reveals a hypochromic microcytic anaemia.
2. Serum iron, low values expected.
3. Barium swallow, reveals an anterior web or pin-hole orifice at the level of the cricoid cartilage.

Treatment

Treatment consists of dilating the web by bougies via an oesophagoscope. At the same time the iron deficiency anaemia should be corrected.

CARCINOMA OF THE OESOPHAGUS

Carcinoma of the oesophagus exists throughout the world, but epidemiological studies have shown great variations in its incidence. Thus, the highest incidence in males is in the South African Bantu, 41 per 100 000, compared to an incidence of 0.6 per 100 000 males in Hungary. In females the highest incidence is again in the Bantu, 36 per 100 000, compared to 3.5 per 100 000 females in the UK.

Certain aetiological factors have been considered responsible in the Bantu, among which are maize beer-drinking, tobacco smoking or chewing, and malnutrition possibly associated with chronic alcoholism. However, in the Transkei the Bantu women smoke and drink little despite a high incidence of oesophageal cancer.

Rarely, there appears to be a genetic association between the possibly inherited condition of tylosis – thickening of the palms and soles – and the development of carcinoma of the oesophagus in adult life.

Pathology

Carcinoma of the oesophagus may exist at any level, its distribution being in part determined by the group who report it: the incidence of upper cervical and hypopharyngeal tumours is always higher in series reported by radiotherapists because radiotherapy has been more commonly used than surgery for this group of tumours.

From the surgeon's point of view the oesophagus can be divided into thirds. Primary cancer of the upper third – in the cervical and supra-aortic oesophagus – is always squamous and is relatively rare. Unlike cancer of the oesophagus elsewhere, it is a disease predominantly of women, especially in the postcricoid region, where it is associated with an iron deficiency anaemia. Cancer of the middle third – behind the hilum of the lung – is more common. Cancer of the lower third – extending from the inferior pulmonary vein down to and including the gastro-oesophageal junction – is the most common site of all; the majority of these tumours arise from the cardia and invade the lower end of the oesophagus chiefly by submucosal spread.

Macroscopic appearance

In the early stages with little growth, carcinoma of the oesophagus may merely appear as a roughened plaque. Later the tumour may be annular, ulcerating or polypoidal.

Histopathology

Nearly all tumours of the upper oesophagus are squamous, varying from highly differentiated tumours with well-formed cell nests to undifferentiated tumours which may be difficult to identify as squamous.

At the lower end of the oesophagus two types of tumour are found:

1. The rare adeno-squamous variety, in which both squamous and glandular elements are found.
2. The adenocarcinoma, which arises from the stomach proper and invades the oesophagus by proximal extension.

A significant pathological feature of all oesophageal tumours is their submucosal spread. This may extend for several centimetres above and below the apparent naked-eye involvement of the oesophagus, and is of considerable importance to the surgeon when he considers the line of transection of the oesophagus should the tumour appear operable on exploration.

Clinical presentation

Nearly 25% of patients have a history of at least 6 months before seeking advice. The symptom complex produced by oesophageal cancer varies from an abnormal sensation behind the sternum to progressive dysphagia, the latter only developing when the tumour has reduced the lumen of the oesophagus by 50%. Symptoms may be produced by involvement of adjacent structures. This may occur early because the thin submucosal and muscular layers of the oesophagus provide little resistance to the invasion of neighbouring structures. The dysphagia normally begins with solid foods, but as the condition progresses so it becomes difficult to swallow liquids. When this stage is reached, there may be overspill into the larynx, with the production of pulmonary complications, including the development of lung abscesses. As the dysphagia worsens, the nutritional state of the patient suffers and secondary anaemia develops. Indeed, by the time the patient comes for an opinion there may already be signs indicating that the tumour is inoperable, including:

1. Vocal cord paresis.
2. Symptoms of tracheobronchial fistula.
3. Enlarged cervical lymph nodes.
4. Enlarged liver due to hepatic metastases.

Investigations

1. *Plain X-rays of the chest.* These may show:
   a. Enlarged mediastinal lymph nodes.
   b. Infective complications in the lung fields due to regurgitation.
2. *Barium swallow.* This may show:
   a. An irregular stricture failing to relax even after the administration of antispasmodics.
   b. Moderate dilatation of the oesophagus proximal to the obstruction.
   c. A filling defect with typical shouldering; if barium passes through the stricture a typical 'rat tail' deformity may be seen.

d. When the growth is advanced a deep ulcer crater develops with an irregular base, and in some cases barium flows into the trachea or bronchus.
   e. Fundal tumours invading the lower end of the oesophagus may cause a soft tissue mass which is interposed between the undersurface of the diaphragm and the cardia.

It should be noted that dilatation of the oesophagus proximal to a malignant stricture is never as great as that seen above the fibrous stricture caused by gastric reflux.

3. *Ultrasonography* plays no part in the assessment of the growth itself but may assist in detecting malignant hepatic secondaries not yet large enough to cause hepatomegaly.

4. *CAT* accurately identifies all patients in whom the tumour is confined to the oesophagus (Stages I and II) but has a limited ability to assess direct organ invasion (Stage III).

5. *Endoscopy*. Endoscopy can be performed using either a rigid or flexible fibre-optic system. The disadvantage of the former is that it requires a general anaesthetic whereas the latter can be carried out under sedation. The advantages of the former method are, however, that it allows a more accurate assessment of the distance of the tumour from the incisor teeth, greater evidence of fixity and, lastly, a larger biopsy and hence greater diagnostic accuracy. Using a fibre-optic instrument the biopsy is small; if the tumour is endophytic rather than exophytic the endoscopist may have to be content with brushings from the strictured area, which may give rise to a false result.

6. *Bronchoscopy*. This investigation is particularly indicated in the presence of chest symptoms and an abnormal chest X-ray. Direct spread, the presence of a fistula, or carinal deformity due to involvement of the mediastinal lymph nodes may all be observed.

If the above investigations suggest that major surgery is feasible the cardiorespiratory status of the patient must be evaluated (see Vol. 1, p. 108).

Management

Regardless of the method of treatment adopted the overall results are poor. Different series obviously report slightly different survival rates but all approximate to a 5-year survival of only 5% for those in whom investigation suggests that the lesion is resectable. However, resection is claimed to have two advantages over palliative treatment:

1. The mean survival time is longer.
2. It is claimed that the quality of swallowing is better than in those patients in whom palliative methods are adopted.

Radical radiotherapy

In squamous tumours involving the upper two-thirds of the oesophagus, radical radiotherapy produces an overall 5-year survival which ranges from 5–10%, the results being somewhat better for tumours situated in the upper third than in the middle third.

Because of the submucosal spread typical of oesophageal tumours the field of irradiation must extend 5 cm above and below the macroscopic level of the tumour. A tumourcidal dose may cause excessive damage to several organs, and indeed Pearson, who was a major protagonist of this method of treatment, found that half the patients to whom a dose of 5–6000 rads was being delivered had to suspend treatment. Damage may occur to the lungs, spinal cord, heart and pericardium and in some patients a tracheo-oesophageal fistula may develop.

Such damage may be limited by the careful placing of the portals but, in the majority of successfully treated patients, strictures develop which require periodic dilatation.

Surgery

Preoperative preparation

Prior to surgery, if there has been a considerable loss of weight (e.g. 10–15%) a period of preoperative nutritional supplementation may be helpful. This can be delivered using a fine-bore Silastic tube introduced into the stomach, or via a peripheral vein where a compound mixture comprising 2500 kcals and up to 14 g of nitrogen can be given if the osmolality does not exceed 800 mosmols/l.

Surgical methods

Tumours of the cardia invading the lower end of the oesophagus. These can be resected using a left thoraco-abdominal approach via the bed of the 7th or 8th rib. The diaphragm is divided to the hiatus and the overall situation examined, after which the stomach is mobilized and divided, the oesophagus is mobilized, and the 'neo-fundus' anastomosed to the oesophagus.

Tumours which are shown to be more extensive or are primarily tumours of the lower oesophagus. The classical approach has been that described by Ivor Lewis, in which the stomach is first mobilized through a midline abdominal incision; a right thoracic incision is then made, through which the oesophagus is mobilized and the intrathoracic anastomosis is performed.

Apart from the cardiorespiratory complications which follow both these procedures, the great danger of all intrathoracic anastomoses is that of leakage leading either to death from mediastinitis or, at best, postoperative stricture formation.

To obviate this difficulty McKeown described a three-stage procedure which begins with total mobilization of the stomach via a midline abdominal incision, followed by a right thoracotomy through which the whole of the intrathoracic oesophagus is mobilized after dividing the azygos vein. This performed, a third incision is made in the neck and the stomach is drawn up into the neck; an anastomosis is then performed between the cervical oesophagus and the apex of the fundus of the stomach. The obvious advantage of this approach is that the dangerous intrathoracic anastomosis is avoided.

However, the principle of radical curative cancer surgery cannot be satisfied in oesophageal surgery because of the proximity of vital organs, which precludes a satisfactory en bloc resection of the oesophagus and its associated local spread.

An alternative procedure, which obviates the necessity for a thoracic incision, is the operation of trans-hiatal oesophagectomy, described by Oringer in 1986. This operation involves the complete mobilization of the stomach through a midline abdominal incision followed by a blunt dissection of the oesophagus via the diaphragmatic hiatus; this dissection is carried up as far as the superior mediastinum, after which an incision is made above the right clavicle and the remainder of the oesophagus mobilized and an anastomosis performed within the neck.

Although the oesophageal dissection is performed blindly, bleeding is not usually a problem because the oesophageal blood supply is derived from feeding arteries at some distance from the oesophagus and only small blood vessels reach the oesophageal wall. However, severe bleeding may occur if the azygos vein is torn and it is generally agreed that the operation should be abandoned if a large, fixed mass is encountered, because this may well mean that the azygos vein, the membranous trachea, the right main bronchus or the thoracic duct may be damaged. Indeed many surgeons would not attempt this approach for tumours occupying the middle third of the oesophagus.

The results obtained by this approach are comparable with the other methods which have been described. Nevertheless despite the theoretical advantages of not opening the thoracic cavity the mortality remains high, as does the incidence of cardiorespiratory complications.

Radical excision carries a hospital mortality of between 12–15%, even in patients below the age of 70.

Palliative treatment

Originally a variety of tubes, including the twisted wire tube developed by Souttar, were used. This particular tube has now been superseded by a variety of other, superior tubes, including the Mousseau-Barbin, Celestin, and Atkinson tubes. One of the disadvantages of the Mousseau-Barbin is that a laparotomy is required for its placement, whereas the others can be introduced directly after passing a dilator through the growth via a rigid oesophagoscope. Interestingly, in the majority of reported series the mortality rate for intubation remains remarkably high, in the region of 10%.

Recently, with the application of laser to surgery, attempts have been made to palliate the condition by means of 'local excision' of the obstructive elements of the tumour by this means. In a series of 190 patients reported by Barr and his co-workers in 1990 they found no significant difference in the quality of life between those patients treated by laser alone and those treated by both laser and intubation. However, other reports record better results, Krasner (1987) found that, after four treatments at 4-weekly intervals, 32% of their patients could swallow any solid, 54% could take most solids, and only 8% had to be maintained on liquids. Swallowing was maintained until death in all but 15% of patients, although 15% required intubation.

Laser fails if the tumour is rapidly growing or if extrinsic pressure on the oesophagus is present as a result of local spread.

DYSPHAGIA ASSOCIATED WITH GASTRO-OESOPHAGEAL REFLUX

It was once considered that gastro-oesophageal reflux only occurred in the presence of a hiatus hernia. The latter condition was originally described by Harrington in 1940 but then separated into two apparently distinct types by Allison in 1951: type 1 or sliding hernia, and type 2 or para-oesophageal hernia; in type 1 hernia the oesophagogastric junction is found in the thorax, whereas in type 2 hernia the gastro-oesophageal junction lies below the diaphragm, and so pathological degrees of reflux do not occur.

The development of newer methods of investigation has led to considerable doubt as to the exclusive role of the sliding hernia as a cause of reflux, since whilst the majority of patients with clinically significant gastro-oesophageal reflux have an associated sliding type of hernia the converse is not true; indeed the majority of patients suffering from a hiatus hernia do not have significant reflux and the hernia itself does not present a major clinical problem. This was substantiated by Palmer, who found that nearly 50% of 1000 patients with a demonstrable hernia had no symptoms, even in the presence of oesophagitis.

Recent investigators therefore suggest that there is only a coincidental role between the two conditions, a hypothesis supported by the fact that in many patients suffering from the symptoms of reflux no hernia can be demonstrated.

Two motor abnormalities, either singly or together, are believed to be responsible for reflux together with a multiplicity of subsidiary factors:

1. The failure of the oesophagus to clear itself of refluxed gastric contents.
2. The failure of the lower oesophageal sphincter to prevent such reflux occurring.

In the great majority of patients the offending material is acid/pepsin but in fact bile and pancreatic juice are equally as irritating and corrosive.

The duration of exposure of the lower oesophagus to acid/pepsin can now be determined by the use of pH probes or by radio pills over long periods of time; by these means it has been shown that some degree of oesophagogastric reflux is present without causing symptoms in 25% of the community – particularly in the postprandial period, when the intragastric contents exceed a critical volume, and at night in the recumbent position – which suggests that the ability of the oesophagus to clear itself of acid is the most important of the two factors.

The factors preventing reflux in the first place are many and the interpretation of their relative importance difficult to define, but they include:

1. *The high pressure zone at the lower end of the oesophagus*, which is a physiological rather than an anatomical concept. Its length

appears to vary between 3–5 cm and its tone appears to arise within the muscle itself. The pressure within this zone is responsive to changes in the intra-abdominal pressure and the intragastric pressure.

2. *The length of the intra-abdominal oesophagus*, which obviously equates with the length of the oesophagus exposed to the positive intra-abdominal pressure.

3. *The acute entry of the oesophagus into the stomach*. The importance of this factor has been demonstrated with ease in dogs, in which species this angle appears to be maintained by a band of muscle fibres originating in the lesser curve and passing over the left side of the cardia. In the dog, division of these fibres results in reflux.

4. *The mucosal rosette*. The bulging of the mucosa into the cardia may produce a valve-like effect when the intragastric pressure is raised.

Clinical presentation

As stated, even in the presence of a radiologically demonstrable hernia no symptoms are necessarily present. Commonly, there is a long history of heartburn before the development of dysphagia due to stricture formation. Even so, when dysphagia occurs it is not necessarily associated with actual stenosis, since either oedema or spasm may produce this symptom. It may also be noted by the patient that as the degree of dysphagia worsens so the severity of the heartburn diminishes.

The typical symptoms actually preceding stricture formation consist of belching, retrosternal burning or even pain, and possibly the regurgitation of gastric contents. All are made worse by physical actions such as stooping, or the development of a massive intra-abdominal mass such as an ovarian cyst, fibroid or pregnancy; the sudden development of obesity may also precipitate symptoms in a hitherto asymptomatic individual.

In addition to these classic symptoms an iron deficiency anaemia may develop due to bleeding from the ulcerating mucosa.

Pathological changes associated with reflux

The pathological changes induced by reflux depend upon the type of epithelium lining the oesophagus. In the majority of individuals the lower oesophagus is lined by squamous epithelium. The introduction of the flexible endoscope and the performance of frequent biopsies in patients complaining of reflux symptoms have led to the finding that, prior to the more overt changes of oesophagitis, subtle changes take place in the mucosa.

The chief changes include: an increasing thickness of the basal cell layer so that it constitutes more than 15% of the total epithelial thickness; and penetration of the papillae of the lamina propria more than two-thirds of the way through the epithelium to the luminal surface. These changes are indicative of an increased rate of epithelial cell turnover and are reliable indicators of excessive reflux.

As the condition progresses the continuity of the mucosal lining of the lower oesophagus is interrupted by multiple shallow ulcers and endoscopic biopsies reveal the classical signs of inflammation, i.e. granulation tissue, polymorphonuclear cell infiltration and granulation tissue. Further progression leads to cicatricial fibrosis.

In the 1950's Barrett drew attention to another type of oesophageal ulceration, which instead of remaining superficial had all the pathological characteristics of chronic peptic ulceration. 'Barrett's oesophagus' is in an oesophagus lined by columnar epithelium, which resembles the mucosa of the fundus of the stomach, but without parietal cells. At first Barrett erroneously thought that this was due to a congenitally short oesophagus with an attenuated intrathoracic stomach. It is more common in males and has been identified in 0.5-4% of the population by endoscopic examination. Allison and Johnstone recognized in 1953 that there was a common association between the columnar lined oesophagus and reflux, and considered that the replacement of the normal squamous epithelial lining was due to the effects of reflux, an opinion now generally accepted. Apart from the propensity to develop deep, penetrating ulcers and strictures, there is a strong association between Barrett's oesophagus and adenocarcinoma.

Investigations

Endoscopic appearances of reflux oesophagitis

Only about 54% of patients with reflux as determined by pH studies have endoscopic changes in the mucosa. In the normal individual the gastro-oesophageal junction is sharply defined, the normal oesophageal mucosa having a pinkish, pearly-white colour, which contrasts with the salmon colour of the gastric mucosa. This junction lies not more than 2 cm above the diaphragmatic hiatus. One of the earliest signs of disease is the disappearance due to oedema, of the tiny, linearly arranged blood vessels in close proximity to one another, normally present in the lower 3 cm of the oesophagus. However, less subjectively, friability and granularity of the mucosa are of greater significance. Erosions, when they develop, may be linear or punctate, composed of a white centre surrounded by a red halo. Although similar erosions occur in monilial oesophagitis, biopsy and cytology lead to easy differentiation.

When a stricture has formed, it is usually smooth although mucosal ulceration may be present, whilst a malignant stricture appears more irregular, friable and necrotic. A biopsy must be taken to exclude malignancy, if possible from the narrowest part of the stricture.

Radiological appearances of benign oesophageal strictures

The barium swallow may demonstrate:

1. Irregular mucosal folds in the lower oesophagus above a gastric pouch.
2. A smoothly tapering, narrowed oesophageal segment running downwards towards the hernial pouch.
3. Concentric narrowing of the oesophagus some distance above the oesophagogastric junction. This appearance suggests a gastric lined oesophagus.
4. Typically, benign strictures have smooth margins and a tapering appearance, and there may be a dilated oesophagus proximal to the stricture. Should the stricture be eccentric and irregular this suggests malignancy.

Treatment

Once an organic stricture has developed, both active as well as medical treatment are required:

Intermittent dilatation (bougienage)

This can be used as a primary method of treatment, remembering that as a severe stricture is dilated so reflux – together with its symptoms and complications – may well begin again. Bougienage may be accomplished by a variety of dilators, including tapered mercury-filled rubber Maloney dilators, dilating the oesophagus to 45 F (1 F = 0.32 mm in diameter). If the stricture is very tight, olive-shaped metal dilators should be passed, but if they are passed without the use of a guide wire perforation of the oesophagus may occur. Other dilators include tapered solid 'neoplex' dilators, also inserted over a guide wire. Although somewhat rigid, these dilators are flexible enough to follow the curve of the pharynx and allow for uniform dilatation of the stricture.

It is essential that dilatation should be followed by efforts to reduce acid secretion, for example using the recently developed drug omeprazole, which is a powerful proton pump inhibitor specifically blocking the enzyme, H^+/K^+-ATPase, inhibiting both the basal and stimulated acid secretion. This drug has been shown to be more effective than the H_2 antagonists, which for so long have been the cornerstone of the treatment of duodenal ulceration. Administered in a dose of 40 mg a day, rapid and sustained healing of oesophagitis can be obtained.

Other surgical procedures

Because of the efficacy of omeprazole, the need for antireflux surgery in the form of Nissen fundoplication, or the Belsey or Collis operations has fallen dramatically and are reserved for the few failures.

ACHALASIA

This condition has been recognized for at least 300 years. It is characterized by a failure of the lower oesophageal sphincter to relax in response to swallowing, combined with a failure of the lower two-thirds of the oesophageal muscle to produce the smooth peristaltic wave normally initiated by deglutition.

Pathology

The smooth muscle of the oesophagus is grossly hypertrophied. Electron microscopic studies show changes similar to those seen in denervated striated muscle with detachment or displacement of the myofibrils. However, the chief pathological change appears to be in the ganglion cells of the myenteric plexus at the lower end of the oesophagus, in which changes in the ganglion cells appear notably in the arygyrophilic ganglion cells as described by Smith in 1972. In addition, Wallerian degeneration has been found in the extra-oesophageal vagus nerves.

The stagnation of food materials in the oesophagus produces mucosal ulceration and severe oesophagitis and, once obstruction has developed and the oesophagus dilated to form a huge reservoir, the oesophageal contents may be aspirated into the respiratory passages producing recurrent bronchopneumonia and lung abscesses.

Clinical presentation

The condition is commoner in women than in men and, although it may occur at any age, it is commonest during the fourth and fifth decades.

Three stages have been described. First there may be dysphagia associated with retrosternal discomfort, and the symptoms may be confused with diffuse oesophageal spasm. In the second stage the pain may diminish and the dysphagia becomes intermittent. Lastly, continuous dysphagia associated with retrosternal discomfort, anorexia and loss of weight develop, with aspiration occurring particularly at night when the patient is recumbent, leading to pulmonary complications.

Carcinoma of the oesophagus is seven times more common in patients suffering from achalasia than in the normal population.

Investigations

Barium swallow

The precise radiological findings depend upon the stage of the disease. Initially, despite considerable dysphagia, there may be no radiological signs, but as the disease progresses the oesophagus dilates, becomes flaccid and tapers to a beak-like narrow distal segment.

Manometry

This is particularly useful in the presence of symptoms without radiological changes in the early stages of the disease, for in achalasia the normal propagated pressure waves are replaced by a series of waves of lower amplitude, and in the area of the lower oesophageal sphincter there is no relaxation on swallowing.

Oesophagoscopy

This confirms the capacious oesophagus, the presence of food retention, and ulceration of the mucosa, and excludes neoplasia in the area of the radiological narrowing.

Treatment

Two methods of treatment are possible. The first, forceful hydrostatic dilatation of the lower end of the oesophagus, is a method which has little place in modern therapy except in the very elderly. It is not without danger since there is a risk of perforating the lower end of the oesophagus. Dilatation is performed inflating the hydrostatic bag to about 35 mm in diameter at a pressure of 300 torr.

The second and generally accepted mode of treatment is by Heller's operation, devised in 1913, in which a myotomy is performed through the muscle of the lower end of the oesophagus for about 5 cm, reaching onto the stomach for about 1 cm. In the past, one of the common complications of this operation was reflux oesophagitis, but this can be avoided in about 97% of patients by dividing the muscle on the lesser curve of the stomach, so that the oblique gastric muscle fibres that serve to maintain the acute angle of entry of the oesophagus into the cardia remain intact. Further care should be taken to avoid the vagus nerves.

Results of treatment. Obviously the results quoted in various series differ in detail, but approximately 70–80% of patients obtain complete relief following a properly performed myotomy. Interestingly the radiological physical signs may remain grossly abnormal even in the presence of clinical improvement.

20. Historical development of duodenal ulcer surgery

Gastric surgery for the relief of peptic ulceration arose from the use of operations that were initially performed to overcome obstructive lesions at the pyloric end of the stomach. The original operation of gastroenterostomy is credited to Wolfler in 1881, but shortly afterwards Rydyier of Poland and Doyen of France described its application for the treatment of cicatricial pyloric stenosis due to duodenal ulceration.

GASTROENTEROSTOMY

In its original form, gastroenterostomy was performed by anastomosing a jejunal loop to the anterior wall of the stomach, and it was not appreciated, at first, that the length of the afferent loop was critical to the proper mechanical working of the operation, too long a loop leading to the syndrome of vicious circle vomiting. The posterior 'no-loop' procedure now in common use was developed by Czerny and was immediately adopted by Mayo and Moynihan.

Until the First World War, gastroenterostomy was regarded as the operation of choice for duodenal ulceration, and in the first decade of the twentieth century individual surgeons were reporting personal series of several hundreds of cases.

Those surgeons who practised gastroenterostomy firmly believed that the anastomosis accomplished three things. First, it diverted food from the ulcer, thus avoiding irritation of the ulcerated surface and allowing it to heal. Secondly, it allowed the influx of bile and alkaline pancreatic juice into the stomach, thus neutralizing the acid contents. Thirdly, it diverted acid from the pylorus, thus abolishing the jet-stream effect on the first part of the duodenum. It was not, of course, appreciated at the time that several effects of gastroenterostomy mitigated against a good result. These include: the damaging effect of bile on the gastric mucosa by destroying the mucosal barrier; the place of continuous antral alkalinity as a stimulus to continuous parietal cell secretion; and lastly, the fact that the stomach drains through the anastomosis only when the pylorus is completely obstructed.

Nevertheless, many surgeons, including Moynihan, reported exceptionally good results. In 1923 Moynihan published his experiences of ten years of ulcer surgery and recorded his results in 531 cases. He reported a low operative mortality and a satisfactory result in over 90% of patients. In his personal series he reported that the incidence of anastomotic ulceration was only a little over 1%. At that time, of course, jejunal ulcers were considered to be caused by faulty operative techniques such as the use of non-absorbable sutures, rather than unsolved physiological problems.

Despite this and many similar reports, it was finally appreciated that gastroenterostomy carried a very high morbidity in the way of jejunal ulceration. Many large series showed that recurrent ulceration, usually situated on the efferent loop, occurred in as many as 50% of patients, the incidence being greatest in males under 50 years of age and within the first 5 years following surgery.

It is also interesting that dumping, which is one of the commoner physiological side-effects of gastric surgery, seems to have gone entirely unrecognized by the earlier surgeons, for the first review of this subject did not appear in the literature until 1920. Today, gastroenterostomy is never used alone for the treatment of duodenal ulceration despite its low mortality, even in patients suffering from severe pyloric stenosis in whom it was once regarded as the treatment of choice.

PARTIAL GASTRECTOMY

In 1881, Bilroth successfully removed the pyloric end of the stomach and restored the continuity of the gastrointestinal tract by a direct gastroduodenal anastomosis (Fig. 20.1A). In 1885, he performed a pylorectomy and then closed the duodenum and restored the continuity of the bowel by anastomosing the jejunum to the stomach remnant (Fig. 20.1B). Following the original description of these surgical techniques, many useless but original anatomical modifications were described. By the end of the First World War both operations were being performed for the treatment of duodenal ulceration and, indeed, the Bilroth II, or Polya gastrectomy, as it came to be known, was the operation of choice from the mid 1930s to the early 1960s.

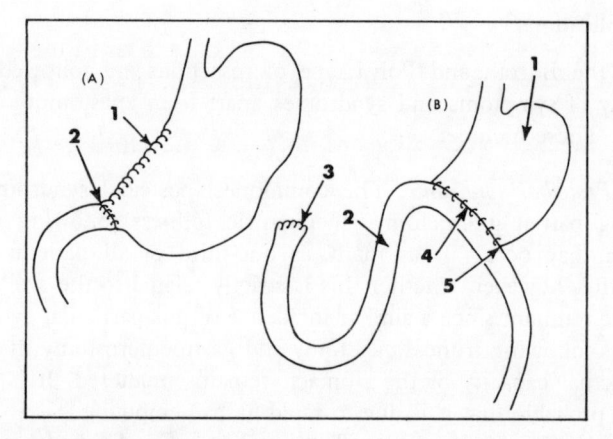

Fig. 20.1 Partial gastrectomy.
(A) Bilroth I operation (described in 1881).
1, reconstructed lesser curve; 2, gastroduodenal junction (angle of sorrow, due to possibility of leakage).
(B) Bilroth II operation (described in 1885).
1, gastric remnant; 2, danger point – too long an afferent loop; 3, danger point – rupture of duodenal stump; 4, gastroduodenal anastomosis; 5, site of recurrent ulceration.

It was soon appreciated that the avoidance of recurrent ulceration depended upon two factors:

1. *Total resection of the antral mucosa.* Incomplete resection of this zone leads to continued high acid secretion due to stimulation of the residual antral mucosa by the regurgitant alkaline duodenal juices.

2. *Adequate resection of the body of the stomach*, thus reducing the parietal cell mass.

However, it was also recognized that too radical a resection produced a gastric cripple. An individual who lost weight and energy due to the small stomach remnant, its rapid emptying and intestinal hurry. Thus most surgeons limit the resection to three-quarters or two-thirds of the stomach.

Several decades passed before it was fully appreciated that the Bilroth I type of resection was not as satisfactory as the Polya for the treatment of duodenal ulceration. The main disadvantage of the former was the high incidence of recurrent ulcers astride the anastomosis, despite apparently adequate resection of the stomach; an incidence as high as 28.6% has been reported from some centres as compared to an incidence of 1–2% following an adequate Polya resection in which two-thirds to three-quarters of the stomach are removed.

Complications

Both the Bilroth and Polya type of resections are followed by a variety of symptoms and syndromes apart from anastomotic ulceration. These include:

1. *Postcibal syndrome.* The commonest postcibal syndrome following partial gastrectomy is epigastric fullness following meals, which may occur in as many as one-third of all patients. It is doubtful, however, whether this is strictly related to the size of the gastric remnant since a similar incidence of this particular symptom occurs following truncal vagotomy and gastroenterostomy in which the actual capacity of the stomach remains unaltered. It is much more probable that it is due to rapid gastric emptying.

Less common but still affecting 20% of individuals is early dumping, which affects approximately one in five patients. Late dumping, specifically associated with a reactive hypoglycaemia occurring 1-2 hours after eating, is a rare postcibal syndrome which can be relieved quite simply by taking carbohydrate in any form.

2. *Bile vomiting.*
3. *Iron deficiency anaemia*, especially in the premenopausal woman.
4. *Weight loss*, probably due to postcibal symptoms.
5. *Megaloblastic anaemia.*
6. *Severe malnutrition* following very radical resection.
7. *An increased incidence of pulmonary tuberculosis.*
8. *Cancer of the stomach remnant.* The incidence of cancer in the gastric remnant is some five times higher than is anticipated in the intact stomach. This risk, however, only becomes evident after 15-25 years. Two major hypotheses have been advanced to explain its occurrence: first, that bile regurgitation produces dysplastic changes which ultimately culminate in the development of gastric cancer; and second, that the hypoacidity which follows partial gastrectomy favours colonization of the gastric remnant by bacteria which produce carcinogens such as the nitrosamines.

Results

Despite this formidable list of undesirable side-effects, approximately 80% of patients subjected to a Polya gastrectomy are highly satisfied with the result. Of the remainder, three-quarters regard their condition as improved, while the rest are dissatisfied.

The degree of dissatisfaction is, in the majority, closely related to the extent of the gastric resection. Visick, a protagonist of radical resection, found that although extensive resection reduced anastomotic ulceration to neglible proportions it was, at the same time, accompanied by a distressingly high incidence of postcibal symptoms.

This suggested to Visick that the results of gastric surgery should be quantified in some way and he divided his results into four groups, the definitions of which were later somewhat modified by Goligher of Leeds as follows:

a. *Group I*: Excellent – absolutely no symptoms.
b. *Group II*: Very good – the patient considers the result as good, but interrogation elicits mild occasional symptoms easily controlled by adjustments to the diet.
c. *Group III*: Mild or moderate symptoms are present and not controlled by care, causing some discomfort, but both the patient and the surgeon are satisfied that they are not interfering with the patient's lifestyle or work.
d. *Group VI*: Moderate or severe symptoms or complications interfering with work and life. All patients with a proven recurrent ulcer submitted to further surgery belong to this group.

Some of the symptoms and syndromes listed above tend to improve with the passage of time. Thus, early dumping can be expected to improve and even completely disappear, although complete remission may take many months. Other conditions such as bile vomiting may improve, but if it persists it can be eliminated in the majority of patients by dividing the afferent loop and re-anastomosing it to the efferent loop at least 25 cm distal to the gastrojejunal anastomosis. If this operation is considered necessary it should be accompanied by vagotomy, otherwise anastomotic ulceration occurs in about 25% of patients. Yet other conditions such as anaemia may require continuous medication and supervision, particularly the rare megaloblastic anaemia.

Mortality

The mortality of partial gastrectomy varies from 1 to 5% according to the series examined. The fatal complication specifically related to partial gastrectomy depends upon the type of operation performed. Following a gastroduodenal anastomosis (Bilroth 1), the major problem is leakage from the junction of the reconstructed lesser curve and duodenum, a point known to the Germans as the 'angle of sorrow'.

Following a Bilroth II or Polya gastrectomy the chief hazard is rupture of the duodenal stump, a complication which may occur 4–21 days postoperatively. When it occurs early, this complication leads to a general peritonitis, and when it occurs later the common manifestation is the development of a right supra- or infrahepatic abscess which, if treated by open drainage, leads to a temporary duodenal fistula.

VAGOTOMY

Truncal resection

The unphysiological nature of partial gastrectomy and the relatively high incidence of unsatisfactory results led to attempts to control parietal cell secretion by section of the vagi. The first subdiaphragmatic vagotomy was reportedly performed by Exner in 1911, but the operation was only seriously advanced as an alternative to gastrectomy by Dragstedt in 1943. However, at this time the operation was almost immediately abandoned because of the undesirable effects of gastric stasis and the development of secondary gastric ulcers in some 10–15% of patients. It was reintroduced, combined of this occasion with a drainage procedure in 1945, again by Dragstedt.

Two methods of drainage have been commonly used, either a posterior gastroenterostomy or a Heinke–Mickulicz pyloroplasty. In the latter operation the antrum, pylorus and duodenum are divided in their long axis over a distance of some 10 cm, i.e. 5 cm on either side of the sphincter. The resulting defect is then repaired by one layer of sutures at right angles to the original incision. Somewhat later it was suggested that antrectomy followed by gastrojejunal anastomosis would not only provide drainage but would also remove one further stimulus to acid secretion.

Results

The results of these three operations have been extensively investigated over the years since their introduction and have been compared to the results obtained by partial gastrectomy. Using the Visick classification, although the results from the various series analysed vary somewhat in detail, those produced by Goligher and others in 1972 may be regarded as typical.

The results derive from a large number of surgeons in the Yorkshire region, who performed a randomized blind trial. In terms of the overall Visick classification, vagotomy and pyloroplasty resulted in 14% of patients falling into Group IV; vagotomy and gastroenterostomy, 11%; vagotomy and antrectomy, 8%; and gastrectomy 6%.

Insofar as recurrent ulceration is concerned, the results of this series of about 200 patients showed that it occurred in approximately 7% of patients following vagotomy and pyloroplasty; 11% following vagotomy and gastroenterostomy; 8% following vagotomy and antrectomy; and 6% following partial gastrectomy.

Regarding the less serious symptoms (excluding severe diarrhoea), there appeared to be little difference between the four operations under consideration. Approximately 40% complained of some epigastric fullness after meals; early dumping occurred in 10–20% – vagotomy and gastroenterostomy, and partial gastrectomy producing the worst figures in this respect. Late dumping occurred in some 5% and some degree of nausea occurred in 10–20%. Somewhat surprisingly, bile vomiting was equal in all groups, occurring in about 14% of patients.

So far as diarrhoea was concerned, this was rare after partial gastrectomy but occurred in 20% of patients subjected to the other three operations, although it was only regarded as severe in 5%. The typical severe diarrhoea associated with truncal vagotomy can in fact be very disabling as the author is personally aware, although strangely it tends to improve with the passage of time. Most investigators believe that post-vagotomy diarrhoea arises because viscera other than that of the stomach have been denervated. Particular attention has been paid to the fact that truncal vagotomy causes gallbladder dysfunction because it interferes with the nerves supplying this organ. It has been shown that, following truncal vagotomy, the gallbladder enlarges and almost doubles its fasting volume, that it contracts poorly after a fatty meal, and that there is an increased incidence of gallstones. In addition, the hypothesis has been put forward that when such a dilated gallbladder does contract it delivers so large a volume of bile into the gut that the small intestine is unable to absorb the bile-salt content, with the result that some bile salts reach the large bowel and there inhibit the absorption of water, salt, and potassium, to produce the watery motion which is so classical of post-vagotomy diarrhoea.

This theory is supported by the fact that in many patients the diarrhoea can be controlled by the drug cholestyramine, which binds the bile salts and, secondly, that the incidence of diarrhoea is sharply reduced by performing a selective vagotomy.

Selective vagotomy

Essentially this operation, as first described in 1948 by Franksson of Stockholm and Jackson of Ann Arbor, consists of dividing the vagi a little lower down on the stomach itself, below the origin of the hepatic branches of the anterior vagus and the coeliac branch of the posterior vagus, so that although the vagal supply to the entire stomach is interrupted the biliary tract and small gut remain innervated.

This operation received enormous attention, particularly from the late Harold Burge in the United Kingdom. The protagonists claimed that it was effective both in terms of a low incidence of recurrent ulceration and a reduced frequency of diarrhoea. However, because this operation is still associated with a drainage procedure, all the consequences of destruction of the pyloric sphincter and rapid emptying of the stomach may follow, such as dumping. It is also interesting to note that not all surgeons are agreed that this operation successfully reduces the incidence of postoperative diarrhoea.

Highly selective vagotomy

In 1957, Griffith and Harkins attempted to denervate, in the dog, the acid-producing parietal cell mass alone, and in 1967 this work was applied to man by Holle and Hart who combined it with a drainage procedure because they failed to realize that when the vagal innervation of the antrum and pylorus is retained, the emptying mechanism of the stomach is unimpaired and a drainage procedure is unnecessary. It was left to Johnson and Wilkinson of Leeds and, simultaneously, Amdrup and Jenson of Copenhagen to realize the true significance of highly selective parietal cell vagotomy or, as some prefer to call the operation, proximal gastric vagotomy.

Essentially, this operation consists of dividing all the branches of the anterior and posterior vagal nerves, commonly known as the anterior and posterior nerves of Latarget, from a point distal to the division of the anterior vagal trunk into its hepatic and gastric branches (Fig. 20.2). This division should start at a point on the side of the oesophagus and continue along the lesser curve of the stomach to a point about 7 cm proximal to the pylorus, at which it can be seen

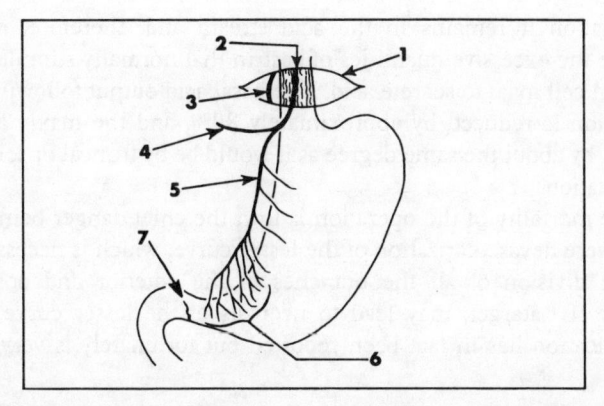

Fig. 20.2 Highly selective vagotomy: start of operation – exposure of main vagal trunks.
1, transverse peritoneal incision exposing lower oesophagus and anterior and posterior vagal trunks; 2, anterior vagal trunk; 3, posterior vagal trunk; 4, hepatic branch; 5, anterior nerve of Latarget; 6, crow's foot; 7, prepyloric vein of Mayo.

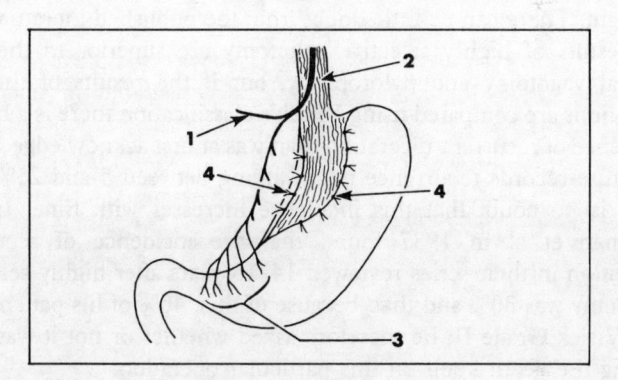

Fig. 20.3 Highly selective vagotomy: final appearance.
1, hepatic branch of anterior vagus nerve; 2, oesophagus; 3, crow's foot left intact; 4, points of division of branches of anterior and posterior nerves of Latarget.

that anterior nerve is dividing to form a 'crow's foot' arrangement as it splits to innervate the antrum (Fig. 20.3).

When performing this operation care must be taken to ensure that the lowermost 5–7 cm of the oesophagus has been completely bared of vagal trunks or nerve fibres running to the stomach and that meticulous haemostasis is maintained throughout.

The advantages of this operation are that by preserving pyloric innervation and, therefore, normal gastric emptying, it should theoretically avoid dumping, and although the antral area retains its innervation it remains in the acid stream and, therefore, cannot release the excessive quantities of gastrin that normally stimulate the parietal cell mass to secrete acid. The basal acid output following this operation is reduced by approximately 80%, and the maximal acid output by about the same degree as it would be by truncal or selective denervation.

The mortality of the operation is low, the chief danger being that the severe devascularization of the lesser curve, which is necessary to ensure division of all the branches of the anterior and posterior nerves of Latarget, may lead to necrosis of the lesser curve. This complication has in fact been reported but fortunately is very rare.

Results

The protagonists of proximal highly selective vagotomy maintained, at least initially, that the incidence of recurrent ulceration was low, not more than 1–2%, that dumping was rare and diarrhoea infrequent. There can be little doubt from the published literature that the results of highly selective vagotomy are superior to those of truncal vagotomy and pyloroplasty, but if the results of the two operations are compared using Visick's classification there is a higher incidence of recurrent ulceration than was at first acknowledged. The literature records recurrence rates varying between 5 and 25%, and there is no doubt that this incidence increases with time. Indeed Hoffman et al in 1987 found that the incidence of recurrent ulceration in their series reviewed 14–18 years after highly selective vagotomy was 30% and that, because of this, 40% of his patients fell into Visick Grade II; he therefore asked whether or not it was time to ring the death knell on this particular operation.

Some investigators have found that recurrence is particularly prone to occur in those patients who have failed to respond, or have relapsed following treatment with the H_2 antagonists such as cimetidine and ranitidine (ranitidine, although more expensive, is preferred because of its lower incidence of side-effects). This has led to the suggestion that the ulcer diathesis is unrelated to the high acid output and is more likely to be genetically determined.

TREATMENT OF THE UNCOMPLICATED DUODENAL ULCER

There is no doubt that the primary treatment of uncomplicated duodenal ulceration is by medical means. In the past, medical treatment was relatively ineffective until the development of the H_2 antagonists, which dramatically altered the ulcer scenario. Using these drugs 90% of all ulcers heal with a relapse rate estimated to be approximately 10%, diminishing with time.

Recently the situation has become even more complicated by the identification of *Helicobacter pylori*. This organism can be identified in nearly all patients suffering from duodenal ulceration; the association, however, is between duodenal ulceration and carriage of the organism in the pyloric antrum rather than in duodenum itself, unless gastric metaplasia has occurred in the latter. What unfortunately is not yet known is whether this organism is present prior to development of the ulcer. Nevertheless it has now been shown that elimination of this organism by a combination of tripotassium-dicitratobisulphate (De-Nol), tetracycline and metronidazole for 2 weeks will free the gastric antrum of the organism and lead to healing of duodenal ulceration, and over a period of 4 years a failure rate of only 25% has been recorded. An alternative drug now undergoing trials is omeprazole, which has just been licensed for prolonged use. This proton pump inhibitor has been shown in double-blind trials to be superior to ranitidine.

These advances in the medical treatment of duodenal ulceration have meant that ulcer surgery – once one of the mainstays of any surgical practice – has become a rarity. Whilst this may represent a very satisfactory state of affairs for the majority of patients, it is exceedingly serious for the small minority of patients in whom surgical treatment becomes mandatory because of the development of complications such as uncontrollable relapses or bleeding which cannot be controlled. The rarity of such surgery unfortunately means that the surgeon's practical experience of dealing with such emergencies may be minute in the extreme. All surgery has a learning curve and repetitive performance of any operation leads to improvement in the results obtained.

21. Gallstones

Gallstones are found incidentally during routine autopsies in about 20% of the adult white population in the Western world, and it is obvious therefore that many must have remained symptomless throughout life. There is some evidence that the incidence of gallstones in a given population is in some way related to dietary factors, since gallstones are rare in developing countries and common in those communities in which the diet contains large numbers of calories and short-chain fatty acids.

CLASSIFICATION

Gallstones can be classified into three principal types:

1. Pure pigment stones.
2. Cholesterol stones.
3. Stones of mixed constitution.

To this list must be added the calcium carbonate stone, which is associated with calcification of the gallbladder wall, and the condition known as 'limey' bile.

The first two varieties are considered to be aseptic formations, a result of derangements of pigment or cholesterol metabolism, whereas the third variety is usually associated with an inflammatory process. Pure pigment or calcium bilirubinate stones are rare, pure cholesterol stones account for about 10% of all stones, and the remainder are 'mixed', but even these contain between 70 and 80% by weight of cholesterol.

Recently, a considerable volume of investigatory work has been carried out in an attempt to understand and localize the precise metabolic derangements associated with stone formation. The stimulus for these investigations has been the frequency of cholelithiasis and its complications in Western society, and the desire to find a medical regimen that might either prevent the disease or lead to the dissolution of stones already formed.

BIOCHEMICAL COMPOSITION OF BILE

Biochemical investigations have shown that the three important constituents of bile related to calculus formation are: the bile acids, the phospholipids, and cholesterol. The bile acids, cholic and chenodeoxycholic acid, are synthesized by the liver and represent the end product of cholesterol metabolism. In man, these acids are immediately conjugated with glycine (75%) or taurine (25%) to form the primary bile salts which account for approximately 80% of the solid matter in bile. In addition, bile also contains secondary bile salts, the deoxycholates, which are formed in the intestine during the enterohepatic circulation of bile when bacterial action converts cholic acid into deoxycholic acid and chenodeoxycholic acid into lithocholic acid. Of the two other major fractions in bile, the phospholipids, mainly lecithin, account for about 15% and cholesterol 5%.

The mixed micelle

The present concept regarding the nature of bile is that cholesterol, which is insoluble in water, is held in solution in normal bile because it is taken into micellar solution by the bile salts and the phospholipids. All three classes of compound possess water-soluble hydrophilic groups and water-insoluble (but oil-soluble) hydrophobic groups. When they are presented with a lipid–water interface, those compounds with a large component of hydrophilic groups orientate themselves so that the latter are, in effect, dissolved in the aqueous phase while the bulky lipophilic steroid nucleus is dissolved in the lipid phase.

The highest number of hydrophilic groups is found on the conjugated bile acids because they possess not only the greatest number of hydroxyl groups but also the negatively charged taurine and glycine radicles. Lecithin and cholesterol also organize themselves in a similar fashion, but neither can be actually dissolved in water. Their solution depends on their ability to combine with the bile acids to form the complex aggregates known as the mixed 'micelles', which are polymolecular aggregates comparable to detergents. The stability of such a chemical system depends wholly on the relative concentration of all three lipid classes.

CHOLESTEROL STONE FORMATION

An unresolved problem concerning the formation of cholesterol stones is whether the primary disturbance is in the liver cell itself or whether the defect lies elsewhere. Evidence supporting both these views has been discovered.

Certainly extrahepatic factors may have a considerable effect on the composition of bile. Thus, patients suffering from Crohn's disease or who have suffered a massive ileal resection have a two- to threefold increase in the incidence of cholesterol stone formation. This is thought to be because of the disturbance of the enterohepatic circulation of the bile salts due to their reduced absorption.

In man, the normal bile salt pool is small, 3–5 g, and it is turned over approximately six times a day. If reabsorption decreases, only a limited compensatory increase in production is possible, amounting to approximately 20%, after which production fails to keep pace with the loss.

In theory, if the bile salts decrease in quantity the relative concentration in the bile should fall, disturbing cholesterol solubilization and producing a lithogenic bile. In practical terms, as in the clinical conditions sited, it would indeed appear that a lithogenic bile is produced. However, experimental evidence is somewhat conflicting because, in the Rhesus monkey, as the concentration of bile salts falls the phospholipid concentration rises. This change would tend to overcome the adverse effects of the falling bile acid concentration because lecithin associates with the cholesterol fraction to form a liquid crystalline phase.

Cholesterol stones are also common in cirrhosis in which the bile salt pool is also reduced and the biliary concentration of bile salts falls. Since no extrinsic lesion is present, this suggests a primary liver cell defect possibly related to the lipoprotein plasma membrane of the bile canaliculi.

Bile obtained from a gallbladder in which cholesterol stones have formed differs both physically and chemically from normal. Ultracentrifuge studies reveal striking changes in the macromolecules and the cholesterol crystals. Chemically, the bile is oversaturated with cholesterol and the bile salt profile is disturbed.

Secondary factors

Stasis

When gallbladder contraction is reduced it is possible that small crystalline deposits may not be flushed from the viscus, allowing more time for the growth of stones. This is probably the reason why cholelithiasis is commoner in women than in men, for each pregnancy, particularly the last trimester, is associated with diminished motility. There is also abundant evidence that truncal vagotomy produces biliary stasis by decreasing the contractility of the gallbladder, and that this operation is associated with an increased incidence of gallstones. Decreased motility may also enable mucoprotein produced by the epithelial cells of the gallbladder to be retained and trapped in the mucosal niches. Such retained mucoprotein would then increase the viscosity of the bile and form a core and a scaffold upon which crystallization could build up.

Infection

In the past, the importance of infection was greatly stressed; Moynihan's dictum was that every gallstone was a monument to a dead bacterium. However, the importance of infection has been stressed less often of late because gallbladders containing stones are nearly always sterile. However, infection, as in acute cholecystitis, does have two important effects on the biliary tree:

a. Mucus production is enhanced and precipitable unconjugated bile acids are formed.
b. Infection with *Escherichia coli* increases the β-glucuronidase activity in the bile with the result that bilirubin glucuronide is hydrolysed to free bilirubin, which is then precipitated as calcium bilirubinate, one of the main constituents of 'infective' stones.

PIGMENT STONES

A pure pigment stone is formed only when excessive quantities of bile pigment are produced by red cell breakdown. Pigment stones are believed to represent the precipitation of non-polar unconjugated bilirubin, although it is difficult to demonstrate this substance in the bile, possibly because it is normally selectively reabsorbed by the liver cell membrane.

The greatest incidence of pigment stones occurs in hereditary spherocytosis in which stone formation is twice as common as in other haemolytic states such as sickle cell anaemia or thalassaemia major. A possible explanation of this difference is that the spherocyte contains a normal complement of haemoglobin whereas in the sickle cell disease there is a diminished red cell mass and in thalassaemia a reduced amount of haemoglobin per corpuscle.

SYMPTOMS OF GALLSTONES

As is clear from the autopsy evidence, the majority of gallstones must remain symptomless throughout the life of the patient, but in the absence of complications the common symptoms of which patients complain are either a dyspepsia of varying degrees of severity or attacks of biliary colic, which may be typical or atypical. Assuming that in such a patient investigation of the stomach and duodenum prove negative, the following means of investigating the gallbladder and its function exist:

1. *Ultrasonography.* This is now the first line of investigation in any patient suspected of biliary disease, since it is cheap, quickly performed and non-invasive and, unlike cholecystography, its efficacy does not depend on liver function. It is possible to confirm that the gallbladder can contract by observing its volume after a fatty meal.

2. *Oral cholecystography.* This investigation is only of use in the non-jaundiced patient since it depends on the intestinal absorption and hepatic excretion of the contrast medium. Furthermore the cystic duct has to be patent, otherwise the dye will not gain entrance to the gallbladder. In general a plain film of the abdomen is taken prior to the administration of the dye, usually iopanoic acid (Telepaque) or calcium iodate (Solu-Biloptin). After this, 3 g of either dye is administered by mouth and some 14 hours later the first films are taken, both in the erect and supine positions.

3. *Intravenous cholangiography.* When oral cholecystography is unsuccessful and there is reason to believe that some technical fault is responsible, intravenous cholangiography can be performed, which will produce satisfactory results provided the serum bilirubin is below 60 mmol/l. The patient is tested for iodine sensitivity after which an intravenous dye concentrated by the liver, e.g. iodopamide, is slowly injected. If films are taken 1–2 hours after the injection, some indication of partial obstruction can be obtained; if no obstruction is present the density of the dye in the duct decreases between these intervals whereas in the presence of obstruction an increase in concentration can be expected.

4. *ERCP.* Prior to treatment the presence of stones in the common bile duct can be confirmed by the performance of endoscopic retrograde cholangiopancreatography (ERCP), which involves

cannulation of the ampulla of Vater. This is of considerable importance when some of the newer methods of surgical treatment of gallstones are adopted since if common duct stones are present they can be treated by sphincterotomy.

TREATMENT OF UNCOMPLICATED BILIARY DISEASE

Non-invasive treatment

Two chemicals have been shown to be effective in causing the dissolution of some stones: chenodeoxycholic acid and urodeoxycholic acid. To be effective:

1. The stones must be wholly translucent, containing no calcium.
2. The stones should be of moderate size, i.e. not more than 2–2.5 cm in diameter.
3. The gallbladder should be functioning normally as shown by cholecystography.

When adequate doses of these drugs are given it has been shown that the cholesterol saturation index of bile obtained by nasoduodenal intubation after the intravenous administration of cholecystokinin falls to 0.8, at which point the dissolution of 'pure' cholesterol stones begins.

The only side-effect following the administration of these drugs is diarrhoea, which can be alleviated in most patients by temporarily reducing the dose for a matter of days.

The disadvantage is the period over which the drugs have to be taken, often as long as 2 years, and that recurrence may follow the cessation of treatment since the conditions causing the gallstones in the first place remain unaltered.

Lithotripsy. This technique has been 'borrowed' from the urologists as also has the technique of percutaneous cholelithotomy.

Invasive treatment

Laparoscopic cholecystectomy

Since this method was introduced in 1989 it has received wide publicity and large series of cases have been reported especially in the American literature. However, the method requires the relearning of hand–eye coordination and is not a technique which is easily learnt. In the US at the time of writing 38 centres have been set up to train surgeons in the technique. The advantages claimed are that the patient need only be hospitalized for one day. In one published series of 1000 cases the average duration of hospitalization was in fact 1.8 days as compared to 4.5 days for a routine cholecystectomy. However, in the learning curve there appears to be a moderately high incidence of complications, especially injuries to the common duct.

Routine cholecystectomy

Although requiring a longer period in hospital the mortality following cholecystectomy is low and the morbidity, given proper pre- and postoperative care, is minimal. In either operation a thorough knowledge of the extrahepatic biliary tree (including its various anomalies) must be appreciated. However, in practice it is probable that these variations and anomalies do not make a significant contribution to the incidence of ductal injuries and that the more important factor is haemorrhage in the operation field, which to the inexperienced operator appears to be uncontrollable, leading him or her to take panic measures – incorrectly applying instruments to control the bleeding when simple packing for several minutes will bring the haemorrhage to a halt. Further, the anatomy may be perfectly normal but the inexperienced surgeon may misinterpret his operative findings; for example, a normal but narrow common bile duct may easily be mistaken for the cystic duct, particularly if it should separate easily from the other structures contained in the right border of the lesser omentum.

The accepted normal anatomy of the ductal system

The commonly accepted description of the normal anatomy of this region is as follows (Fig. 21.1).

The right and left hepatic ducts emerge from the liver and join to form the common hepatic duct, in the great majority of individuals in an extrahepatic situation. At a somewhat lower level, the cystic duct enters the common hepatic duct, and below this level the duct, now known as the common bile duct, which is approximately 1 cm in diameter, proceeds inferiorly, posteriorly, and slightly laterally. It passes behind the duodenum and through the head of the pancreas to enter the medial surface of the duodenum at the ampulla of Vater. Recognition of both the common hepatic and common bile ducts is made easier by the presence on their surface of a venous network. The cystic duct is usually easily recognized near its junction with the

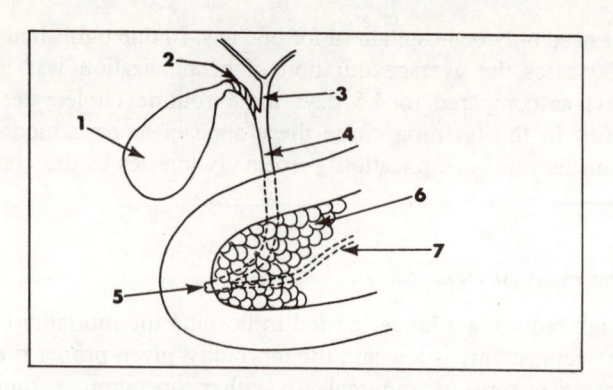

Fig. 21.1 Accepted 'normal' anatomy of the extrahepatic biliary system. 1, gallbladder; 2, cystic duct with valve of Heister; 3, common hepatic duct; 4, common bile duct; 5, ampulla of Vater; 6, pancreas; 7, duct of Wirsung.

common hepatic by the presence of the cystic duct lymph node and, in addition, this point also becomes more obvious once tension has been exerted on the gallbladder by cholecystectomy or sponge forceps. The level of the conjunction may be considered 'neutral' if a reasonable length of the common hepatic and common bile ducts can be identified above and below it.

Variations in the ductal system

1. Rarely, the cystic duct joins the right hepatic or the common hepatic at such a high level that an apparent trifurcation is produced (Fig. 21.2A). Either of these anatomical anomalies may cause difficulties at operation, particularly if a stone is impacted at the points of conjunction.

2. The cystic duct may run parallel with the course of the common hepatic for a considerable distance before joining the common bile duct (Fig. 21.2B), occasionally in the retroduodenal position or even within the pancreas. The cystic may be so tightly bound to the common bile duct that the only indication of the presence of this variation is a shallow groove between the two structures. A second indication that this anomaly exists may be the obvious presence, from the external appearance of the cystic duct, of the spiral valve of Heister which causes, when marked, a series of 'ripples' on the surface of the cystic duct.

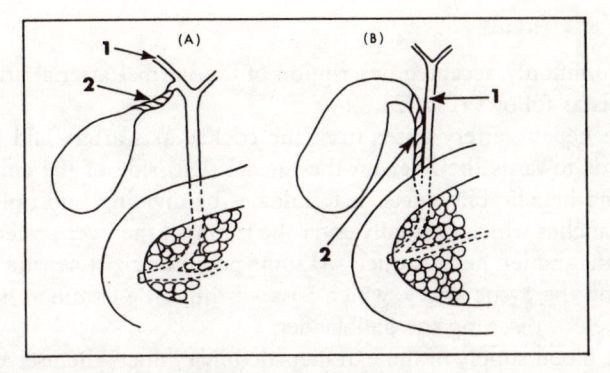

Fig. 21.2 Variations from normal in ductal system.
(A) Cystic duct joining the right hepatic duct.
1, right hepatic duct; 2, cystic duct entering right hepatic duct.
(B) Cystic duct running parallel with common hepatic duct for an abnormal distance.
1, common hepatic duct; 2, cystic duct running parallel to and usually adherent to common hepatic duct over an abnormal distance.

True anomalies

The cholecysto-hepatic duct. Such ducts are rare and are often unrecognized at the time of surgery because they emerge from the gallbladder bed and immediately join the gallbladder. During the dissection of the gallbladder from its bed a duct of this kind can easily be overlooked unless the operator is astute enough to recognize the presence of bile issuing either from the raw surface of the liver or from a small orifice on the hepatic surface of the gallbladder.

The importance of this rare anomaly is that, should it go unrecognized and the duct is left unligatured, in the early postoperative period it may cause an unexpectedly large loss of bile from the wound. Alternatively, it may cause biliary peritonitis or, at a later stage, lead to the development of a subphrenic abscess.

Accessory hepatic ducts. These are also rare and, if present, usually enter the common hepatic duct proximal to its junction with the cystic duct. As with a cholecysto-hepatic duct, inadvertent damage may lead to postoperative biliary leakage. However, unlike the former, this anomaly should be more easily recognized during the course of dissection.

Fusion of the cystic duct with the right hepatic duct. Fortunately, this anomaly is also rare, because if it is unrecognized a number of surgical misadventures, including ligation of the right hepatic duct, may await the unwary.

Vascular anatomy

The commonly accepted description of the normal arterial arrangement is as follows (Fig. 21.3):

The hepatic artery arises from the coeliac axis artery and passes upwards towards the liver on the medial (left) side of the common bile and hepatic bile ducts. It terminates by dividing into right and left branches which normally enter the hilum of the liver posterior to the right and left hepatic ducts. At some point the right hepatic artery gives off the cystic artery, which passes behind the common hepatic duct before reaching the gallbladder.

The blood supply of the extrahepatic biliary ducts themselves was virtually ignored until the appearance of a classic paper on the subject by Northover and Terblanche. They found that these ducts were supplied by two small arteries positioned at the 3 and 9 o'clock positions.

Anomalies of arterial supply

The arterial anomalies are important to the surgeon because unanticipated and unrecognized vascular anomalies may be the cause of severe bleeding if such a vessel is inadvertently divided before a ligature has been applied. If this should happen, damage to the biliary system could result if attempts to control the haemorrhage are misdirected. Furthermore, although a normal healthy individual is usually unaffected by division and ligation of the right hepatic artery,

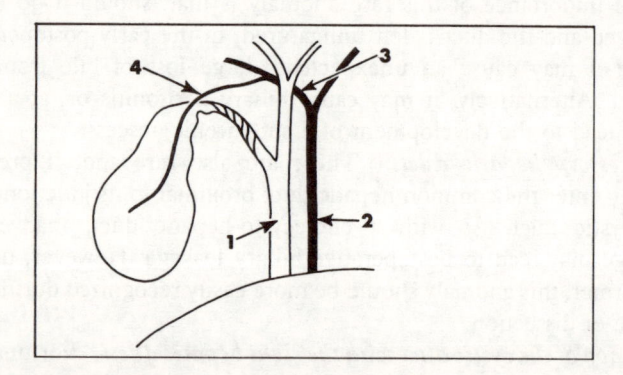

Fig. 21.3 Normal arrangement of hepatic arteries.
1, common bile duct; 2, hepatic artery; 3, right branch of hepatic artery passing behind bile duct; 4, cystic artery.

which is the vessel in greatest danger, in the presence of cirrhosis the result may be fatal.

The common anomalies of the vascular supply to the liver and biliary system in order of frequency are:

1. *The presence of an accessory cystic artery.* These arteries always arise from the right hepatic artery. Unrecognized, such an artery may be avulsed from the main artery causing severe haemorrhage with all its attendant dangers.

2. *Anterior transposition of the right hepatic artery* (Fig. 21.4) and hence of the cystic artery. Such an anatomical arrangement should be of little importance, but if the artery crosses the common bile duct at a relatively inferior level it may interfere with its exploration, i.e. cholodochotomy, should this be considered necessary.

3. *The 'caterpillar hump' right hepatic artery.* This is the least common of the arterial anomalies. The artery, instead of proceeding directly into the hilum, forms a loop which bulges laterally beyond the right hepatic duct in either an anterior or posterior position. This anomaly is frequently associated with a short, stubby, cystic artery so that the application of a ligature becomes technically difficult. An alternative source of danger is failure to recognize the anomaly at all, with the result that the vessel is ligated and divided after which the two cut ends may slip from the ligature and cause torrential bleeding.

Causes to injury to the extrahepatic biliary system

The common causes of injury to the extrahepatic biliary system include:

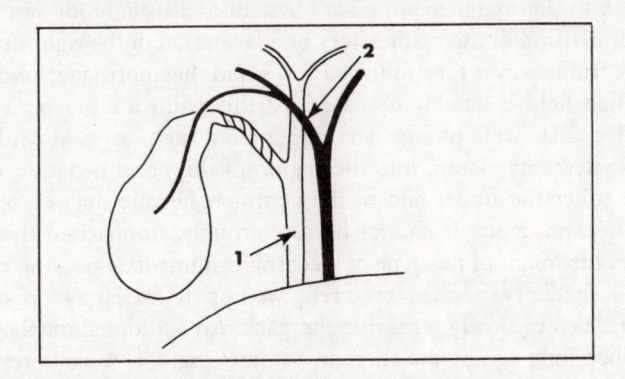

Fig. 21.4 Transposition of right hepatic artery.
1, common bile duct; 2, anterior transposition of right hepatic artery.

1. Failure to recognize the common duct even in the presence of negligible pathological changes. This can only be defined as 'ham-handed' surgery and should seldom, if ever, occur. Cholecystectomy demands the proper visualization of all parts of the biliary tract before any ligature or clamp is applied, or structure divided, and a large part is played in this by the assistants. Remember Moynihan's dictum, it is the assistants who perform the operation. This was, of course, particularly true in his day in which relaxants were unknown. Then, exposure of the biliary tree demanded a full-scale Kocher's incision from the tip of the tenth rib on the right to the costal margin on the opposite side, the incision being placed two fingers' breadth below the costal margin.

2. 'Tenting' of the common bile duct at its junction with the cystic duct. This type of injury, in which a cholecystectomy forcep is placed across the right lateral face of the common duct, occurs only if excessive traction is used when attempting to identify and ligate the junction of the cystic with the hepatic ducts. It is also more common when there is little or no pathology of the common duct. An absence of inflammatory change allows it to be more easily displaced laterally by traction from the right free border of the gastro-hepatic omentum.

3. Northover and Terblanche concluded from their work on the blood supply of the extrahepatic ducts that in some cases overenthusiastic exposure of the junction of the cystic duct with the common hepatic duct, particularly if followed by a 'flush tie', might produce avascular necrosis and later stricture formation in a small number of patients.

4. Injury caused by inadvertent clamping during the arrest of unanticipated bleeding. This is now the most common cause of damage to the extrahepatic biliary system and usually follows avulsion or division of the cystic artery or a laceration of the right hepatic artery. Either event is followed by rapid haemorrhage, and the operation field is quickly obscured. At this point the inexperienced operator may well plunge an instrument, such as a Moynihan's cholecystectomy clamp, into the region of the porta hepatitis, damaging either the upper end of the common hepatic duct or one or both hepatic ducts. It cannot be too strongly emphasized that the correct treatment of this type of bleeding is immediate packing of the wound. Patience is then required, waiting if necessary up to 30 minutes before slowly removing the pack. An additional manoeuvre, described long ago by the surgeon Seton Pringle, is to compress the hepatic artery in the free border of the hepatoduodenal ligament. The latter has not been found by the author to be of great value.

Less common causes of injury include:

a. Damage during the performance of a partial gastrectomy. This was commoner in the past when this operation, which involves mobilization of the first part of the duodenum, was in general use for the treatment of severe duodenal ulceration.
b. Operations designed to remove diverticuli from the second part of the duodenum.

How to avoid injury

1. *Obtain an adequate exposure* of the area by a generous incision and good retraction when performing 'orthodox' cholecystectomy.
2. *Define all structures*; in particular clearly demonstrate the junction of the cystic duct with the common hepatic duct and the hepatic and common bile ducts proximal and distal to this point.
3. Should the anatomy of the region be so distorted by disease that 2. above appears impossible, then retrograde cholecystectomy should be performed, removing the gallbladder from the fundus towards the cystic duct. Unfortunately, this may be far from easy because of bleeding from the liver bed which, however, can be controlled by a second assistant putting pressure on the raw surface with a retractor well padded with gauze, and advancing the retractor progressively as the dissection proceeds.
4. In cases presenting overwhelming technical difficulty the inexperienced surgeon should retire from the scene after first performing a cholecystotomy and extracting those stones present in the gallbladder.
5. Do not open the common bile duct unless previous investigation or operative cholangiography demonstrates the necessity for this manoeuvre.
6. Transduodenal exploration. Several papers have appeared recently suggesting that transduodenal exploration of the common bile duct accompanied by sphincteroplasty is a viable alternative to supraduodenal exploration. The mortality of this operation is variously reported as being between 0.5 and 2%. However, two dangers are associated with this procedure: postoperative pancreatitis and leakage from the duodenum. The protagonists of this manoeuvre, however, claim that in their hands the mortality is no greater than supraduodenal exploration of the duct. No controlled trial comparing the morbidity and mortality of the two methods of exploration has been reported.

Clinical signs of inadvertent injury

Injuries recognized at the time of operation

Inadvertent division of the common bile duct at the time of the operation, if recognized immediately, should be followed by repair. A one-layer anastomosis of the cut ends is performed, leaving a T-tube inserted through a separate opening in the duct in place for 3 weeks. Anastomotic breakdown, which will cause the escape of bile from the wound, inevitably means the subsequent development of a stricture. Such an event can be demonstrated by postoperative cholangiography performed via the T-tube on the 10th and 16th days. Immediate repair is not, however, necessarily followed by long-term success. In Blumgart's recent paper, of 78 common duct strictures 15 had followed immediate repair.

Injuries unrecognized at the time of operation

Unfortunately, the majority of injuries are nowadays afflicted on the hepatic ducts themselves or occur high in the common hepatic duct, and it is this type of injury that may go unnoticed, particularly by a relatively inexperienced surgeon.

The common postoperative course, if such an injury occurs, is as follows:

1. There is a profuse discharge of bile from the wound in the early postoperative period.
2. Intermittent fever develops.
3. The biliary discharge may stop and the subsequent development of either a right supra- or infra-hepatic collection of bile will require drainage.
4. Increasing jaundice, associated with intractable pruritus, anorexia and rapid loss of weight may develop.
5. In many patients, after an illness associated with jaundice and intermittent fever lasting for several weeks, resolution apparently occurs, the fever abates, and the jaundice diminishes, although it seldom disappears. This is a sign that the upper end of the damaged duct or ducts is in communication with the duodenum via a fistulous tract lined by granulation tissue. Unfortunately, such tracts do not usually remain open or uninfected for very long, hence recurrent fever and jaundice can be expected after a variable interval of time.

6. At any time, the following serious consequences may follow the development of a stricture:
   a. Biliary cirrhosis.
   b. Multiple cholangitic abscesses.
   c. Portal hypertension.

MAJOR COMPLICATIONS OF GALLSTONES

The major complications of gallstones are:

1. Complications within the gallbladder:
   a. Acute cholecystitis.
   b. Carcinoma of the gallbladder.
2. Complications within the common duct and liver:
   a. Obstructive jaundice.
   b. Obstructive cholangiohepatitis.
   c. Biliary cirrhosis.
3. Complications affecting other viscera:
   a. Spontaneous cholecystoduodenal fistula.
   b. Gallstone ileus.
4. Metabolic complications:
   a. Steatorrhoea in the presence of obstructive jaundice.
   b. Hepatorenal failure.

Complications within the gallbladder

Acute cholecystitis

Although acute cholecystitis can occur in the absence of gallstones, even in these circumstances the disease becomes obstructive at an early stage due to oedema of the cystic duct. The initial description of the sequence of events following the sudden impaction of a stone in the cystic duct or the neck of the gallbladder was made by Rutherford Morrison. Following impaction, the gallbladder becomes distended with mucus, bile and blood due to exudation associated with acute chemical inflammation and transudation secondary to congestion of the gallbladder wall. As the gallbladder becomes distended, so the intraluminal tension interferes with the blood supply to produce necrosis and rupture of the gallbladder wall.

As the chemical phase advances, there is a secondary bacterial infection with coliforms and bacteroides. In the author's personal series of 200 consecutive cases of acute cholecystitis, there was perforation of the gallbladder in 16, but this produced a generalized biliary peritonitis in only 4 patients because, in the remainder, the effects of perforation were masked by the rapid isolation of the gallbladder from the peritoneal cavity by the omentum.

Clinical features. The chief clinical manifestations of acute cholecystitis are pain in the right upper quadrant of the abdomen and a fever that usually rises to 38–39°C. Examination reveals extreme tenderness, rebound tenderness, and rigidity. If the gallbladder perforates before the viscus is sealed from the general peritoneal cavity, the whole abdomen is rigid.

Some observers state that acute obstructive cholecystitis can be distinguished from the non-obstructive variety by the presence of a mass in the former which is not observed in the latter. This is a dubious distinction because the ability to palpate a mass is, in large measure, dependent on the presence or absence of rigidity.

Differential diagnosis. The common conditions from which acute cholecystitis must be distinguished are as follows:

1. *Perforated peptic ulcer.* In this condition there is usually a previous history of ulcer dyspepsia and only rarely do the signs of peritonitis remain limited to the upper abdomen. In the early stages, there is no fever, and a plain X-ray of the abdomen in the erect position shows air under the diaphragm in 40% of patients.
2. *Acute pancreatitis.* This may be difficult to distinguish, but in severe cases there is nearly always severe backpain and hypotension due to plasma loss. Although the serum amylase may be elevated in acute cholecystitis it never reaches the levels seen in acute pancreatitis, i.e. 1000 Somogyi units and above.
3. *Miscellaneous conditions.* See Non-surgical causes of acute abdominal pain.

The investigations required to establish an absolute diagnosis of acute cholecystitis are:

1. *Plain X-ray of the abdomen and chest.* The latter is necessary to exclude pneumonic conditions. The former yields evidence supporting the diagnosis in over 60% of patients. The radiological physical signs observed include (*a*) an absence of gas under the diaphragm, (*b*) a soft tissue mass, (*c*) presence of opaque gallstones, and (*d*) gas in the gallbladder itself.
2. *Serum amylase.* In acute cholecystitis this is usually less than 500 Somogyi units.
3. *Differential white count.* The white count should be elevated with a relative polymorphonuclear leucocytosis.

4. *Serum bilirubin.* Jaundice may occur in acute cholecystitis due either to oedema in the region of Hartmann's pouch compressing the common duct, or the presence of concomitant common duct stones.
5. *Ultrasonography.* In the presence of calculous cholecystitis this investigation may reveal an increased diameter of the gallbladder, thickening of its wall and, lastly, the presence of a calculus.
6. *Cholescintigraphy.* This investigation, performed using ^{99m}Tc-HIDA demonstrates blockage of the cystic duct.

Treatment of acute cholecystitis. Much controversy surrounds the question of the treatment of this disease; the major dilemma is whether early or delayed surgery produces the best results.

Du Plessis states that if operation is performed on the basis of clinical diagnosis alone a number of mistakes will be made due to faulty diagnosis. He gives as examples of possible incorrect diagnoses acute pancreatitis, secondary carcinoma of the liver, or primary carcinoma of the gallbladder. It would seem logical to argue that these 'mistakes' are of little ultimate consequence to the patient. He also states that, in approximately 10% of patients suffering from acute cholecystitis, there may be a stone in the common bile duct difficult to diagnose and technically difficult to remove in the presence of acute inflammation. The latter is a more cogent argument. Other authors such as Glenn favour early operation. There is, in fact, no great advantage in rigid adherence to one method or another. Much depends on the skill and experience of the surgeon under whose care the patient is admitted. Those who claim that early operation is time-saving, particularly of hospital beds, are probably wrong, for careful examination of a personal series showed that complications of acute cholecystectomy could delay the discharge of patients for so long that the mean duration of hospital stay became equal to the two separate admissions required to treat the patient conservatively and then readmit for further elective surgery. In the author's series of 200 patients, 100 treated by operation and 100 treated conservatively, 4 patients died in each group. All were over 75 years of age. It became obvious from studying this and other series that acute obstructive cholecystitis is only mortal in the elderly. Of those who died in the author's series, two patients in each group might have been saved by the alternative treatment regimen.

Technical difficulties associated with acute cholecystectomy. Occasionally, operation in the acute stage becomes difficult due to oedema, fibrosis, or distortion of the anatomy. In these circumstances two alternatives exist. First, cholecystectomy can be abandoned and a cholecystostomy alone performed. If this is done all the stones must be removed, otherwise a mucous fistula tends to develop. Alternatively, the cholecystectomy can be performed from the fundus proximally so that, finally, the gallbladder is left attached to the hepatic artery by the cystic artery and the common duct by the cystic duct. If either of these methods is adopted, damage to the common duct should not occur.

Complications of acute cholecystectomy. Apart from damage to the common bile duct itself the chief complications of this operation are:

1. Pulmonary atelectasis and embolus.
2. Prolonged bile drainage.
3. Wound infection.

Conservative management. Conservative management of acute cholecystitis demands bed rest, restricted oral fluids, and analgesics to reduce pain. An appropriate antibiotic is probably helpful but not mandatory.

The abdomen should be repeatedly examined and the abdominal tenderness should be greatly reduced within 48–72 hours. As it does so, an inflammatory mass becomes palpable which should then slowly disappear.

Conservative treatment should be immediately abandoned if there is rapid progression, as opposed to resolution, of the physical signs indicating the development of biliary peritonitis, or increasing systemic disturbance indicating uncontrolled infection.

Occasionally, an acute attack ends in the development of a mucocele of the gallbladder. A large pear-shaped palpable mass develops in the right upper quadrant which at operation is found to contain colourless mucus. If a patient is treated conservatively and the gallbladder is left in situ after an acute attack, approximately 30% of patients will suffer further attacks of acute inflammation, suggesting the advisability of interval cholecystectomy.

Carcinoma of the gallbladder

This is infrequent, and is rare in the absence of gallstones. The commoner tumour is an adenocarcinoma, but occasionally, in the presence of gallstones, squamous metaplasia appears, with the later development of a squamous cell carcinoma. In most patients the disease is inoperable when first seen. The common presenting signs are a mass in the right upper quadrant and obstructive jaundice.

Complications of stones within the common duct

The presence of gallstones in the common duct does not necessarily lead to the development of jaundice. This is proven by postmortem statistics which show that cholelithiasis is present in 25% of patients dying of intercurrent disease and that stones are found in the common bile duct in 25% of these patients. It is obvious, therefore, that most common duct stones are symptomless. When, however, there are symptoms, the various clinical syndromes that may follow are obstructive jaundice, obstructive cholangiohepatitis, multiple liver abscesses and biliary cirrhosis.

Obstructive jaundice

When obstructive jaundice is due to the presence of stones in the common bile duct it is usually intermittent. The jaundice usually follows an acute attack of abdominal pain, the conjunctivae are noted to be yellow, the urine becomes the colour of cold tea, and the stools putty-coloured. In the absence of gross infection the jaundice commonly fades and disappears within a few days. If there are no contraindications to operation or, alternatively, the jaundice persists, surgical treatment is required. In the absence of jaundice an intravenous cholangiogram may confirm the presence of choledocholithiasis. In the presence of jaundice this investigation is useless. Ultrasonography may be helpful if the common duct is grossly dilated, but this is not an invariable accompaniment of obstructive jaundice due to stones. Furthermore, gallstones lodged at the lower end of the common bile duct may remain undetected.

Of greater effectiveness is endoscopic retrograde cholangiopancreatography if this is available, performed following a prophylactic dose of a broad spectrum antibiotic to prevent endotoxaemia if the biliary tree is infected, or alternatively, percutaneous transhepatic cholangiography using the skinny-needle technique described by Okuda and others in 1974. Using such a needle the dangers associated with biliary leakage following withdrawal of the needle from the liver are much reduced. When the ducts are dilated they can nearly always be cannulated and the cause of obstruction of the biliary tree established. In a jaundiced patient the prothrombin time should be estimated prior to the investigation and if it is elevated it must be reduced to normal levels by the administration of vitamin K prior to investigation.

Treatment. During routine cholecystectomy an operative cholangiogram should be performed. In many centres this is regarded as a routine procedure performed during every operation whereas in other centres this added investigation would be performed if the common duct is found to be greater than 10 mm in diameter, the accepted upper limit of normal. False positive results may be obtained if the lower end of the duct is in systole at the time the examination is performed and following dilatation of the lower end of the duct by Bake's dilators an abnormal appearance, difficult to interpret, may be seen.

When stones remain in the common duct following cholecystectomy an attempt can be made to relieve the situation by sphincterotomy performed via a fibreoptic endoscope. The chief danger of this procedure is haemorrhage, which contributes in greater part to the mortality associated with this condition, approximately 1%.

Cholangiohepatitis

This is caused by a combination of obstruction to the common bile duct, usually by stone, together with infection. The infecting organisms are both aerobic and anaerobic and include the coliforms, of which *Escherichia coli* is the most common, the bacteroides, and the anaerobic streptococci. If the infection is acute, a bacteraemia may develop leading to the onset of chills and fever, mental confusion, dyspnoea, and, possibly, hypotension. The latter usually develops within 10–16 hours of the onset of the disease and may lead to secondary renal failure. Initially, in bacteraemic shock the peripheral skin is warm and dry, but as the condition progresses, peripheral circulatory failure ensues with the development of cold cyanotic limbs. Even in the absence of overt clinical infection, organisms are commonplace in a common duct that contains stones. A further clinical syndrome associated with cholangitis is Charcot's intermittent hepatic fever, a combination of intermittent jaundice, pain and fever.

Route of infection. The precise route by which the biliary tree becomes infected is still open to question. Three alternative hypotheses have been advanced: the haematogenous, lymphatic, and direct intraluminal. Each of these theories has its protagonists and antagonists. When the jaundice rapidly deepens and there is severe fever there is an absolute indication to drain the biliary tree.

The precise operation depends on the anatomical findings at operation; the minimum required is the performance of a cholecystostomy and choledochostomy. In practice, every effort should be made to extract the obstructing stone from the common duct, which will be found to be grossly dilated, thick-walled, hyperaemic, and filled with purulent bile-stained fluid. Prior to, and immediately after drainage, the patient must receive a suitable antimicrobial drug. At the time of the operation, swabs should be taken for the culture of both aerobic and anaerobic organisms and the determination of their sensitivity. At initial microscopic examination *E. coli* cannot by Gram staining be differentiated from any other Gram-negative organism and, therefore, culture and a variety of biochemical tests are necessary. However, the majority of *E. coli* are sensitive to ampicillin and gentamicin or the cephalosporins and these compounds form a suitable starting point for antimicrobial therapy. On theoretical grounds, rifampicin, which is concentrated in the bile, should be the ideal agent, but without drainage or the spontaneous relief of obstruction antibiotics cannot actually reach the infected area in high concentration. The development of multiple liver abscesses is an ever-present danger if a conservative policy is adopted, hence the danger of accepting the dictum that Charcot's intermittent hepatic fever is always intermittent. When an abscess forms secondary to cholangitis the clinical condition of the patient deteriorates. The liver itself becomes enlarged, and scattered through it are numerous greenish-yellow areas. Some of these are soft, others solid. If there has been cavitation the pus is deeply bile-stained.

Biliary cirrhosis

Although biliary cirrhosis is more common in association with simple or malignant strictures of the common bile duct it is still occasionally seen in patients who have suffered intermittent obstruction due to stones. There are histological changes around the central bile canaliculi, which rupture due to the increased biliary pressure. When an infective element is present a dense concentration of inflammatory cells accumulates in the portal zone which will, in the absence of progressive infection, later be replaced by fibrosis and bile duct proliferation. As the fibrous tissue bands grow in size and coalesce, the lobules are reduced in size. In the later stages, biliary cirrhosis may be difficult to distinguish from portal cirrhosis although foci of liver cell hyperplasia are less conspicuous in the former.

A patient suffering from biliary cirrhosis usually remains in reasonable health, and in the absence of infection physical deterioration is slow to develop. In the late stages of the disease, however, the patient appears very ill, the skin coloration becomes greenish, and there will be portal hypertension and associated hepatic failure. There may be various physical manifestations, which include hepatic failure, pruritis, xanthomata, enlargement of the liver and spleen, steatorrhoea, and osteomalacia. Since the hepatic changes may well be reversible, every effort must be made to relieve the obstruction.

Complications affecting other viscera

Fistula formation

Acute inflammatory change complicating stones in the gallbladder or common duct may result in adherence of either viscus to the duodenum, with the production of a fistulous tract between the two. Once the acute inflammatory process has resolved the patient may become symptomless. In these circumstances the diagnosis is sometimes made by a plain X-ray of the abdomen which will show air outlining the biliary tree.

Treatment. In general all that is required to deal with a cholecystoduodenal fistula is blunt separation of the two viscera by pressure between the finger and thumb. The gallbladder is removed and the duodenal defect which is never more than a few millimetres in diameter is closed by two layers with catgut.

Gallstone ileus

Very rarely, a large gallstone passes from the gallbladder into the duodenum and makes its way down the small bowel. Normally, it impacts in the distal ileum where the lumen of the bowel is narrowest. The obstruction, being of a simple variety, may be present for several days and is associated with intermittent vomiting, small bowel colic, and slowly increasing distension. A preoperative diagnosis may be made if air is present in the biliary tree and a gallstone can be seen lying in the lumen of the bowel. Treatment consists of resuscitation followed by laparotomy. The stone, if possible, is milked proximally away from the site of impaction and removed through a small enterostomy. The primary condition of the biliary passages may or may not be explored immediately, a decision which depends upon the age, general condition of the patient and the accessibility of the gallbladder, which is usually surrounded by adhesions.

Metabolic complications

Steatorrhoea

In the presence of obstructive jaundice steatorrhoea occurs because of the absence of bile salts from the intestine. In general, the severity of malabsorption is related to the degree of obstruction, which can be assessed by measuring either the serum bilirubin or the faecal stercobilinogen content.

If the obstruction is of long duration, which is unlikely when the cause is due to stone, there may be nutritional deficiencies due to lack of absorption of the fat-soluble vitamins A, D and K. Lack of vitamin A produces night blindness and hyperkeratosis, lack of vitamin D, osteomalacia with its associated kyphosis and fractures, and lack of vitamin K produces a prolonged prothrombin time associated with spontaneous bruising.

Hepatorenal failure

The mortality of operations performed for the relief of obstructive jaundice is abnormally high, approaching 10%. At least half these patients develop increasing jaundice and progressive renal failure, the hepatorenal syndrome, which is particularly likely if the patient suffers from hypotension during or immediately after operation. It was thought at first that jaundiced patients suffered from a reduced blood volume, but this has been disproved. Current experimental evidence suggests that high circulating levels of bilirubin glucuronide sensitize the cells of the renal tubules to the adverse effects of ischaemia. The glucuronide reaches the tubules after passing through the glomeruli. Such evidence suggests that every effort should be made to avoid hypovolaemic hypotension during operations on the obstructed biliary tree and that renal function should be assisted by the routine use of mannitol infusion daily following surgery.

22. Acute pancreatitis

The Marseille symposium on the aetiology and pathology of pancreatitis agreed that acute pancreatitis should be subdivided into two main types, acute pancreatitis and relapsing acute pancreatitis, in both of which conditions morphological and functional recovery of the gland can be expected once the cause or factor responsible has been eliminated. This variety never progresses to the chronic form, even though the pancreas may be scarred. The incidence of both conditions is extremely variable. In the UK it is as low as 5 per 100 000 of the population, with a mean age of 50 at onset, whereas in the US the incidence varies from 4 per 100 000 in persons below the age of 30 to 62 per 100 000 of the population in persons over the age of 70. It is believed that this variation is accounted for by the greater degree of alcoholism in the latter country. Similarly, in the UK the incidence is far higher in Scotland than in England, again possibly due to the higher consumption of alcohol north of the border.

AETIOLOGY

Certain well-recognized associations have been identified even though the exact relationship and mechanism by which they produce the acute changes in the gland remains an enigma.
  They include:

- Gallstones.
- Alcholism.
- Drugs, e.g. thiazide diuretics, azathoprine, 6-mercaptopurine and corticosteroids.
- Infections, e.g. mumps, *Mycoplasma pneumoniae* and coxsackie B virus.

- Metabolic conditions, e.g. aminoaciduria, Types I and IV hereditary lipoproteinaemia.
- Postoperative, especially after Polya gastrectomy, ERCP or forceful dilatation of the sphincter of Oddi.
- Post-traumatic, usually after closed abdominal injury.

Of these the two most important are gallstones and alcoholism. The latter is a common association in France, the US and Scotland, in all of which the intake of alcohol is excessive in certain areas and within certain groups of the population.

Although the association between gallstones and acute pancreatitis is clear – cholelithiasis being present in as many as 70% of cases of pancreatitis in some series – the mechanism by which gallstones cause pancreatitis remains unclear. The probability, however, that they are of aetiological significance is strengthened by the finding of gallstones in the stools of patients suffering from acute pancreatitis, suggesting that at the onset of the attack a gallstone was passing from the biliary system into the gastrointestinal tract. In 1901 Opie described his classical case involving a small gallstone impacted in the ampulla of Vater. This led to the 'common channel theory' in which it was postulated that a stone impacted in the distal end of the common biliopancreatic duct allowed the reflux of bile from the biliary tree into the pancreatic ductal system, the bile triggering pancreatitis either by activating pancreatic enzymes or by injuring pancreatic cells directly. However, this theory has been rejected on the basis that only in a small minority of patients is the conjunction of the biliary and pancreatic ducts of sufficient length to permit outflow obstruction. Further, since the pancreatic secretory pressure exceeds the biliary secretory pressure distal obstruction would favour a flow of pancreatic juice into the bile duct rather than the reverse. Furthermore bile itself does not activate pancreatic enzymes, and experimental surgical procedures that direct bile flow through an unobstructed pancreatic ductal system do not result in pancreatitis.

A second theory is that acute pancreatitis is caused by the reflux of activated digestive enzymes or even bile and trypsin into the pancreatic duct via an incompetent sphincter of Oddi, an incompetence caused by the recent passage of a stone through the ampulla. This theory could explain those cases of acute pancreatitis which follow afferent loop obstruction after a Polya gastrectomy. This suggestion was supported by the fact that this situation can be produced in an experimental animal such as the dog by forming a closed loop of duodenum, the Pfeffer loop, and then restoring continuity of the gastrointestinal tract by anastomosing the stomach to the jejunum. If this is done, acute haemorrhagic pancreatic necrosis occurs, although if at the same time the pancreatic duct is ligated no pathological changes occur in the gland; also, in a normal animal, ligation is merely followed by atrophy.

A third theory is that the offending stone triggers pancreatitis by obstructing the ductal system, leading to rupture of the smaller ducts and hence extravasation of pancreatic juice into the parenchyma of the gland. The objections to this theory are that ligation of the pancreatic duct causes atrophy and that pancreatic ductal fluid normally contains inactive digestive enzymes and that these would be released unactivated.

The known effects of alcohol on the pancreas which may be of importance in the pathogenesis of acute pancreatitis are:

1. It stimulates the secretion of pancreatic juice and increases the intraductal pressure.
2. It increases the protein concentration in the pancreatic duct. This may then coagulate to produce plugs which cause ductal obstruction.
3. It reduces the tone of the ampullary sphincter, a factor which might allow reflux into the pancreatic duct, thus activating the pancreatic enzymes which then might diffuse through the wall of the ducts and cause destruction of the parenchyma.

Whatever the mechanism the onset of severe pancreatitis leads to the rapid release of a 'toxic broth' into the interstitial tissues of the gland, the peripancreatic tissues and the bloodstream. Within the 'broth' are:

1. *A variety of proteolytic enzymes including chymotrysin, carboxy-peptidase, elastase, phospholipase A and lysolecithin.* The proteolytic enzymes recovered from the pancreas in experimental pancreatitis, trypsin and chymotrysin, can cause pancreatic inflammation when injected into the pancreatic duct. It is probable that the chief action of trypsin is to activate the enzymes elastase and phosphatase A, and possible kallikrein. Elastase, which causes the dissolution of elastic fibres in blood vessels, appears to be important in the transition from oedematous to haemorrhagic pancreatitis and concentrations of high levels of elastase have been found in the pancreas of patients dying of haemorrhagic pancreatitis. Phospholipase A is important in the development of pancreatic necrosis by promoting production of lysolecithin from bile lecithin.

2. *Unidentified short-chain peptides* which produce myocardial depression and shock lung.
3. *Endotoxins.*

PATHOLOGY

Once damage has occurred to the acinar cells a series of changes occurs within the gland. The role of the various pancreatic enzymes remains a matter of conjecture. In the transition from an oedematous form to the haemorrhagic elastase liberated by the action of trypsin from pro-elastase appears to be important causing the dissolution of the elastic fibres of the blood vessels and thus bleeding into the parenchyma of the gland and beyond. Phospholipase A also activated by trypsin is important in the development of necrosis by converting bile lecithin to lysolecithin and in addition ischaemia caused most probably by a variety of vasoactive substances not only promotes haemorrhage but also necrosis.

It is usual to distinguish three grades of acute pancreatitis, each of increasing severity according to the pathological changes in the gland: the interstitial or oedematous, haemorrhagic, and gangrenous. In oedematous pancreatitis the gland itself is swollen and oedematous and surrounded by exudate. It has been estimated that 20–30% of the circulating blood volume may leak within 6 hours of the onset of the disease, a finding which has given rise to the expression 'pancreatic burn'. In the more severe haemorrhagic and gangrenous varieties of the disease the circulating blood volume is further reduced by pooling of blood in the splanchnic bed.

In haemorrhagic pancreatitis the gland is not only swollen but is also bright red in colour due to bleeding. This may be patchy or involve the whole gland. In this variety of pancreatitis clotting in the small vessels in and around the pancreas may be found, thus impairing the microcirculation. In addition, areas of fat necrosis are found in the region of the pancreas, in the mesocolon and omentum. Although it has always been assumed that this was directly due to the liberation of lipase it is now considered to be due to the combined effects of both lipase and a phospholipase.

In gangrenous pancreatitis tissue necrosis destroys the entire structure of the gland, both exocrine and endocrine, the supporting tissue, and the blood vessels. At the margin of the necrotic areas, collections of polymorphonuclear cells are found but there is now general agreement among pathologists that this is not a truly inflammatory lesion and for this reason the term 'acute pancreatic necrosis' is being increasingly used. However, once death of tissue has occurred infection commonly follows so that not only large sloughs of pancreatic tissue may be found but also purulent exudate.

CLINICAL PRESENTATION

Acute pancreatitis presents as an 'acute abdomen', pain being present in over 90% of sufferers. Cases associated with alcohol tend to occur in younger patients whereas those associated with gallstones affect an older group. The onset may follow excess of either food or alcohol. The pain in a typical case is band-like, the pain in the back being as severe or even more severe than that felt in the epigastrium, although so concerned may be the patient with the severity of the abdominal pain that he or she fails to describe the girdle-like nature of the pain. In addition to pain nausea, vomiting and hiccup may occur. On physical examination the abdomen is usually rigid, especially in the upper quadrants, and occasionally there may be discolouration in the loins or around the umbilicus – Cullen and Grey Turner's signs – although both are more common following the rupture of an intra-abdominal aneurysm. In addition there may be slight fever. In areas in which the incidence of the disease is low the condition may not even be considered and a mistaken diagnosis of perforated peptic ulcer, acute cholecystitis, myocardial infarction or infarction of the bowel may be made, the situation being further confused by the fact that the serum amylase, the commonest diagnostic indicator used, may well be elevated in any of the above conditions.

CLASSIFICATION OF THE SEVERITY OF THE DISEASE

The initial clinical examination only identifies one-third of patients in whom severe disease is present; after 24 hours recognition of severity is possible in 78%, and after 48 hours in 83%.

A classification of the disease into three categories – mild, moderate and severe – may be based on the clinical features found on examination, i.e. the presence of 'shock', adequacy of peripheral perfusion, urine output, the presence of respiratory distress, fever, body wall staining, degree of abdominal wall staining, degree of abdominal tenderness, distension and, lastly, the presence of ileus. Using more precise indicators the Glasgow Prognostic Score takes the following eight factors into consideration:

1. White cell count $>15 \times 10^9/l$.
2. Blood glucose >10 mmol/l.
3. Blood urea >16 mmol/l and not falling on rehydration.
4. Serum calcium < 2 mmol/l.
5. Serum albumin < 32 g/l.
6. Serum LDH >600 U/l.
7. Serum SGOT or SGPT >200 U/l.

The presence of more than three factors is indicative of a severe attack.

Even more complex systems have been evolved by applying the APACHE II system to the disease, APACHE standing for *a*cute *p*hysiological *a*nd *c*hronic *h*ealth *e*valuation, this system permitting a division of those cases in which a severe attack is occurring within a few hours of the onset of the disease. In this system the following parameters are taken into account: rectal temperature, mean arterial blood pressure, heart rate, respiratory rate, oxygenation, arterial pH, serum sodium, serum potassium, serum creatinine, haematocrit, white cell count, and the Glasgow coma scale as well as the age and general health of the individual concerned.

INVESTIGATIONS

The commonest diagnostic indicator used in the initial stages of the disease is *serum amylase*. The upper limit of normal is 300 IU/l; in acute pancreatitis this value is usually exceeded and often rises to levels well in excess of 1200 IU/l. The level itself gives no indication of the severity of the disease although persistent elevation indicates that complications may well occur. Only occasionally does the amylase remain normal throughout the course of the disease. Amylase is estimated rather than lipase because the estimation of the former is easier. In the majority the amylase falls to normal values within 48 hours of the onset of the disease making retrospective diagnosis by means of this test virtually impossible.

Other enzyme measurements have been advocated from time to time but none have come into routine clinical use. These include:

1. Estimation of the P-type isoamylase, which cannot be detected after total pancreatectomy and is therefore only of pancreatic origin.
2. Radioimmunoassay of trypsin.
3. Serum ribonuclease.
4. Serum deoxyribonuclease.

Serum calcium. The normal range of serum calcium is 2.25–2.60 mmol/l. In severe acute pancreatitis the level may fall below 2.0 mmol/l. Originally it was thought that the simple combination of ionic calcium with fatty acids formed by the digestion of neutral fat by circulating lipase was responsible for the fall, but recently other factors have been suggested including the release of glucagon causing secondary hypocalcitonaemia and hypomagnesaemia as well as impairment of parathyroid function. Regardless of the precise cause the magnitude of the fall parallels the severity of the disease, and when the level falls by more than 30%, i.e. to a value of 1.75 mmol/l or below, death is probable.

Blood sugar. If the disease is severe, islet cell function is disturbed and a temporary rise in the blood sugar occurs.

Serum bilirubin. Any swelling of the head of the pancreas is liable to compress the common bile duct, leading to a rise in the serum bilirubin and, possibly, clinical jaundice.

Serum methaemalbumin. As necrosis and vascular disruption occur in the pancreas, haemoglobin is liberated into the circulation. In the presence of proteolytic enzymes, haematin is formed which is bound with albumin to form methaemoglobin. This compound is formed only when free haemoglobin liberated into the plasma by the breakdown of red cells has used up the haptoglobin to which it is normally bound. Methaemalbumin is not usually present in the circulation and its presence in pancreatitis indicates that the pathological changes in the gland are haemorrhagic rather than oedematous. A continuing high circulating level of this compound usually signifies the development of complications.

Serum methaemalbumin is nonspecific since any other condition in which necrosis of tissue is occurring will produce the same effect.

Plasma fibrinogen. The normal fibrinogen level in the plasma is 200–400 mg/dl. The fibrinogen level increases in a number of surgical conditions in which there has been tissue injury, including acute pancreatitis. Normally the value rises towards the end of the first week and in the uncomplicated case falls to normal within 2 weeks. Although the magnitude of the initial elevation bears little relationship to the severity of the disease, an elevation of the fibrinogen level extending into the third and fourth weeks is highly suggestive of complications.

Blood counts and sedimentation rates. The total white count is elevated, together with an absolute polymorphonucleocytosis in the early stages of pancreatitis. Persistent leucocytosis or a late rise indicates complications. The sedimentation rate rises in acute pancreatic necrosis because the condition is associated with tissue necrosis. A persistent rise continuing into the third week is again indicative of complications.

Electrocardiography

ECG changes are common in acute pancreatitis and commonly simulate those occurring in acute myocardial infarction with S-T segment depression or elevation, inversion of T waves, and extended T wave negativity. Such changes are made worse by the presence of pre-existing coronary artery disease. The changes probably result from vagally mediated reflexes from the pancreas as well as subsidiary factors such as fluid and electrolyte disturbance.

Radiological investigations

Plain radiology

The place of radiological investigation is initially restricted to plain X-rays of the abdomen in the erect and supine positions. These may show either a single fluid level in the duodenum, the sentinel loop, or, in severe disease, multiple fluid levels in the upper left abdominal quadrant suggesting a more generalized paralytic ileus. Occasionally, opaque gallstones may be seen, and there may sometimes be a generalized hazy opacity over the abdominal cavity due to a collection of peritoneal fluid. Later, a number of radiological investigations may be required. Particularly important, however, once the disease is quiescent, is ultrasonography to eliminate or confirm the presence of gallstones.

Ultrasonography

Ultrasonography is most useful in patients who are thin (with little or no fat planes) and is of greatest value in identifying lesions chiefly involving the head and body of the pancreas rather than the tail.

Computerized axial tomography

The changes which can be demonstrated by computerized axial tomography include:

1. Thickening of the parietal peritoneum due to oedema.

2. Thickening of the anterior pararenal fascia, eponymously known as Gerota's fascia.
3. Swelling of the pancreas accompanied by blurring of its outline.
4. Decreasing density in the region of the pancreas indicates either early cyst formation or pancreatic necrosis.

In a recent series reported by London and his co-workers in 1989 it was found that the use of CAT did not improve the prognostic ability of modified Glasgow criteria described above. They used as their index of severity the maximum A/P measurement of the head and body, together a pancreatic size index in cm^2; they found that the latter index was 12.8 cm^2 and 6.0 cm^2 in severe and mild attacks, respectively.

ERCP

ERCP can be used to identify gallstones within the common duct, which can then be released by sphincterotomy. Neoptolemos and his co-workers adopted this policy in a series of 121 patients and found that fewer complications of the disease occurred in those patients so treated and that sphincterotomy itself was associated with few complications although others have found a significant number, particularly bleeding.

Peritoneal tap and lavage

Peritoneal tap has been used to assess the severity of the disease for many years. In severe attacks free peritoneal fluid is present; increasing discolouration indicates more severe disease.

In addition to visual observation the following estimations are of value: albumin content (>39 g/l indicates severe disease); SGOT (>10 IU/l indicates severe disease); and total protein (>7.5 g/l indicates severe disease).

MANAGEMENT

The mortality of acute pancreatitis is related to the severity of the disease. In various large reported series the overall mortality varies between 6–10%. However, when the condition progresses from the oedematous to the haemorrhagic and then onwards to the gangrenous form the mortality rises to as high as 50%.

The majority of deaths used to take place within the first 48 hours indicating that the cause must have been either overwhelming 'toxaemia' or failure to control the hypovolaemic shock, or both.

In part the hypovolaemia is readily explained in terms of the massive plasma leak which takes place into the pancreas itself and into the surrounding tissues. It has been estimated that there may be a 30–40% loss of plasma volume, the whole being known as the 'pancreatic burn'. However, more subtle changes are at work.

The preliminary measures that must be taken are, therefore, to relieve pain and restore the intravascular volume by plasma or plasma expanders; controlled trials using fresh frozen plasma have been shown to confer no benefit. If necessary a central venous pressure line should be inserted. The stomach should be kept empty and the urine output monitored so that incipient renal failure can be recognized.

Even despite adequate resuscitatory measures refractory shock may develop suggesting that unidentified vasoactive substances are contributing to the failure of response.

In elderly patients, because of the myocardial depressant effect of the 'toxic broth', the patient should be fully digitalized if ECG changes are present. When associated ileus is prolonged and it is becoming clear from both clinical and biochemical parameters that the disease is severe, total intravenous feeding should be commenced.

Specific measures of dubious value

A large number of measures have been proposed over the past two decades, most of which have been found to be useless:

1. *The administration of aprotinin (Trasylol)*. This drug inhibits the action of trypsin and chymotrypsin. It was first introduced into clinical practice in 1958 and, at first, reports appeared which suggested that it was highly effective in reducing the initial mortality of pancreatitis. However, in the late 1960s a rather less optimistic view was taken as controlled trials showed little benefit from the administration of the drug, and its use has been gradually abandoned.

2. *Corticosteroids*. There is no 'hard' evidence that corticosteroids alter the prognosis of this disease although in general terms it has been shown that corticosteroids assist in maintaining the integrity of

the microcirculation in animals suffering from experimental endotoxaemia.

3. *The routine use of broad-spectrum antibiotics* has now been abandoned unless the disease is associated with acute cholecystitis, pulmonary infection or 'shock' lung.

4. *Glucagon*. The use of this drug in the treatment of pancreatitis was first suggested in 1973, its theoretical value being to rest the gland. However, an MRC trial in the late 1970s showed in a double-blind trial that no reduction in mortality followed the use of this drug.

5. *Peritoneal lavage*. This treatment was first suggested by Wall of Australia in 1956 but, more recently, carefully controlled trials have shown that it fails to reduce morbidity or mortality.

Operative intervention

Laparotomy

Many older surgeons were convinced that laparotomy had a definite place in the treatment of pancreatitis and various series showed that at the very least it did not contribute to mortality, but there is no evidence that it is beneficial. The typical findings are:

a. Blood-stained ascites.
b. Retroperitoneal oedema.
c. Scattered areas of fat necrosis.
d. A swollen pancreas, possibly infiltrated with blood if the condition has progressed to the haemorrhagic stage.
e. Gallstones.

The general consensus now appears to favour the performance of an immediate cholecystectomy if gallstones are found to be present, with exploration of the common duct.

Transduodenal sphincterotomy is not recommended because of the danger of producing a duodenal fistula.

ERCP with endoscopic sphincterotomy

Papers are now appearing in the literature that convincingly show that if common bile duct stones are demonstrated by means of ultrasonography an early endoscopy and sphincterotomy should be performed.

Complications of acute pancreatitis and their management

1. *Tetany.* The onset of tetany usually occurs within a few days of the onset of the disease and, as previously stated, a serum calcium below 1.75 mmol/l carries a grave prognosis. However, in the presence of overt symptoms calcium supplements should be given in the form of calcium chloride.

2. *Renal failure.* Severe pancreatitis is associated with hypovolaemic shock; therefore intravascular haemolysis and unidentified toxic factors organic renal damage may occur. Treatment should be as described in Volume 1, Chapter 14.

3. *Shock lung* (see Vol. 1, Ch. 13).

4. *Consumptive coagulopathy and diffuse intravascular coagulation* (see Vol. 1, Ch. 14).

5. *Post-pancreatitis mass.* Three pathological lesions may result in a palpable abdominal mass following an acute attack:

a. *Pancreatic swelling.* This term is used to describe a condition of the pancreas accompanied by oedema and an inflammatory infiltrate of the pancreas and peripancreatic tissues. The importance of this condition lies in the fact that it will usually spontaneously resolve without surgical interference. In clinical terms the patient, having recovered from the acute attack, continues to complain of malaise, nausea and upper abdominal discomfort. A slight fever may be present together with a leucocytosis. Depending on the build of the patient and the degree of abdominal tenderness a mass may or may not be palpable. A definitive diagnosis can be reached by a CAT scan but if this is not available simple clinical observation noting the gradual improvement of the patient eventually leads to the correct diagnosis.

b. *Pancreatic pseudocyst.* A pseudocyst is an accumulation of exudate within the lesser sac which persists after the acute attack has subsided. This condition is usually more easily diagnosed than a multilocular abscess because with the passage of time a very easily palpable swelling develops under the left costal margin. A characteristic feature of a pseudocyst is its tendency to vary in size. This is because, for a time at least, a communication may be present between the cyst and a major pancreatic duct, making spontaneous drainage a distinct possibility. For this reason, when the cyst first makes its appearance it is advisable to wait and see if spontaneous resolution will occur.

The diagnosis is confirmed by ultrasonography and a barium meal produces a typical picture showing the cyst lying between the spine and the stomach, pushing the latter forwards.

The treatment of such cysts are revolutionized by the development of the transgastric approach and internal drainage first described by Jedlucka in 1923. At the present time interventional radiologists are able, using ultrasonic control, to place drainage tubes directly into the cyst and hence save the patient from open operation. Various series report success in up to 90% of cases using either repeated aspiration or continuous drainage over a period.

c. *Pancreatic abscess.* The incidence of this complication varies between 1 and 9% according to the series studied, and the mortality between 14 and 67%. It occurs only following acute pancreatic necrosis, which leads to sloughing of some or all of the pancreas. Colonization of the slough and the surrounding tissues takes place with both aerobic and anaerobic organisms producing an abscess. Clinically the patient, initially severely ill, partially recovers only to develop a high swinging fever, a marked leucocytosis, hypoalbuminaemia and a falling haemoglobin, all of which persist unless adequate surgical drainage is achieved and the slough removed. Once formed the abscess tends to spread within the retroperitoneal tissues as well as into neighbouring organs and blood vessels so that a variety of complications may develop, including a massive fatal haematemesis. Operative treatment is necessary, removing the slough and inserting numerous drains through which the abscess cavity can be irrigated. The exploration can be by an anterior transperitoneal approach or via a retroperitoneal approach utilizing a left subcostal incision. Following recovery an external pancreatic fistula may develop but the majority will close spontaneously and therefore should be treated conservatively. It is in this type of patient that parenteral nutrition is of great assistance, combined with control of the orifice of the fistula to reduce autodigestion of the skin to a minimum.

6. *Duodenal ileus.* This complication usually develops within 14 days of the onset of an acute attack. A barium meal shows that the stomach empties slowly if at all, the duodenal mucosa is irregular and the duodenal loop widened. In the majority of patients the condition resolves spontaneously but in a small minority a gastrojejunostomy is required.

7. *Haematemesis.* Severe upper gastrointestinal haemorrhage following an attack of acute pancreatitis may be due to:

a. Multiple gastric erosions in the acute stage of the disease, a condition which should be treated with H_2 antagonists.

b. Erosion of a major vessel in patients in whom an 'expanding' pancreatic abscess is present. This condition may be fatal.

8. *Burst abdomen.* The incidence of abdominal dehiscence, if a laparotomy is performed, is approximately three times higher than the generally accepted level following surgery. The cause is presumably leakage of pancreatic enzymes and the early digestion of catgut sutures in the wound. Wounds should therefore be closed with non-absorbable sutures.

23. Chronic pancreatitis

Chronic pancreatitis is a condition in which structural and functional changes are present in the pancreas, even in the symptomless patient. Using the Marseille symposium the condition can be classified into:

- Recurrent chronic pancreatitis.
- Chronic pancreatitis.

The difference between the two groups is clinical rather than pathological since in the recurrent type of the disease the patient suffers from intermittent abdominal pain whereas in the latter variety the pain is constant.

Both types of pancreatitis are rare in most parts of the United Kingdom.

AETIOLOGY

Unlike acute pancreatitis, which is associated with an abnormally high incidence of gallstones, chronic pancreatitis is more commonly associated with a high alcohol and high fat intake.

In an experimental animal such as the rat the histological changes associated with chronic pancreatitis can be reproduced if the animal is allowed to drink unrestricted quantities of 20% alcohol and, in the same animals, if to the high alcohol intake is added a diet rich in fat and protein. In these conditions intracanalicular precipitation of protein plugs develops, which many investigators think may be the underlying cause of the disease.

Chronic pancreatitis may also develop when the pancreatic duct is blocked either by an inflammatory stricture of the ampulla or occasionally by an underlying carcinoma of the head of the pancreas. A rare cause is hypercalcaemia due to primary or secondary hyperparathyroidism.

PATHOLOGY

Macroscopic appearance

A severely diseased gland is so fibrosed that it is often contracted to about half its normal size. The pancreatic margins, so clearly defined in the normal gland, are indefinite due to the associated peripancreatic fibrosis. The gland is hard, fixed and may impart a gritty sensation to the palpating fingers highly suggestive of malignant disease.

Histological appearance

Histological examination may show ductal dilatation, cyst formation and periductal and periacinar fibrosis with little derangement of the lobules and acini or there may be pronounced fibrosis accompanied by duct ectasia. In the latter condition there is squamous metaplasia of the lining epithelium together with periductal round cell infiltration. Islet cell destruction is possible and is responsible for diabetes in 5% of the so-called mild cases and 75% in the more severe.

An additional pathological change, rarely seen in the UK, is glandular calcification, the exact significance of which remains unknown since routine radiology of the abdomen sometimes reveals gross pancreatic calcification in the absence of any clinical symptoms.

The cysts seen in chronic pancreatitis may be small but as coalescence occurs so larger cysts are formed which may either remain confined to the organ or burst into the peripancreatic tissues to form pancreatic pseudocysts.

In the early stages of the disease the major ducts may appear normal but as the disease progresses so the ducts may become dilated by the development of strictures, calculi or both.

CLINICAL PRESENTATION

The common presenting symptoms of this disease include:

1. Abdominal pain.
2. Symptoms due to reduced or absent exocrine function, i.e. steatorrhoea.
3. Symptoms due to endocrine dysfunction, i.e. diabetes.
4. Symptoms due to associated disease:
   a. Biliary tract disease.
   b. Carcinoma of pancreas.

c. Alcoholism.
d. Narcotic addiction.

Pain

The pain of chronic pancreatitis may be continuous, remittent and, occasionally, colicky. It is distinguished from cardiac pain in that it seldom, if ever, radiates to the neck and arms. It may be relieved by sitting up, which may lead to increasing exhaustion if the pain begins in the late evening. When chronic and continuous it can easily be mistaken for ulcer pain but, unlike the latter, it is not relieved by vomiting or alkalis.

The pain may be precipitated by eating or drinking and, apart from the specific metabolic disturbances associated with pancreatitis, e.g. loss of exocrine function which may itself lead to weight loss, patients may literally starve themselves to death in an effort to avoid painful episodes.

Steatorrhoea

As increasing deterioration of exocrine function develops steatorrhoea eventually follows and is found in over half the patients. Clinically this condition is recognized by the changing quality of the stools, which become paler, bulkier, loose, and perhaps watery. Such stools are often offensive and may be difficult to flush.

Diabetes

The onset of diabetes is usually heralded by the development of thirst and polyuria. This condition is common in the severe cases and less frequent in the milder type.

Symptoms due to associated disease

1. *Gallstones.* The incidence of gallstones, and therefore symptoms due to gallstones, is much rarer in chronic than acute pancreatitis. A review by Berman showed that stones were present only in about a fifth of patients suffering from chronic disease.

2. *Carcinoma of the pancreas.* Although the two diseases are not commonly associated there are numerous reports in the literature of chronic pancreatitis secondary to carcinoma of the head of the gland.

3. *Alcoholism.* The published literature makes it clear that pancreatic calcification is commoner in alcoholics suffering from pancreatitis than non-alcoholics. The majority of physicians would also agree that undue amounts of alcohol will often precipitate pain and renewed activity but the converse is not necessarily true and total abstinence may still be associated with attacks of pain.

4. *Narcotic addiction.* The pain of chronic pancreatitis may be so severe and prolonged that eventually narcotic addiction develops. This is not difficult to believe when one has the opportunity of observing such a patient at first hand.

INVESTIGATIONS

Biochemical

1. *Serum amylase.* So long as functioning exocrine tissue remains the serum amylase will rise with each attack of severe pain above the upper limit of normal.

2. *Pancreatic function studies.* The duodenum is intubated under X-ray control, after which the pancreas is stimulated by the administration of secretin, 1.0 U/kg and pancreazymin, 1.7 U/kg. As the functioning exocrine tissue is destroyed so the total volume, bicarbonate and enzyme secretion falls. At the time of injection of secretin the patient may develop pain and an elevated serum amylase.

3. *Glucose tolerance test and plasma insulin levels.* Either of these studies may reveal the presence of latent or overt diabetes.

4. *Investigation of the stools.* A simple microscopic examination of the stools may show undigested meat fibres or fat globules. More sophisticated (and much more expensive) is a fat balance; a daily excretion of fat in excess of 6 g/day on a diet containing 100 g of fat clearly indicates steatorrhoea.

Radiological investigations

The following radiological investigations are of assistance:

1. *Plain abdominal X-rays.* These may show pancreatic calcification, gallstones and, at times when the patient is complaining of severe pain, a sentinel loop.

2. *Oral cholecystography.* This may demonstrate loss of biliary function, gallstones or both.

3. *Hypotonic duodenography*. First introduced by Liotta in 1951 this may show deformity of the duodenal mucosa.

4. *Retrograde pancreatography*. The normal pancreatic ductal system was first investigated by radiological means by Birstingl in 1959 who injected radio-opaque dyes into 150 necropsy specimens. In 1968 the ampulla was first cannulated endoscopically in the living and various studies have shown that normally:

   a. The main pancreatic duct tapers smoothly from head to tail.
   b. The mean length of the main duct is 15.4 cm (12.2–19 cm).
   c. The mean diameter of the main duct in the head is 3.2 mm (1.7–6 mm); in the body, 2.4 mm (1.4–3.4 mm); and in the tail, 1.2 mm (0.7–3 mm). The branches of the main pancreatic duct enter at right angles in the body and tail but follow no set pattern in the head. In chronic pancreatitis the changes which develop may be *minimal*: irregularity, dilatation and minimal stenosis of some major ducts; *moderate*: marked tortuosity associated with greater degrees of dilatation alternating with increasingly severe stenosis; or *advanced*: gross tortuosity, cyst formation and pancreatic calculi. A review of the literature shows that in the great majority of patients the diagnosis of chronic pancreatitis can be made with certainty by the use of this investigation, although it is generally agreed that the radiological changes do not correlate with the severity of symptoms.

5. *CAT*. This may demonstrate a small shrunken pancreas, unsuspected calcification and cyst formation.

MANAGEMENT

Essentially the treatment of chronic pancreatitis is medical rather than surgical.

Medical treatment

When alcoholism is a contributing factor every effort must be made to persuade the patient to abstain. Diabetes, if present, should be controlled by insulin, and exocrine deficiencies producing steatorrhoea can be partially alleviated by the use of pancreatic extracts, the dose of which will nearly always require considerable adjustment in the early period.

Surgical treatment

The indications for surgical treatment are nearly always relative rather than absolute. They include:

1. Recurrent attacks of pain, increasing in frequency and severity.
2. Continuous pain after meals.
3. Marked weight loss due to fear of eating.

In general the pain of chronic pancreatitis tends to lessen with the passage of time rather than become worse, and for this reason – assuming that the pain can be controlled to give a reasonable quality of life – surgery should be delayed as long as possible. Unfortunately it remains impossible to identify that group of patients in whom improvement rather than worsening of the condition will occur and thus the decision to operate on patients remains one of clinical judgement.

Indirect surgery

Cholecystectomy with or without choledochotomy. The literature suggests that even relapsing pancreatitis will sometimes respond to cholecystectomy if stones are present in the biliary tree. On the other hand, cholecystectomy should never be performed in the absence of demonstrable gallbladder disease.

Ampullary sphincterotomy. In 1948, Doubilet and Mulholland published the first article presenting the rationale for this operation and by 1956 they were able to review their results in 319 patients, 190 of whom had been followed up for more than 2 years. They reported an operative mortality of 7 per cent and excellent clinical results in 88%. Prior to the division of the sphincter, radiological studies were used to confirm that the pancreatic and common bile ducts passed through a common channel. This they regarded as an extremely important step before performing sphincterotomy because Doubilet's concept of the aetiology of chronic pancreatitis was that the basic cause was the reflux of bile into the pancreatic duct. Obviously this can happen only if a common channel exists so that spasm or stricture can result in such reflux.

In their series, a higher than average proportion of patients were shown to have such anatomical arrangement. They claimed that sphincterotomy abolished acute attacks or chronic pain and allowed regeneration of the damaged pancreas. However, in 214 patients a diseased gallbladder was also removed and this could, of course, also explain some of their success.

It is interesting that no other surgeons were able to reproduce such good results, that experimental work indicates that fibrosis and stenosis tends to follow sphincterotomy, and thirdly, that any decrease in pressure within the biliary tree after sphincterotomy is only temporary.

Coeliac ganglionectomy. This operation, either unilateral or bilateral, has been performed by a number of surgeons for the relief of pancreatic pain. The largest reported series is that of Mallet-Guy who reported his results in 42 patients who were followed for a variable period of between 1 and 9 years. He found that approximately 80% of his patients were relieved of pain although no other surgeon has obtained such a degree of success.

Direct pancreatic surgery

Two rather different types of operation have been described:

Puestow's operation. The aim of this operation is to retain as much pancreatic tissue as possible and to decompress the gland by opening the duct widely along its anterior surface. The basic concept behind this operation is the belief that sphincterotomy fails due to a multiplicity of strictures along the length of the pancreatic duct. The basic steps of this operation are as follows:

1. The abdomen is opened and the diagnosis confirmed.
2. The spleen is removed and the pancreas is dissected free from the peripancreatic fibrous tissue as far medially as the superior mesenteric vessels.
3. The tail is removed from the gland so that the pancreatic duct can be identified.
4. The duct is now opened along its whole length and a segment of the anterior part of the body is removed.
5. A Roux en Y is fashioned and the jejunal loop is then brought over the pancreas and its serosa is stitched to the peripancreatic tissues.
6. The abdomen is closed.

Puestow described the results in 25 patients: there was 1 death, 2 were not improved and 22 were relieved of pain. The author has also found that this operation gives good results but in about half the patients the pancreas is so shrunken that the operation is not technically possible.

Pancreatectomy. This operation involves removal of all the remaining pancreatic tissue except for a small cuff of the head lying within the lesser curve of the duodenum. This not only preserves some pancreatic tissue and the common bile duct, but also the superior and inferior pancreaticoduodenal arteries so that necrosis of these various structures is rare.

Fry, who has written extensively about this form of surgery in chronic pancreatitis, has performed the operation 25 times. A quarter of his patients were narcotic addicts and 14 had had one or more unsuccessful operations. Of the 25 patients, 13 had an excellent result, being free from pain, gaining weight and able to return to work, and the remainder had an indifferent or a poor result. Fry concluded that if the entire head of the pancreas is left recurrent pain is almost inevitable, a conclusion with which most other authors would agree. The natural extension of this procedure would, of course, be total pancreaticoduodenectomy but the mortality rate of this procedure is high and the postoperative condition leaves much to be desired.

Following direct interferences with the pancreas it is important to abstain from alcohol, correct the diabetic state and, if possible, control the steatorrhoea.

Miscellaneous procedures. Rarely, chronic pancreatitis is associated with a parathyroid adenoma. Removal of the adenoma then results in total relief so long as the pancreatic pathology has not progressed to complete destruction.

Vagotomy and partial gastrectomy have also been advocated but the rationale seems extremely doubtful.

24. Crohn's disease

Crohn's disease has been recognized as a clinical entity since 1932 when it was described by Crohn and his colleagues. In their original description these authors defined the condition as a regional ileitis, acknowledging the inflammatory nature without being able to specify a cause. The position remains the same today except that it is now realized that the disease may affect any part of the gastrointestinal tract from the mouth to the anus.

AETIOLOGY

The following suggestions have been put forward:

1. *Genetic factor.* The evidence in favour of a genetic factor is based on the following:

a. Family aggregations.
b. The unexpected frequency of the disease in monozygotic but not dizygotic twins.
c. The frequency of the disease in patients who also suffer from ankylosing spondylitis; in such patients Crohn's disease is 30 times commoner than in the general population.

Even despite the above features the genetic factor involved certainly cannot be one of straightforward Mendelian inheritance.

2. *Food.* Crohn's disease is commoner in Europe than elsewhere and the reported incidence of this condition has also increased in Scotland and Sweden. The importance of manufactured foods with chemical additives has aroused considerable speculation.

3. *Immunological.* Consideration has been given to possible sensitization to exogenous antigens or to the tissues of the gastrointestinal tract provoking an autoimmune type of response. No clear-cut evidence exists, however, and the fact that complement, often an

important factor in cell-mediated immunity, is not taken up is regarded as an important negative finding.

However, an immunological basis for the disease would serve to explain the extragastrointestinal manifestations such as uveitis and arthritis which occur in Crohn's disease.

4. *Infective.* The suggestion has frequently been made that the disease is infective, and for many years an intensive search was made for *Mycobacterium tuberculosis*. This was finally abandoned, but recently the theory has been revived by the finding of a comparable disease in animals caused by a mycobacterium. The therapeutic effectiveness of sulphasalazine in Crohn's disease could be explained on an infective basis. Recent work has also suggested that an agent similar to that causing sarcoidosis may be responsible, for in both conditions the Kveim test is positive.

Finally, an RNA virus has recently been isolated from the gastrointestinal mucosa and lymph nodes in patients suffering from both Crohn's disease and ulcerative colitis which cannot be found in normal individuals.

5. *Lymphatic obstruction.* A lesion similar to Crohn's disease can be produced in experimental animals by feeding powdered glass or, alternatively, by injecting iron particles into the mucosa. Either procedure results in a granulomatous lesion.

PATHOLOGY

Gross appearance

The disease may be acute, in which case the bowel appears congested and the bowel wall thickened and turgid. In the commoner chronic form the bowel has been likened to an eel in rigor mortis. The affected bowel and its mesentery are thickened, and enlarged mesenteric glands can be seen or palpated in the mesentery.

Although great importance was attached to the latter finding by earlier writers, recent investigations have shown that the nodes are equally enlarged in ulcerative colitis. When the bowel is opened, the wall is seen to be thickened, and oedematous. The lumen is generally narrowed and long narrow linear ulcers run along the mucosa. The ulcers have swollen, overhanging edges of inflamed mucosa. From the ulcers fissures may extend deeply into the wall of the bowel. The changes described give rise to the classic cobblestone appearance observed on X-ray.

One of the most characteristic features of Crohn's disease is the presence of skip lesions, long intervals of apparently normal bowel separating the diseased areas. The bowel proximal to a lesion may be dilated due to the obstructive nature of the diseased portion. Multiple adhesions, internal fistulae, and abscess formation are common.

Microscopic appearance

The chief histopathological feature of Crohn's disease is the formation of non-caseating granulomatous lesions that resemble sarcoidosis. Each is composed of large mononuclear cells and foreign-body giant cells. There is considerable oedema of the mucosa and submucosa. Lymphoid follicles may be seen in the submucosa and deeper layers. The mucosa itself may appear fairly normal, apart from fissures lined by epithelioid cells, but as the ulceration continues the exudate of polymorphonuclear leucocytes, lymphocytes, epithelioid cells and mononuclear cells increases.

Since Crohn's disease can involve the whole of the large bowel it is obvious that one difficulty may be to distinguish this disease from ulcerative colitis. The main distinguishing pathological features upon which reliance can be placed are:

1. Presence of the confluent linear ulcers.
2. Deep fissures.
3. Sarcoid-like granulomas, which appear not only in the bowel wall but also in about half the involved lymph nodes.

CLINICAL PRESENTATION

The symptoms of Crohn's disease are in large measure related to the site of the disease. The frequency of the various sites of involvement as determined by the examination of several large reported series are as follows:

a. Terminal ileum and ascending colon, 60%.
b. Small bowel, 20%.
c. Large bowel alone, 20%.

The disease may occur in childhood but is more common in early adult life. Once the disease is sufficiently severe to produce symptoms they are nearly always progressive.

The common presenting symptoms are:

- *Abdominal pain* due to intestinal obstruction caused by either oedema or fibrosis of the affected bowel, in which case the pain is intermittent and colicky in nature, or constant abdominal pain due to peritoneal irritation.
- *Diarrhoea* due to:
  a. Destruction of the mucosa of the terminal ileum leading to defective fat absorption or inability to absorb bile salts. The latter spill over into the colon and produce a typical watery diarrhoea.
  b. Internal fistulation, producing blind loops and functional shortening of the bowel.
  c. Stricture formation leading to alteration in the bacterial flora of the bowel.
- When the large bowel alone is involved, particularly when the involvement is total, *severe diarrhoea accompanied by blood and mucus* is a prominent feature of the disease.
- *Weight loss* or, in childhood disease, failure of growth. This is due to malnutrition brought about by loss of the absorptive capacity of the small bowel due to the disease itself, failure of absorption due to bile salt deconjugation by the abnormal intestinal flora, by fear of pain following eating and lastly, loss of protein in the form of mucus.

In addition to these specific symptoms of gastrointestinal disease the following general manifestations of the disease may be present:

1. Fever.
2. Anaemia, hypoproteinaemia, hypoprothrombinaemia, vitamin deficiency disorders, and gross fluid and electrolyte imbalance.
3. Polyarthritis of the rheumatoid type, especially in childhood.
4. Pyoderma gangrenosum.
5. Uveitis.
6. Oropharyngeal ulceration.
7. Finger clubbing.

In addition, perianal disease – fissures, fistulae or recurrent abscesses – occur in about 15% of all patients and about 90% of all those suffering from colonic involvement.

As the disease progresses so entero-enteral and enterovesical fistulae may develop, the latter causing frequency, dysuria and the passage of flatus per urethra.

The clinical progress of a patient suffering from Crohn's disease can be followed by means of the Harvey–Bradshaw Disease Activity Index described by these authors in 1980.

Five aspects of the clinical condition of the patient were considered and a points systems allocated to each, the general wellbeing of the patient, the presence and severity of abdominal pain, the number of stools passed daily, the presence of an abdominal mass, and lastly the number of complications, giving one point for each of the following recognized complications:

a. Arthralgia.
b. Uveitis.
c. Erythema nodosum.
d. Aphthous ulceration of the oropharynx.
e. Pyoderma.

These latter features appear to be commoner with diffuse small bowel disease than with distal small bowel disease alone.

Physical examination

This may reveal little, but in an advanced case the following signs may be present:

1. A palpable abdominal mass, frequently in the right iliac fossa.
2. Signs of intestinal obstruction.
3. Evidence of anaemia, hypoproteinaemia or vitamin deficiency.
4. Cachexia.
5. Perianal disease.
   a. The most common finding is the presence of oedematous skin tags or fissures, neither of which are as painful as they would appear.
   b. Perianal abscesses.

INVESTIGATIONS

Proctoscopy, sigmoidoscopy and colonoscopy

Biopsy of anal lesions is frequently disappointing in that the typical granuloma may not be found even when gross perianal lesions are present.

Depending on the degree of involvement and the chronicity of the disease small aphthous-like ulcers 1–4 mm in diameter, surrounded by normal or hyperaemic mucosa, or large, round serpiginous or longitudinal mucosal defects may be present; the latter may be solitary or in clusters. The mucosa between the defects may appear normal or nodular. If possible any biopsy taken should include the submucosa, otherwise the histological changes associated with Crohn's disease may be missed.

According to Price and Morson the presence of specific histological changes depends on the extent of the distal spread of the disease. If disease is present distal to the splenic flexure a positive biopsy showing unequivocal signs of Crohn's disease is obtained in about 50% of patients whereas when there is no involvement of the large bowel mucosal changes will only be found in 12% if there is co-existent anal disease.

Haematology and biochemistry

1. *Full blood count and ESR.* A raised ESR is always an indication of activity although the best single marker appears to be the platelet count.
2. *Serum Fe, vitamin B_{12} and folic acid.*
3. *Examination for acute phase reactants, C-reactive protein, orosomucoids, and cytokine interleukin 6 (IL6).*

Radiological examination

This is performed by means of a 'small bowel enema' unless the large bowel is being investigated, in which case a normal barium enema is performed.

The following radiological signs have been described:

a. In non-stenotic lesions: blunting, flattening and thickening of the valvulae conniventes.
b. Fusing of the mucosal folds.
c. Evidence of ulceration, deposition of barium in the linear ulcers leading to the typical 'cobblestone' appearance.
d. Further destruction of the mucosa leads to loss of the cobblestone appearance and its replacement with an irregular network of barium.
e. Palpation of the barium-filled loops reveals their lack of pliability and their rigidity.
f. Stenosis. When the lesions are small in length the radiological appearances are not dissimilar to those produced by multiple

tuberculous strictures; when of greater length, the 'string sign' of Cantor is created.
g. Proximal to the stenotic areas gas and fluid filled distended loops may be seen.
h. Sinuses or internal fistulae may be demonstrable.

The most valuable radiological physical signs, according to Dyer, are contraction and rigidity of the bowel wall.

Faecal fat

At least one-third of all patients suffering from Crohn's disease have steatorrhoea and numerous investigators have shown that the degree of malabsorption correlates with the site and extent of the disease. Cooke put great emphasis on the presence of steatorrhoea before and after surgery, claiming that a continuation of steatorrhoea after resection indicated a high recurrence rate, although this has since been disproved.

MANAGEMENT

Unless demoralizing symptoms or complications are already present the treatment of Crohn's disease is medical, since it has now been appreciated that Crohn's is not, as originally described, an inflammatory disease limited to the terminal small bowel and ileocaecal region, but is in fact a pan-intestinal disease in which spontaneous remissions and acute flare-ups occur, and in which surgery plays only a limited role and is never curative.

The medical management may involve:

1. *The correction of anaemia and vitamin deficiency states by appropriate means.*
2. *The use of elemental diets.* It has been shown that such diets will reduce the acute inflammation within 2 weeks, but after the cessation of treatment improvement is not maintained. In one reported trial, an elemental diet alone produced improvement regardless of age, sex and the severity of the disease and associated complications. Using Vivonex (Norwich Eaton) as the only source of nutrition, treatment began with feeds of 1800 ml at one-third strength, and within 3 days osmolality had been increased to full strength of 550 mmol/l. Of 113 patients treated in this manner for 2–12 weeks, the disease failed to remit in 17 patients; remission occurred in 33 out of 35 patients who

entered the trial with symptomatic strictures, but within 6 months 22% required an operation.

3. Considerable relief from the associated diarrhoea can be achieved by the use of the following drugs: *codeine phosphate* 20–30 mg daily; *diphenoxylate* 5–20 mg daily; *loperamide* 4–16 mg daily.

4. The specific drugs which have been used in Crohn's are:
   a. *Sulphasalazine.* The active principle of sulphasalazine, (sulphapyrine) is 5-amino salicylic acid. The oral dose is 1–2 g q.d.s. by mouth. This treatment may be continued for 2–3 weeks and as remission occurs the dose can be gradually reduced to 1.5–2 g daily. Although effective in the treatment of the acute phase of the disease it appears to be of little value in maintaining remission, and trials indicate that the simultaneous administration of corticosteroids does not increase the overall benefit.
   b. *Glucocorticoids.* The administration of prednisolone in doses as high as 40–80 mg given over a short period will produce a remission in the majority of patients. However, in patients who have been treated surgically by means of total colectomy and ileorectal anastomosis endoscopic inspection of the ileum proximal to the anastomosis showed no improvement and there was no decrease in phospholipase A_2 in the mucosa, which is believed to be a major contributor to the inflammatory process. However, the European Co-operative Crohn's Disease Study, the results of which were published in 1984, came to the conclusion that prednisolone was the single most effective drug in the treatment of this disease and that prednisolone combined with salazopyrine was most effective in the treatment of previously untreated patients or when the disease was localized to the colon. They also concluded that there was no significant benefit to be obtained by treating quiescent disease.
   c. *Immunosuppressive agents*, both azathioprine and the newer drug cyclosporin, have also been used but neither have been found to be effective in the long term. Whilst a short-term remission may be achieved, relapse occurs in nearly all patients.
   d. *Immunostimulants.* The drug levamisole hydrochloride 2.0–2.5 mg/kg/day has also been used but, compared to a placebo and azathioprine, little beneficial effect has been recorded.

Thus many patients suffering from Crohn's disease eventually come to surgery.

Indications for surgical intervention.
1. Intractable abdominal pain caused by stricture formation resulting in intermittent obstruction.
2. Severe haemorrhage as occurs in Crohn's colitis.
3. The development of either internal or external fistula.
4. Abscess formation – although occasionally presenting as a spontaneous discharge into the bladder or vagina presenting on the surface and demanding drainage – automatically leads to the development of an external fistula.
5. Growth retardation in childhood.

Surgical treatment
Following the initial description of the disease by Crohn in 1932 and the failure to recognize the pan-intestinal nature of the disease, the operation normally performed was resection of the distal ileum and ascending colon followed by an ileocolic anastomosis. Indeed Crohn insisted that all the affected bowel should be removed with a margin of healthy bowel 12 inches (30 cm) on either side of the lesion together with the enlarged mesenteric lymph nodes. Gradually – as it was appreciated that recurrent symptomatic disease was common (as high as 65% of patients after long-term follow-up) – it became common surgical practice to limit the resection but to examine by frozen section the planned level of the anastomosis to make certain that this site was free of disease. However, it was soon apparent that microscopic disease might be present without necessarily jeopardizing the integrity of the anastomosis or in fact altering the frequency of recurrence.

A second method commonly practised in the past was to perform a bypass in continuity or with exclusion. Again, long-term statistics proved that this was even more prone to recurrence than resection although the operative mortality was reduced. However, this operation was also dropped when it was found that carcinoma developed with relatively greater frequency in the excluded small bowel.

With these facts in mind, Bryan Brooke of Birmingham performed in 1961 an operation which has become known as stricturoplasty. It is possible that the idea for this operation in Crohn's disease originated in India where surgeons had found that the alleviation of tuberculous strictures could be achieved by dividing the strictured bowel along its antimesenteric border in a longitudinal manner and then suturing it transversely.

In 1981 Alexander Williams, also of Birmingham, began to employ this operation, and between 1981 and 1984 reported a series of 106 stricturoplasties performed on 37 patients, most commonly in the ileum and jejunum. The mean duration of the disease in this series was 15.9 years and the indications were recurrent obstruction (34) and enterocutaneous fistula formation (3); whilst 19 patients had a single stricture, multiple strictures were present in 18. He found on follow-up that, when re-operation was necessary because of the development of a stricture at a new site, the original stricturoplasty was still patent, a 25 mm balloon catheter passing through the area treated with ease. Alexander Williams pointed out that when treating the disease in this manner it is essential to rule out the presence of other strictures, either proximal or distal, by the passage of a balloon catheter; otherwise a missed distal stricture could lead to the breakdown of the suture line and the formation of an enterocutaneous fistula. In 1982 Lee of Oxford reported similar results, but in a smaller series of cases. Although most commonly performed in the presence of short strictures, long strictures several centimetres in length can also be dealt with by performing an enteroenterostomy and resuturing the bowel in a similar fashion to constructing a Finney pyloroplasty.

Large bowel disease

Unlike ulcerative colitis, Crohn's disease involves all layers of the bowel and therefore radical surgery in this disease demands total protocolectomy with the formation of a permanent ileostomy. However, prior to such radical surgery and in the absence of specific indications such as severe haemorrhage or perforation, a diversion of the ileal contents from the large bowel by means of a split ileostomy may improve the patient's condition. It has been shown in many series that this operation in the majority of patients will improve the patient's general condition with a corresponding gain in weight. It has also been shown that if ileal contents are instilled into the ileal fistula a symptomatic exacerbation occurs, but that if the ileal fluid is first subjected to ultrafiltration no such effect occurs – suggesting that some constituent of the ileal fluid is responsible for the initiation of the inflammatory condition. However, in many series it has been shown that this relatively minor procedure is only successful in about half the cases, and that on restoration of continuity of the bowel the disease once more becomes symptomatic and the patients come to proctocolectomy. In some patients with limited strictures on the left side of the colon, local excision may be of value.

Perianal disease

This should be treated as conservatively as possible, although simple fissures may be treated in the usual manner. Complex fistulae should be treated by placing a seton. Fortunately, in the author's exprience, even though the anus appears horrific the symptoms are not as severe as one might expect.

Late results of major resections

If repeated resections of the small bowel have been performed the patient may develop the symptoms typical of the small bowel syndrome, although the majority of patients suffering from this condition do so because of a massive resection performed for some acute catastrophe, e.g. mesenteric thrombosis or complete small bowel volvulus. In general, ileal resections produce greater degrees of metabolic derangement than jejunal and may lead to a megaloblastic anaemia, fatty degeneration, and gastric hypersecretion due to the defective inactivation of gastrin. Clinically, if an acute massive resection is performed the condition of the patient passes through three stages:

1. In the *immediate* postoperative period there is a severe loss of fluid and electrolytes in which hypovolaemia, tetany, magnesium depletion and hypoalbuminaemia may occur.
2. In the *intermediate* period the severe watery diarrhoea diminishes and nutritional problems begin.
3. In the *late* stages a balance is achieved between the absorptive capacity of the bowel that remains and the degree of physical activity, by which time the total loss of body weight may be as much as 25–30 kg.

Thus the acute symptoms gradually subside coincident with structural and physiological adaptation of the residual small bowel. Reports have appeared in the literature showing that this adaptation process can be facilitated by the use of growth hormone. The long-acting analogue of somatostatin, octreotide, can be used in the early stage to control the profound watery diarrhoea because of its inhibitory action on the exocrine secretion of the gut, especially gastric secretion; there is also evidence that, at least in vitro, it inhibits the proliferation of enterocyte crypt cells. Further evidence suggests that patients suffering from the short bowel syndrome should continue luminal nutrition even though this may increase diarrhoea. Experimental work performed by Dowling and others in 1976 showed that, in greyhounds subjected to a 50% proximal small bowel resection, if the animals were exclusively fed intravenously even though they remained well nourished, no evidence of functional adaptation occurred and a significant fall in the mean ileal villous height occurred from 823 ± 48 μm to 732 ± 57 μm within 6 weeks.

25. Tumours of the large bowel and rectum

Colorectal cancer is the second commonest epithelial cancer in England and Wales, and in Western society as a whole it accounts for 9–20% of all cancer deaths. However, even in the industrialized nations the incidence of colorectal cancer varies considerably; for example, it is three times commoner in Scotland than in Finland. The actual prevalence of colorectal cancer in Great Britain is probably of the order of 3 per 1000 of the population over the age of 40 years.

The most disappointing aspect of colorectal cancer is that virtually no improvement in survival has occurred over the past two decades, the overall 5-year survival rate of both cancer of the colon and rectum being of the order of 20–25%. Adjuvant chemotherapy has failed to alter the picture, and trials of pre- and postoperative irradiation have yielded differing results according to the series examined. The prognosis in colorectal cancer is ultimately determined by the stage and the histological grade of the tumour. Nevertheless the quality of life for many sufferers of carcinoma of the rectum has been improved by improved surgical techniques.

AETIOLOGY

Genetic factors

In some patients the genetic factor is patently obvious. Thus the polyps characteristic of familial polyposis coli, Gardner's or Turcot's syndrome almost inevitably become malignant, giving rise to multiple tumours in the colon and rectum. Of these syndromes the most common is familial polyposis, which is inherited as an autosomal dominant and affects males and females in equal numbers. Symptoms of bowel disturbance begin at an average age of 16 years and overt malignancy develops within 15 years in most untreated victims by the time they reach early adult life.

To date there exists, however, no 'hard' evidence that the majority of colonic cancers are due to a genetic cause, although without doubt families exist in whom generation after generation of colorectal cancers develop. Studies in Utah, Ohio and Scotland confirm that among the many aetiological factors a genetic predisposition to colorectal cancer exists.

Dietary factors

The fact that the incidence of colorectal cancer is greatest in the higher economic groups and in countries where a Western diet has been adopted supports the hypothesis that diet plays a role in the aetiology of this tumour.

However, whilst most authorities accept this hypothesis, there is little agreement concerning which specific dietary item is implicated. In 1969 Aries postulated that colonic cancer was caused by metabolites produced in the colon from some benign substrate by bacterial flora. Diet would, therefore, control the concentration of substrate and the composition of the flora would determine the amount of metabolite. This would explain both the fact that the risk of colorectal cancer is related to diet and the complexity of the relationship.

The hypotheses relating a dietary factor to colonic cancer focus on the enzymatic activity of the intestinal bacteria. The suggestion has been made that these enzymes could either activate an ingested carcinogen and/or produce a carcinogen from dietary components or intestinal secretions.

The majority of investigators have pursued the suggestion that the important substrates are the bile acids which, secreted by the liver, are extensively metabolized by the colonic bacteria, the major metabolites being deoxycholic acid and lithocholic acid. Evidence that the bile acids may act as promoters is derived from animal studies.

Suspensions of deoxycholic acid in croton oil produce skin tumours when painted on mouse skin, the croton oil being the initiator and deoxycholic acid the tumour promoter. In animals also, the direct diversion of bile into the colon causes the development of tumours. However, at present there is no evidence in humans that bile acids can cause the formation of precursor adenomata but they may be implicated in the development of increasing degrees of dysplasia.

TUMOURS OF THE LARGE BOWEL AND RECTUM

Bacterial population

It is still a matter of disagreement as to whether the anaerobic or the aerobic population of the gut is of greater significance. Some investigators have found that anaerobes predominate in communities with a high incidence of colonic neoplasms and there is no doubt that in vitro anaerobes can produce carcinogens from bile acids.

However, other investigators have found that aerobic bacteria predominate and postulate that the aerobes metabolize choline to secondary and tertiary carcinogenic amines, choline being present in the gut from the bacterial degradation of lecithin, a major component of animal fats.

Fibre intake

It is also possible that a high-fibre diet influences the production of nitrosamines by diminishing the normal intake of animal fat or by decreasing the aerobic bacterial population which is capable of producing secondary and tertiary amines.

Specific precancerous conditions

The most important of these is ulcerative colitis. The incidence of malignancy in this condition is related to the length of the history. Cancer of the rectum and colon is approximately 20 times higher in patients who have suffered for 20 years as compared to 5 years. However, the risk of cancer is almost exclusively related to those patients suffering from total colitis; patients suffering from distal proctitis or proctocolitis appear to have only a slightly increased incidence of malignancy.

PATHOLOGY

Polyps

The term polyp has been generally discarded by the histopathologist but retained by the clinician to imply the presence in the colon and rectum of a circumscribed tumour which projects above the surface of the colonic mucous membrane and which may be sessile or pedunculated.

Juvenile polyps

These tumours, whether single or multiple, are hamartomas in which there is an excess of lamina propria enclosing tubules lined by normal epithelium. Unlike the polyps of the Peutz–Jeghers' syndrome they contain no smooth muscle. Such tumours are covered by a single layer of epithelium which is easily damaged leading to secondary infection. Whilst found in any part of the gastrointestinal tract the colorectum is often the only region involved. In some polyps the epithelium is dysplastic and in keeping with this finding it is now considered that some juvenile polyps have a malignant potential which appears to be greater among those families in which several members are affected.

Symptoms usually begin in the first decade and the average age at diagnosis is 18 years.

The common presenting symptoms are:

1. Recurrent rectal bleeding, frequently severe.
2. Prolapse with auto-amputation.
3. Recurrent prolapse.

Metaplastic polyps

These occur with increasing frequency with advancing age. They are widely distributed throughout the large bowel although they occur with greatest frequency in the rectum. They are seldom more than 0.5 mm in diameter and form plaque-like excrescences projecting from the mucosa, particularly on the crests of the mucosal folds. They are composed of elongated tubules in which cystic dilatation occurs. Epithelial dysplasia does not occur and isotopic techniques have shown that their development depends upon quantitative rather than qualitative changes in the epithelial cells.

Adenomas

These can be graded according to their structural appearance into:

1. *Tubular adenomas*, previously known as adenomatous polyps. These tumours are composed of proliferated epithelial tubules.
2. *Villous adenomas*, previously known as villous polyps. These have a villous pattern, and are composed of finger-like papillary villi which may branch. These tumours are commonly single and are attached by a broad base often extending over a wide area of the

mucosal surface. They are most frequently found in the rectum and sigmoid.
3. *Tubulo-villous adenomas*, which have the structural features of both tubular and villous adenomas.

In all three structural variants, epithelial dysplasia occurs, varying from mild to severe, the latter approximating to the changes seen in invasive carcinoma. Different grades of dysplasia may be seen in one adenoma; the characteristic histological features seen in the different grades are:

1. *In mild dysplasia*, the nuclei are elongated and slightly hyperchromatic. Pleomorphism and loss of nuclear polarity does not occur. The glandular arrangement is irregular with some branching.
2. *In moderate dysplasia*, the nuclei are round rather than elongated, and there is a loss of nuclear polarity with some increase in the nuclear:cytoplasmic ratio. The amount of mucin in the cells is decreased. Nuclear pleomorphism is common.
3. *In severe dysplasia*, the changes are very similar to those of invasive adenocarcinoma. Marked pleomorphism is associated with loss of nuclear polarity and an increase in the number of mitotic figures.

Grading of adenomas into those showing mild, moderate or severe dysplasia has shown that regardless of the histological growth pattern their malignant potential increases with the degree of dysplasia. The severity of dysplasia is also related to size. Thus in small adenomas, less than 1 cm in diameter, only mild dysplasia is normally present, and therefore they have a low malignant potential, whereas in adenomas greater than 2 cm in size severe dysplastic changes are present in some 50%. Structural type also bears a close relationship to potential malignancy, for whatever their size, villous adenomas are the most potentially malignant.

The hypothesis has been advanced therefore that there exists an adenoma–carcinoma sequence – a gradual change occurring from a benign to a malignant tumour. This sequence appears to take on average some 10–15 years to complete and can be followed most accurately in patients suffering from familiar polyposis coli in which the time interval between the diagnosis of polyposis without cancer and of polyposis with cancer is approximately 12 years.

Specific syndromes associated with colonic adenomas are familial polyposis, Gardner's syndrome and Turcot's syndrome.

Overtly malignant tumours of the colon

The gross morphological features of colonic primary adenocarcinoma have considerable influence on the symptomatology of the disease. Ulceration developing in an adenoma showing severe dysplastic changes results in the typical lesion in which an ulcer with rolled edges develops, and all signs of the original benign epithelial tumour rapidly disappear.

Other types are described as polypoidal, nodular, scirrhous and colloid. In general, tumours on the right side of the colon tend to be polypoidal and to ulcerate later than tumours on the left side. Tumours on the left side of the colon tend to be scirrhous, annular and circumferential, the tumour being intramural rather than intraluminal and in consequence infiltrating and thickening the bowel wall.

Distribution of colorectal neoplasms

The distribution of large bowel tumours is as follows:

a. Caecum – 10%.
b. Ascending colon – 8%.
c. Transverse colon – 12%.
d. Descending colon – 6%.
e. Sigmoid colon – 6%.
f. Rectum – 28%.

The frequency of synchronous tumours of the large bowel has been variously reported as 1.7–2.7%, excluding tumours occurring as complications of familial polyposis and chronic ulcerative colitis.

Tumour spread

1. *Locally in the bowel wall*, both in a vertical direction and towards the peritoneal surface.
2. *By the lymphatics.* Lymphatic spread occurs via the lymph vessels of the bowel wall to related lymph nodes in the proximal part of the large intestine. Lymph nodes are especially numerous in the mesocolon and adjacent retroperitoneal tissues.
3. *By the venous system.*
4. *Transcoelomic spread.* Gravitational metastases may occur at any time after the tumour has penetrated the bowel to involve the

serosal surface, after which cells may be detached and seeded in the peritoneal cavity. Such seedling deposits eventually result in a shelf of malignant tissue developing in the pouch of Douglas or, in the female, secondary deposits in the ovaries which are known as Krukenberg tumours.

Pathological staging

In 1932 Dukes presented a pathological staging system for carcinoma of the rectum, which was later applied to colonic tumours as well.

In his classical description he divided the progress of the tumour into three stages:

1. *Stage A.* Spread by direct continuity into the submucosa or muscles but not beyond, and without lymph node involvement.
2. *Stage B.* Spread beyond the muscle coat into the paracolic or pararectal tissues, but without lymph node involvement.
3. *Stage C.* As with A and B, but with metastasis to the regional lymph nodes. Stage C has been further subdivided into:
   a. Stage C1, where the involved nodes do not extend up to the point of surgical ligature of the vascular pedicle.
   b. Stage C2, where the node at or immediately below the ligature is involved.

The relative frequency of patients in these categories when the condition is first diagnosed is: Stage A, 15%; Stage B, 40%; Stage C, 45%.

In the absence of lymph node metastases the 5-year survival may be as high as 80%, but with involvement of lymph nodes the 5-year survival falls dramatically; of course, in the presence of distant metastases, which occur most commonly to the liver, peritoneum and lungs, the 5-year survival is zero.

It is of interest to note that the mortality statistics for carcinoma of the colon have remained depressingly constant over the past 25 years.

Other factors which influence the prognosis are:

1. *Venous involvement.* If veins in the immediate vicinity of the tumour are involved the 5-year survival falls to 64% and if thick-walled veins in an extramural situation are involved it has been shown that the 5-year survival falls to only 20% since in this group Talbot et al (1980) found that liver metastases developed more frequently.

2. *Degree of tumour differentiation.* Originally described by Broders in 1925, the degree of differentiation is based on microscopic features such as tubule formation; variability in size, shape and staining of nuclei; orderliness of arrangement of their nuclei within the tubules; and the number of mitotic figures. In large series the majority of tumours are only moderately differentiated.

3. *The presence of lymphoplasmocytic infiltration* around the tumour is associated with a more favourable prognosis.

More accurate than the Dukes classification, but more complex, is the TNM classification.

SYMPTOMS ASSOCIATED WITH COLONIC TUMOURS

Right-sided tumours

The symptoms associated with tumours of the right colon are determined by:

1. The gross pathological features of tumours in this area; the majority of tumours in this segment of the colon tend to be polypoidal and ulcerating.
2. The liquidity of the faecal stream.
3. The large calibre and distensibility of the right colon.

Thus, with the exception of tumours situated in the region adjacent to the ileocaecal valve, tumours in the ascending and transverse colon rarely cause intestinal obstruction. The more common symptoms are:

a. Vague abdominal pain, 80%.
b. General malaise and lassitude associated with anaemia, 20%.
c. Palpable abdominal mass, 67%.
d. Symptoms and signs suggesting the development of an appendix mass – this is particularly common if subacute perforation occurs or should the tumour act as the obstructing agent to the appendix itself, 20%.
e. When the tumour is situated at the hepatic flexure, or the caecum has failed to descend, it is possible to mistake a perforating carcinoma for acute cholecystitis.
f. Melaena, 8%.
g. Weight loss, 48%.

Left-sided tumours

Due to the frequency with which tumours of the descending colon tend to be circumferential and because the faeces are semisolid, the common symptoms associated with left-sided growths are:

a. Intermittent lower abdominal colic, present in 50–70% of patients.
b. Loss of appetite, a symptom often induced by the fear that eating may precipitate the onset of pain.
c. Change in bowel habit, 60%.
d. Recognizable blood intimately mixed with the faeces, 10%.
e. Right iliac fossa swelling, due to intermittent obstruction causing distension of the caecum.
f. Weight loss, 14%.
g. Palpable mass, 45%.

In addition to the symptoms listed above, left-sided tumours may also result in:

1. *Acute large bowel obstruction*, which is usually ascribed to one of three causes:
   a. Superadded infection resulting in a rapid increase in size of the tumour and sudden occlusion of the lumen.
   b. Faecal impaction.
   c. Intussusception.
2. *Peritonitis*. This is due to perforation at the site of the growth or perforation of the bowel proximal to an obstructing lesion due to stercoral ulceration.

Physical signs associated with colonic carcinoma

1. A *palpable mass* is most commonly associated with right-sided tumours, a tumour in this situation being palpable in approximately 50–75% of patients compared with only 30–45% of patients suffering from tumours of the descending colon. Lesions of the sigmoid colon may be palpable per rectum as an extra rectal mass.
2. *Anaemia*. This is normocytic and hypochromic and associated with a low serum iron. A history of failure of such anaemia to improve following the administration of oral iron therapy is relatively common.
3. *Abdominal distension and borborygmi* if chronic large bowel obstruction is present.
4. *Signs of local or general peritonitis* will follow perforation of the tumour or a stercoral ulcer if obstruction should occur.

INVESTIGATIONS

Sigmoidoscopy and biopsy

Because approximately 50% of colorectal cancers occur within the terminal 25 cm of the large bowel, inclusive of the rectum, sigmoidoscopy is mandatory. It should be performed, if possible, without any preliminary bowel preparation since even when the tumour itself cannot be seen the character of the contents of the bowel may be very suggestive of a lesion at a higher level. When a lesion is seen, a biopsy should be taken to establish the precise pathology of the lesion. The differential diagnosis of carcinoma of the lower sigmoid includes protocolitis, large bowel Crohn's disease, amoebic dysentery, and benign or malignant villous papilloma.

The common appearance of a visible lesion is one of an ulcer surrounded by an edge that is everted and the base of which is commonly greyish in colour. Less commonly, colloid cancers form large soft, friable, gelatinous ulcerating tumours which may produce mucous in such large quantities that the lesion cannot be distinguished from the papillary type of adenocarcinoma; the malignant counterpart of the villous papilloma.

Barium enema

When sigmoidoscopy is negative, a barium enema is the next logical investigation. The accuracy of this examination has been greatly increased by the introduction of double contrast techniques by which the radiologist is able to demonstrate lesions in areas which are difficult to visualize, such as the overlapping parts of the sigmoid colon. Lesions of the caecum are also better delineated and polyps can usually be distinguished from faecal masses.

The radiological appearance of a carcinoma of the colon depends upon its site and its type. Classically, the common ulcerating tumour causes a filling defect with a typical fingerprint deformity or 'shouldering' at its margins. The more scirrhous types of tumour may cause an annular constricting lesion extending for a variable distance along the bowel to produce the characteristic 'napkin-ring' appearance. Both types are associated with mucosal destruction at the site of the lesion.

Colonoscopy

This investigation is extremely useful when:

[History, examination, PR, E scope, Ba enema, Colonoscopy, CXR, Rectal ultrasound, liver USS,]

1. The diagnosis remains uncertain following a barium enema.
2. Barium enema has demonstrated a polypoid lesion. In such cases polypectomy during colonoscopy has virtually replaced open laparotomy and if subsequent pathological examination indicates the polyp is benign or that no infiltration of the stalk has occurred, this is regarded as definitive treatment.

The only contraindication to colonoscopy is severe mucosal ulceration or the presence of peritonism.

The only limitation of its usefulness are the relative technical difficulty of manipulating the instrument around the colon to the caecum.

The chief complications are:

1. Haemorrhage: significant bleeding only occurs after removal of large polyps, greater than 2 cm in diameter.
2. Perforation: incidence 0.1%.
3. Death: normally a complication of perforation.

Haematological examination

There are no specific haematological tests to enable a distinction to be drawn between the various causes of diarrhoea, but since any case of blood loss will eventually result in anaemia, the haemoglobin and red cell count should be determined in order that the anaemia, if found, can be corrected before operation. In tumours of the right colon an anaemia refractory to iron is a highly suggestive feature of the disease.

FBC

Tumour markers

Carcino-embryonic antigen (CEA)   Oncofetal antigen

One of the most exciting developments relating to colorectal cancer has been the discovery of CEA, more correctly known as the oncofetal antigen, i.e. an antigen associated with both fetal material and tumour tissue, perhaps because both are composed of rapidly dividing cells. This antigen can now be estimated by radio-immunoassay techniques. It was named CEA because an apparently identical antigen can be detected in normal embryonic and fetal gut, pancreas and liver during the first two trimesters.

Thereafter it disappears, only to reappear in appreciable quantities in patients suffering from carcinoma of these organs. It is a

RIA

E-scope - Mucosa.

glycoprotein with a molecular weight between 200 000 and 370 000 daltons. Its appearance in malignant disease of the gastrointestinal tract is believed to be due to de-repressive de-differentiation, the antigen having been repressed during the course of differentiation of the normal bowel.

A positive CEA test with an absolute concentration greater than 2.5 µg/ml is found in 70–80% of patients suffering from carcinoma of the colon and rectum. The level tends to be higher with large tumours and higher still in the presence of hepatic secondaries. If the tumour is wholly removed, the CEA level falls to normal, only to rise if recurrent disease develops.

The estimation of CEA, therefore, is of no value as a diagnostic tool but if it is elevated when the patient is first seen it normally indicates that the condition is incurable. In 68% of patients in whom residual disease is present following surgery, the CEA level may be normal, although if it is followed by serial examination elevation is inevitable.

TREATMENT OF COLONIC CANCER

Preoperative bowel preparation

In the absence of complications, or general contraindications to surgery, the treatment of all colonic cancers is surgical resection. This must be preceded by suitable preoperative preparation, one of the most important aspects of which is local preparation of the bowel itself.

The most suitable method of cleansing the bowel is still a matter for debate.

1. The conventional method of bowel preparation consisted of a low residue diet, oral magnesium sulphate, repeated enemas and washouts.

2. In 1975, Crapp and others described the method known as 'whole bowel irrigation' in which, on the day before operation, normal saline is infused through an indwelling nasogastric tube until the fluid passed per rectum is clear for at least 30 minutes.

Such mechanical cleansing reduces the mass of faeces so that although the number of bacteria per gram of faeces remains unchanged the total bacterial content of the colon is reduced. The efficiency of mechanical cleansing has recently been shown to be still further improved by the use of an elemental diet such as Vivonex for periods of up to a week preoperatively.

3. As an alternative to this regime the following somewhat simpler method has been described. Three pints of water (1.7 l) are taken by mouth, followed by 100 g of mannitol in 500 ml of water. To control nausea 10 mg of metoclopramide are given.

4. The majority of surgeons would use, in addition to mechanical cleansing, antimicrobial drugs. Those commonly in use at the present time and which have been found highly effective in reducing the incidence of postoperative sepsis in colorectal surgery are neomycin and metronidazole, the former being particularly active against *Escherichia coli* and the latter against *Bacteroides fragilis*, both organisms commonly found in wound infections.

Controlled trials have shown that the incidence of wound infection following colonic surgery is significantly reduced by the introduction of antimicrobial drugs into the pre- and peri-operative regime. The following regime can be recommended:

    a. Neomycin 1 g: 12, 5 and 1 hour preoperatively.
    b. Oral metranidazole 400 mg: 12, 5 and 1 hour preoperatively.
    c. Cephradine 500 mg: by injection 1 hour preoperatively.

Resection

The essential operative principles underlying definite surgery for colonic cancer are:

1. *Wide removal of the cancer-bearing segment of bowel.* Before proceeding with resection, the whole colon must be carefully examined to exclude the presence of a second tumour, after which the abdominal cavity as a whole is examined to determine the presence or absence of:

    a. Lymphatic metastases.
    b. Peritoneal seedlings.
    c. Hepatic metastases.

Thereafter, attention is paid to the tumour itself, noting particularly the presence of extracolonic invasion and adherence of the tumour to the abdominal wall or other viscera.

2. *Wide excision of the lymphatics draining the involved segment.* In general terms the lymphatics of the right and transverse colon accompany the tributaries of the superior mesenteric vein, whereas those of the left colon, from the splenic flexure downwards, are associated with the tributaries of the inferior mesenteric.

3. *The performance of the resection.* This must be carried out with a minimum degree of contamination of the peritoneal cavity by both bacteria and malignant cells.

Extent of resection

The following are the normally accepted limits of resection for tumours in various parts of the colon:

1. *Carcinoma of the right colon including tumours of the hepatic flexure.* These are treated by right hemicolectomy. The terminal ileum is removed, together with the colon as far as the junction of the right two-thirds with that of the left one-third. The branches of the superior mesenteric artery, including the middle colic, right colic and inferior colic, together with the terminal branches of the ileocolic vessel itself, are ligated and divided at their junction with the main trunk.

2. *Carcinoma of the transverse colon.* These are treated by excision of the whole of the transverse colon and mesocolon. The middle colic artery is divided at its origin from the superior mesenteric, and if the tumour lies at the level of the splenic flexure the ascending branch of the inferior mesenteric artery will also require division.

3. *Carcinoma of the descending colon.* This is normally treated by left hemicolectomy, the left third of the transverse colon, and the descending and sigmoid colon up to the junction of the rectosigmoid junction being excised. This extensive resection involves division of the inferior mesenteric artery proximal to the origin of its branches.

4. *Carcinoma of the sigmoid.* This is treated by sigmoid colectomy, the first, second and third sigmoid branches of the inferior mesenteric artery being divided close to their origin from the inferior mesenteric artery.

5. *Polyposis coli.* This condition, in the absence of malignant change in any of the rectal polyps, is commonly treated by total colectomy followed by ileorectal anastomosis. Prior to the colectomy the rectal polyps are first destroyed by diathermy, several sessions usually being required. This is performed before resection because it is relatively easier to accomplish when the faecal stream is solid.

The anastomosis

1. Following right hemicolectomy, the continuity of the bowel may be restored by end-to-end, side-to-end, or side-to-side anastomosis.

The potential long-term complication of the last mentioned method is the eventual development of the 'blind-loop' syndrome.

2. Following all other types of resection end-to-end anastomosis should be performed.

3. Technique of anastomosis. Some disagreement exists as to the best method of actually performing the anastomosis and whether or not this should be carried out by single-layer inverting or everting technique, or by the standard two-layer technique. The argument arises because anastomotic dehiscence is responsible for at least 10% of deaths following colonic resections.

Comparisons have been made in both the experimental animal and the human.

In the rabbit a single-layer inverting type of suture appears to be superior to the standard two-layer technique or the everting type of suture judged on the incidence of anastomotic dehiscence and perianastomotic leakage.

In the human, however, randomized trials comparing single-layer and two-layer anastomoses have shown that a similar incidence of anastomotic dehiscence and obstructive complications occurs after both types of anastomosis. In addition to clinical evidence of anastomotic dehiscence, subclinical dehiscence, as judged by post-operative barium enema examination, also occurs following either technique. Thus, it would seem that a single-layer inverting anastomosis is in no way superior to the standard two-layer.

The frequency of anastomotic dehiscence appears to depend upon several factors including:

1. The adequacy of bowel preparation. A significant correlation exists between faecal loading and anastomotic dehiscence.

2. Faecal soiling and peritoneal sepsis can be shown in the experimental animal to impair significantly the healing of colonic anastomoses, but in the human such factors tend to be minimized by the use of broad-spectrum antibiotics.

3. Nutritional status. A significant correlation exists between hypoproteinaemia and anastomotic disruption in both the experimental animal and the human.

Mortality

The immediate mortality following colonic resection, in the absence of obstruction or perforation, varies between 5 and 10% according to the series examined. The major causes of death include:

a. Anastomotic dehiscence, followed by intra-abdominal sepsis.
b. Cardiovascular complications.
c. Pulmonary embolus.

COMPLICATIONS OF COLONIC CANCER AND THEIR TREATMENT

The two major complications of colonic neoplasms are:

1. Intestinal obstruction.
2. Perforation followed by local abscess formation or general peritonitis.

The frequency of these two complications varies somewhat according to the series examined, but in a group of 700 patients reviewed by the author the incidence of each was as follows:

1. *Intestinal obstruction.* This occurred in 28% of patients when the tumour was situated in the caecum, ascending colon or hepatic flexure; 26% in tumours involving the transverse colon; and 40% in tumours involving the transverse colon; and 40% in tumours arising from the splenic flexure, descending colon and sigmoid.

2. *Peritonitis.* This complication arises as a result of perforation of a stercoral ulcer in association with intestinal obstruction, or from perforation of the growth itself. The former nearly always results in general peritonitis whereas when perforation of the growth itself occurs a local peritonitis follows, particularly when the tumour involves the right colon.

The incidence of peritonitis in patients suffering from obstruction is remarkably low, in this series accounting for only 1.5% of all cases, the majority occurring in left-sided tumours. In non-obstructed patients the overall incidence of peritonitis was 10%, general peritonitis being somewhat commoner than local. However, local peritonitis is a particular feature of caecal tumours whereas general peritonitis occurs much more frequently when the tumour involves the descending colon and sigmoid.

Treatment of the complications

Intestinal obstruction

1. When the obstructing lesion is proximal to the distal third of the transverse colon a formal right hemicolectomy should be performed.

TUMOURS OF THE LARGE BOWEL AND RECTUM

The presence of a degree of small bowel dilatation is technically helpful since it increases the ease with which an end-to-end ileocolic anastomosis can be performed.

2. When the obstructing lesion lies in the descending colon or sigmoid a number of alternative procedures are possible, including:
   a. A transverse colostomy, inserting a Paul's tube into the proximal limb in order to deflate the colon as rapidly as possible.
   b. A colostomy immediately proximal to the growth is particularly applicable to growths in the sigmoid; the singular advantage claimed for this manoeuvre is that at the time of the definitive resection the colostomy can be included in the resection and the operative management is, therefore, reduced to a two stage procedure.
   c. A Paul-Mikulicz procedure. This operation should be reserved for the treatment of obstructing lesions of the sigmoid colon in which hepatic metastases are already present.
   d. Caecostomy. In the series reviewed by the author this operation was found to be associated with a high incidence of complications and was abandoned.

The overall mortality, i.e. immediate deaths following the relief of obstruction is high, approximately a third of all patients dying in the immediate postoperative period.

Peritonitis

Of the 95 patients in the series reviewed, 22 were already moribund on admission and surgical treatment was withheld. In the remainder the best results were obtained when the growth involved the right colon, probably because in this group the causative lesion could be removed. Perforation of a tumour on the left side was normally treated by proximal colostomy and drainage of the affected area.

The mortality of perforated large bowel growths is naturally high because of the Gram-negative septicaemia that ensues. In addition, it is now considered that the anaerobic *Bacteroides* group play a considerable part in contributing to the overall morbidity and mortality of this condition. However, the use of the newer, broad-spectrum antibiotics, together with metronidazole, can in the future be expected to produce a decrease in mortality from the levels of the past which, in the immediate postoperative period, were as high as 70%.

RECTAL TUMOURS

The number of deaths from carcinoma of the rectum is approximately 5000 per annum, equivalent to one-fifth of the total dying from carcinoma of the bronchus.

Symptomatology

The common symptoms of rectal cancer include:

- Bleeding, especially on defaecation.
- Passage of mucus. (villous adenoma)
- Alteration in bowel habit.
- Early morning 'explosive' motion.
- Continuous rectal discomfort.
- Tenesmus.
- If the tumour infiltrates the anal canal, fissure-like pain.
- If there is pelvic infiltration, sciatic pain.
- Occasionally, rectal cancers of the upper third present with acute intestinal obstruction or perforate, causing pelvic peritonitis.
- Occasionally, urinary obstruction.

The diagnosis of rectal cancer is made by a combination of digital examination, sigmoidoscopy, and biopsy.

1. *Digital examination*. This gives some indication of the size of the tumour, its fixation and possibly the presence of pararectal lymph node involvement. In general it is accepted that the only treatment for the great majority of tumours which can be felt by the examining finger is an abdominoperineal resection. However, recently there has been a suggestion that small tumours palpable by the finger or in the lower third of the rectum which are mobile on the underlying rectal muscle and in whom no pararectal lymph nodes are palpable can be treated by local excision if multiple biopsies show that the tumour is well differentiated. This type of tumour with the characteristics described only account for about 10% of all tumours in any series.

2. *Sigmoidoscopy and biopsy*. The former aids in establishing the level of the tumour and this enables the surgeon to decide on the type of resection required. However, it should be observed that in an intact patient the lower limit of the tumour may appear to be at 8 cm whereas when the rectum is fully mobilized and the lateral ligaments divided the tumour margin may lie as high as 11–12 cm above the anal margin. Whether it is now possible to perform a sphincter-saving operation depends upon both the sex and the build of the patient.

Biopsy, particularly if multiple biopsies of the tumour are taken, allows the surgeon to predict the downward submucosal spread. This is very important since it has been classically taught that the line of resection should be 5 cm proximal and distal to the tumour. It has now been established that adequate clearance of the tumour only requires a resection 2 cm from the tumour margin and recently the importance of the mesorectum has been appreciated.

Staging

Recently preoperative staging of rectal tumours has become more accurate with the development of rectal ultrasonography and the use of CAT and NMR. By means of transrectal ultrasound the bowel wall can be visualized as three layer: a superficial (mucosal) layer, separated from a hypoechoic layer which corresponds to the muscularis propria, and a deep serosal echogenic band. Whilst the use of ultrasound permits an evaluation of the degree of penetration of the rectal wall and possibly invasion of the bladder, prostate, and mesorectum, it is of no use in detecting lymph node metastases. For this purpose CAT or NMR is required, and an accuracy of over 90% can be obtained. However, it should be noted that lymph nodes less than 1.5 cm in diameter can still be reactive rather than infiltrated with neoplastic cells. So far as the identification of hepatic metastases is concerned there is little to choose between the three diagnostic modalities, all having an accuracy of 80–90%.

Treatment

After diagnosis and staging the bowel must be prepared in the same manner as described for colonic surgery.

Local excision

Local excision of rectal cancers should be reserved for those tumours classified as Duke Class A, which are shown by biopsy to be well or moderately differentiated. If the tumour has not spread deeper than the muscularis propria there is only a 10% chance of metastases already having taken place to the regional lymph nodes. Excluding the snaring of polyps, only about 1–20% of rectal tumours can be treated in this manner, for in addition they must be: *accessible*, less than 10 cm from the anal verge; and *small*, less than 3 cm in diameter.

Two methods of local excision have been described:

1. **Per-anal submucous resection**, in which the wound is left open. This method can be used when the tumour rises from the wall of the bowel; the submucosal layer is infiltrated with 1:300 000 adrenaline in saline.

2. **Per-anal full thickness excision**, described by Parks, in which a full thickness disc of normal rectal wall is removed surrounding the tumour and the wound in the rectum is closed.

Major surgical procedures

Anterior resection. This operation is used when the tumour involves the upper end of the rectum or rectosigmoid. Tumours in this situation can be resected without dividing the peritoneum of the pouch of Douglas or rectovaginal fold, and without mobilizing the rectum from the hollow of the sacrum. The lateral ligaments are left intact and so a rectal stump some 10 cm in length remains viable.

Low anterior resection. This operation is indicated for tumours situated in the upper or middle third of the rectum. The rectum must be mobilized from the hollow of the sacrum and the lateral ligaments divided. When the tumour lies in the upper third there is relatively little difficulty in performing either a double or single layer anastomosis by hand, but when the tumour lies in the middle third the restoration of continuity may represent a problem.

This can be overcome:

1. The use of a stapling device.
2. Parks' operation of abdominotransanal resection, in which the sutures connecting the rectum to the anal canal are inserted via the dilated anus by means of a modified Turner Warwick urethroplasty needle. Because the needle is in the same axis as the handle of the instrument there is little problem with angulation, such as exists using an ordinary needle holder and needle.
3. A further technique for dealing with tumours of the middle third is to use a transphincteric approach to the rectum. This type of rectal surgery was described in the earlier part of this century, abandoned, and then modified in the early 1970s by York Mason. The approach to the rectum is made by placing the patient on the operating table in the inverted V position, after which an incision is made extending from the anus just to the left of the midline posteriorly, passing obliquely upwards lateral to the coccyx and the lower part of the sacrum. The posterolateral aspect of the rectum is

divided together with the sphincters and the puborectalis mass, all of which are carefully resutured when closing the lumen of the bowel. Primarily used for the excision of villous papillomas, York Mason has also used this method for the treatment of Duke Class A tumours on a highly selected basis.

Hartman's operation. Essentially this operation consists of a radical abdominal excision of the tumour without the perineal resection required of an abdominoperineal resection. It is particularly valuable in the very elderly.

Abdominoperineal resection. This synchronous combined operation leaves the patient with a permanent colostomy and is therefore to be avoided if at all possible.

Recently evidence has been gathering that preoperative radiotherapy both in non-fixed and fixed tumours will reduce the incidence of local recurrence after resection and increase survival times in low rectal tumours subjected to either sphincter saving operations or perineal resection.

Complications of surgical excision

1. *Immediate*. Shock, reactionary haemorrhage, ureteric injury.
2. *Intermediate*. Intestinal obstruction due to prolapse of a small gut loop through the pelvic peritoneum. Infection, both in the perineal or abdominal wound. Necrosis of the colostomy.
3. *Late*. Persistent perineal sinus, sacral herniation, local recurrence. Metastatic disease. Stenosis of the colostomy, which is now rare due to direct mucosa-to-skin suture. Paracolostomy herniation appears to be much less common since the general adoption of the operative technique of extraperitoneal colostomy.

When an anterior resection or abdomino-anal pull-through has been performed, a major cause of complications is the breakdown of the anastomosis. This is more likely when the resection is 'low', i.e. carried out below the level of the pelvic peritoneum.

Both abdominoperineal and anterior resection are followed by bladder disturbances. There can be a true neurogenic bladder only when the parasympathetic ganglia on both sides of the pelvis have been excised. This probably is more common in the 'easy' than the difficult case. Painless retention with incontinence develops.

Minor bladder disturbances are frequent (35%) but are usually circumvented by leaving an indwelling catheter in situ for longer than the usual period of 4–5 days.

Ancillary methods of treatment

Because of the relatively poor results obtained by surgery alone various ancillary methods, none of which have led to striking improvement in the results, have been tried. These include:

1. *HER*. This has been given preoperatively or postoperatively and whilst there is some doubt as to its efficacy as a form of adjuvant therapy there is little doubt that as a palliative treatment in the rare inoperable tumour it will cause relief of pain, if only temporarily in a proportion of cases.

2. *Chemotherapy*. Many trials proceed using a large number of drugs preoperatively. No positive results are yet available.

3. *Immunotherapy*. Many agents have been used to attempt to increase immunity to the tumour. These include BCG and its methanol extraction residue (BCG-MER), *Corynebacterium parvum* and levamisole, but none appears to delay recurrence or alter the ultimate prognosis.

Despite these various manoeuvres the mortality from carinoma of the rectum has shown little improvement; the overall corrected 5-year survival for all rectal cancers is 30%. The best prognosis is obviously obtained in Duke Class A tumours in which a 92% 5-year survival can be expected. Of interest is the fact that tumours of the lower third of the rectum do less well than those of the middle and upper third.

26. Complications of colostomy and ileostomy

COMPLICATIONS OF COLOSTOMY

Early

Necrosis (sloughing)

An important early complication of terminal or end colostomy is necrosis of the bowel wall proximal to the mucocutaneous suture line. The cause of this complication is a poor blood supply brought about either by faulty ligature of blood vessels supplying the gut, or to early thrombosis in arteries or veins that are possibly constricted by the tension exerted on a short loop in the obese patient, or by the external oblique aponeurosis.

If unrecognized, this can be a serious complication because, as the bowel wall sloughs, coliform and *bacteroides* infection of the subcutaneous fat may lead to extensive cellulitis and, possibly, gangrene of the abdominal wall.

In most patients the treatment of this condition demands reopening of the original abdominal incision and preparation of a new loop from within.

Lateral space obstruction

This form of early small bowel obstruction was relatively common prior to routine closure of the intraperitoneal space that lies on the lateral side of an end colostomy. Following recognition of this form of obstruction, the space was routinely closed (Fig. 26.1) and the complication became extremely rare. It was finally completely eliminated by the use of the extraperitoneal technique (Fig. 26.2).

However, early small gut obstruction may still come about because of kinking, and obstruction of a small bowel loop on the cut edge of the peritoneum or prolapse through the repaired pelvic peritoneum.

331

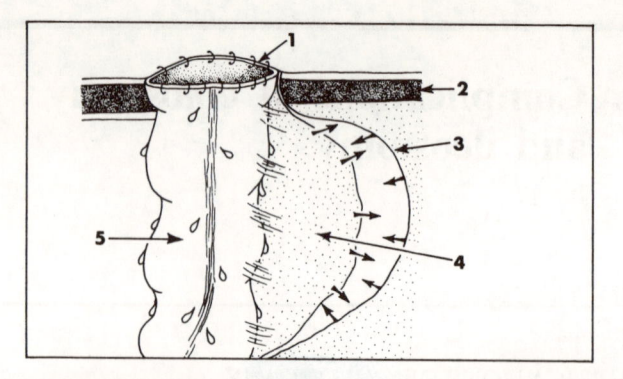

Fig. 26.1 Closure of lateral space by suture.
1, Direct muco-cutaneous suture; 2, Abdominal parietes; 3, Peritoneal covering of lateral abdominal wall; 4, Mesentery of descending colon united to peritoneum of lateral abdominal wall by either single purse string suture or multiple sutures according to preference of surgeon; 5, Sigmoid colon.

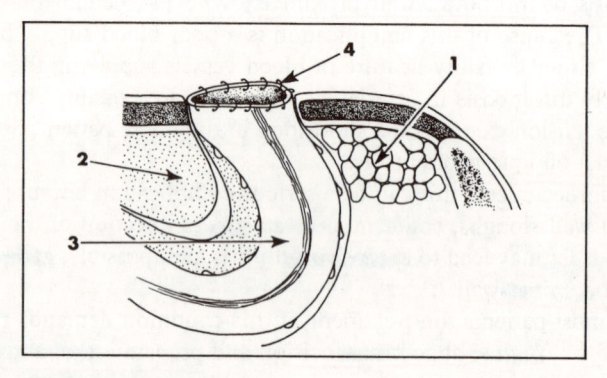

Fig. 26.2 Extraperitoneal colostomy.
1, Extraperitoneal fat; 2, Parietal peritoneum; 3, Sigmoid colon; 4, Direct muco-cutaneous suture.

Late

Stenosis

This complication was once the most common after colostomy operations, but following the introduction of immediate direct muco-cutaneous stitching it is now rare. When stenosis occurs it can be treated in one of two ways. The stenotic area of skin can be divided and excised, after which the skin and mucosa are resutured. This is a minor procedure which may, if necessary, be performed using local anaesthesia. It will not, however, result in a long-term cure of the condition which can be achieved only by completely refashioning the colostomy. It may be sufficient to excise the skin around the whole circumference of the stoma, then to deepen the dissection, even into the peritoneal cavity, so that the loop can be brought to the surface with plenty of slack, after which a direct mucocutaneous suture is performed. Occasionally, however, refashioning demands reconstruction of the loop from within.

Herniation

There is nearly always gross herniation if a colostomy is brought out through a major abdominal incision, and it was also common when brought out through a left iliac fossa stab wound. Although minor degrees of herniation are still relatively common, the adoption of extraperitoneal construction has led to the herniae being smaller and less obtrusive.

Massive herniae of long duration may produce sufficient disability to demand repair. This should be approached with caution. Non-absorbable materials are contra-indicated because of the possibilities of infection followed by chronic sinus formation. If the hernia is large, the return of the contents may lead to embarrassment of the cardiorespiratory system, or occasionally precipitate the development of a sacral hernia.

Prolapse

This complication is rarely seen following the construction of a terminal colostomy but it is commonplace following loop colostomy, and it is especially troublesome in the neonate, in which the commonest indications for loop colostomy are anorectal agenesis and Hirschsprung's disease. Before considering amputation of the prolapse in an infant the surgeon should remember that this may later lead to great technical difficulties in performing a definitive operation such as the Svenson abdomino-anal pull-through operation.

Whereas an ileostomy that is continent can be constructed, it has long been accepted that a colostomy is inevitably incontinent because all the various surgical manoeuvres that have been tried have proved unavailing.

In 1975, however, Feustel and Henning of Erlangen introduced an entirely original idea in the form of a magnetic closing device consisting of a ring and cap, both magnetized. The ring consists of samarium–cobalt coated with an acrylate, which is implanted in the abdominal wall around the emerging colon, and the cap consists of a plastic disc with a central protruding spigot enclosing a samarium–cobalt core.

However, the results published by the originators of this technique in a relatively large series, i.e. 105 patients, showed that the ring had to be removed in about one-fifth of all patients because of sepsis, and that only a quarter were fully continent for both flatus and faeces.

Other surgeons have also had relatively disappointing results following this procedure and it seems probable from the literature that in terms of age and build alone at least 50% of patients should never be considered for the insertion of such a device and that in the remaining patients many would do just as well without this device as with it.

COMPLICATIONS OF ILEOSTOMY

Early

Necrosis

If the blood supply to an ileostomy is inadequate, the projecting bowel becomes purple and an offensive serosanguinous discharge occurs instead of the normal early non-offensive fluid motion.

This complication requires immediate exploration and, if necessary, total reconstruction of the ileostomy loop from within the abdomen.

Late

Recession

The ideal ileostomy should project 2.5–3.5 cm beyond the abdominal wall; it may, however, recede either intermittently or permanently. This relatively common complication is important because severe recession is nearly always associated with difficulties in controlling the ileostomy outflow, part or all of the effluent being discharged at the skin level. Problems arise with the management of the ileostomy flange which cannot be made to adhere to the moist skin and this almost immediately causes skin excoriation. Treatment is determined by the severity of the condition. When the outflow cannot be managed by conservative means the ileostomy must be reconstructed by means of an intra-abdominal approach.

Stenosis

This complication, which was once common at the skin level, has virtually disappeared following the general use of direct mucocutaneous suture after eversion of the projecting bowel. Before the introduction of this technique by Brookes (1952), stenosis affected approximately 30% of stomas. Rarely, the bowel may be constricted at the level of the parietal peritoneum. An early symptom of ileostomy stenosis is an increase in the volume of the outflow together with intermittent colicky abdominal pain. Severe malfunction may lead to electrolyte and water depletion, and because the discharge is watery, there may be temporary mechanical difficulties with adhesion of the flange. The diagnosis can usually be made by digital examination of the stoma, and confirmed by erect X-rays of the abdomen, which show the classic fluid levels of small-gut obstruction. Internal obstruction requires intra-abdominal correction with the fashioning of a new ileostomy. Obstruction at the skin level will respond, at least temporarily, to the removal of the constricting band.

Prolapse

Prolapse of the bud, as with recession, may be fixed or sliding. It is associated with emotional difficulties because the prolapsed stoma is ugly, and mechanical problems arise because the protruding bowel pushes the ileostomy appliance away from the abdominal wall, thus producing leakage followed by excoriation.

Treatment. A fixed prolapse can easily be treated by amputation. The mucocutaneous junction is dissected free and the two layers of bowel separated. The latter manoeuvre is simple because the layers are usually bound together by flimsy adhesions. Once separated, sufficient length of bowel is removed to restore the bud to a reasonable size.

If the prolapse is sliding, a major intra-abdominal procedure is necessary in order to refix the mesentery and the bowel to the abdominal wall.

Fistula

This is a wholly avoidable complication usually caused through wearing an ill-fitting ileostomy ring or one that has ridden across the abdominal wall and ulcerated through the wall of the bowel. All fistulae form at skin level (Fig. 26.3) and once they have formed skin excoriation followed by difficulties in controlling the effluent occurs. Local treatment is useless, and an intra-abdominal reconstruction of the ileostomy is required.

Herniation

This is a relatively rare complication which could demand, if difficulty arose with the ileostomy apparatus, resiting the ileostomy on the opposite side of the abdomen and closure of the defect.

Skin excoriation

Any mismanagement or disturbance, however temporary, of an ileostomy may lead to contamination of the surrounding skin followed by excoriation. This is generally ameliorated by using Karaya gum powder (Pulv. Sterculis B.P.C.), which functions as an adhesive even in the presence of skin ulceration, thus protecting the involved skin. The powder may be applied by dusting it over the skin around the ileostomy, adding water, and then following with more powder, the process being repeated several times until a thick glue-like layer has been produced. An alternative dressing to use is Squibb's Stomahesive, which has the appearance of a wafer of thin toffee. A hole is cut in the wafer to the exact dimensions of the ileostomy, the wafer is then applied to the excoriated abdominal wall, after which the flange is applied. This is a neater, but more costly way of achieving healing.

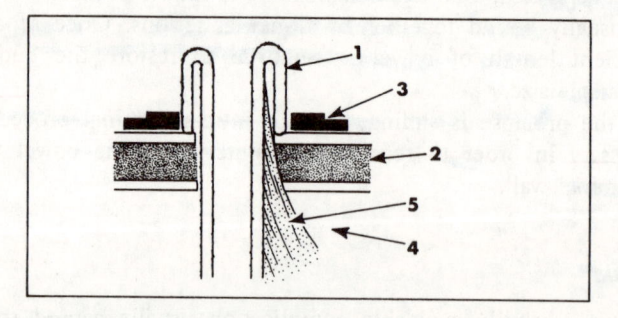

Fig. 26.3 Formal ileostomy as described by Brooke.
1, Ileostomy bud; 2, Abdominal parietes; 3, Adhesive ring; 4, Lateral space; 5, Mesentery of small bowel.

27. Non-malignant conditions of the anal canal

HAEMORRHOIDS

Classification

- *External*. External haemorrhoids arise from the skin-covered lower third of the anal canal.
- *Internal*. Internal haemorrhoids arise from the veins of the haemorrhoidal plexus in the upper two-thirds of the anal canal.

Internal haemorrhoids are classically divided into first, second and third degree, according to the degree of prolapse. A first degree internal haemorrhoid normally reveals its presence only by bleeding on defecation whereas a second degree haemorrhoid prolapses through the external sphincter on defecation only to retract spontaneously. Third degree piles, however, may spontaneously prolapse through the external sphincter or prolapse through the sphincter on defecation, but having prolapsed they remain so until manually replaced – which is usually possible unless some complication such as strangulation has occurred.

Piles arise in three main areas, situated (when looking at the anus with the patient in the lithotomy position) at the 3, 7 and 11 o'clock positions. These sectors were once considered to be the anatomical distribution of the chief haemorrhoidal arteries, but Thompson believes that they represent the location of the submucosal veins which form the anal cushions. He believes that in normal circumstances these cushions assist in maintaining continence, the internal sphincter squeezing the pads to seal the outlet from gaseous or liquid escape. Internal haemorrhoids, he suggests, result from the failure of the anal submucosal muscle, the musculus submucosae ani of Treitz, to prevent the anal cushions from prolapsing during defecation.

Complications of internal haemorrhoids include:

1. Severe chronic anaemia which, in the elderly patient, may lead to heart failure or angina.
2. Prolapse followed by strangulation.
3. Thrombosis followed by the development of a fibrous polyp.
4. Infection followed by the development of a submucous abscess.

Aetiological factors

1. Local obstruction of the venous plexus by a low rectal neoplasm.
2. Increased intra-abdominal pressure, e.g. pregnancy. Many women date the onset of their piles to a pregnancy, when a variety of factors may combine to produce the condition such as increased intra-abdominal pressure, increased pelvic vascularity, and disruption of the supporting structures at parturition.
3. Constipation.
4. Lack of support of the haemorrhoidal plexus due to previous operations which disturb or destroy the sphincter mechanism, e.g. operations for the cure of fistulae.

Symptomatology

Social uncleanliness, bleeding, prolapse and pruritus. Occasionally there may be severe anaemia.

Diagnosis

This requires inspection, digital examination, proctoscopy, and sigmoidoscopy.

External haemorrhoids must be distinguished from a carcinoma of the anal canal. Internal haemorrhoids must be distinguished from a prolapse of the rectum. When the main symptom is bleeding, the differential diagnosis includes proctitis and carcinoma of the rectum.

Treatment

The treatment of external haemorrhoids is simple surgical excision of the skin tags which form and which cause difficulties with anal hygiene. The treatments described for internal haemorrhoids are many and include:

Injection

The material used is normally 5% phenol in almond or arachis oil. Four or five ml is injected into the submucosal areolar tissue above each internal haemorrhoid. The effect is to produce a mild inflammatory foreign-body type of response. Such treatment is most effective when the piles do not prolapse and are not associated with large skin tags. One suggestion in the surgical literature following injection of the pile-bearing area at various intervals prior to excising the rectum suggests that the inflammatory response is minimal and that the effect of injection is chiefly a mechanical one, the bolus of oil temporarily stopping bleeding by pressure on the haemorrhoidal veins. Complications of injection therapy are uncommon but include:

a. Ulceration at the site of injection; this does not occur after a single, but only after repeated, injections.
b. Chemical prostatitis leading to perineal pain, frequency, and dysuria due to injecting the sclerosant into the prostate.

Strangulation by rubber bands

This method of treatment was introduced by Blaiseall in 1952 and has gained considerable popularity, since it can be performed as an outpatient procedure. It is applicable to both second and third degree haemorrhoids, in both of which situations the strangulating band can be passed over a definite pedicle. Follow-up studies have shown that this method is as effective as traditional surgical haemorrhoidectomy and, if recurrence occurs, there is nothing to prevent further treatment by the same method. The patients should be warned that pain is likely to follow banding and therefore they should be supplied with an ample supply of analgesics; in the elderly male such pain may induce acute retention of urine which, if not relieved by simple methods, may require catheterization. When the strangulated pile separates some bleeding will also occur and this again may be sufficient to necessitate admission to hospital.

Lord's procedure

In 1968 Lord put forward the hypothesis that internal haemorrhoids were caused by circular constricting bands in the anal canal which, by causing difficulty in defecation, led to straining at stool and increased venous pressure in the haemorrhoidal plexus of veins. He therefore suggested that piles would be cured if these bands were broken down by dilating the anal canal. The basis of Lord's procedure is that four fingers of each hand are inserted as far as possible into the anus.

After dilatation, a large sponge is inserted into the anal canal to prevent the development of a haematoma. This is removed as soon as the patient has recovered from the anaesthetic and thereafter the patient dilates the anus with a 4 cm diameter perspex dilator, at first daily and then less frequently. Few surgeons have, however, been able to reproduce the excellent results achieved by Lord himself. The following complications of this procedure have been described: rectal prolapse, continued prolapse of the haemorrhoids themselves and incontinence. So far as the latter is concerned Lord attributed this to fibrosis. Investigation, however, has shown that the external sphincter tone may be poor at rest; that the anal squeeze pressure is lower than normal and that the anorectal angle may be reduced all as a consequence of the procedure, all leading to incontinence, as a late complication, in as many as 20% of patients treated in this manner.

Cryosurgery

The cryoprobe is applied to the mucosa overlying the dilated venous plexus until the surface is frosted. Considerable pain and mucous discharge follows this method of treatment and the slough takes approximately 3 weeks to separate. Many surgeons would reserve this method of treatment for true internal haemorrhoids considering that the mixed intero-external type associated with large skin tags are best treated by surgical excision.

Surgical excision

A variety of different operations have been described for the treatment of second and third degree haemorrhoids. The common operative technique requires dissection of the pile-bearing areas and ligation of the pedicles at the level of the internal sphincter. This operation is particularly associated with the names of Milligan and Morgan. Other well-known procedures include Parks' submucous resection and Farquharson's clamp and cautery method. In addition, second and third degree haemorrhoids may be destroyed by freezing with liquid nitrogen, although most exponents of this technique admit to difficulties with the residual skin tags.

Complications of haemorrhoidectomy

Immediate

1. Reactionary haemorrhage.
2. Pain, which normally abates following the first bowel action.
3. Retention of urine.
4. Secondary haemorrhage, which is rarely severe but may on occasion require packing of the anal canal and transfusion.

Delayed

1. Loss of sphincter control, which may be sufficiently severe to produce social difficulties, particularly should the patient develop diarrhoea.
2. Stricture formation, either internal at a mucosal level or external at skin level due to the removal of too much perianal skin at the time of the operation.
3. Residual skin tags.

FISSURE-IN-ANO

Primary fissures-in-ano most commonly occur in the midline, most commonly posteriorly but occasionally anteriorly. They are the commonest cause of severe anal pain. Characteristically the pain associated with a fissure begins at the time of defecation and may in severe chronic cases continue for several hours. The severity of the pain induces secondary constipation. There may be a little bleeding but it is rarely excessive and is usually only sufficient to mark the toilet paper.

The cause of primary fissures is unknown, secondary fissures commonly complicate ulcerative colitis and Crohn's disease but, unlike primary fissures, this variety may cause little pain or discomfort despite the appearance of gross ulceration and oedema.

The pain associated with a fissure is due to abnormal spasm of the internal sphincter during defecation. Anal pressure studies show that the resting pressure of the internal sphincter is similar in patients with and without a fissure. Following dilatation reflex relaxation of the internal sphincter occurs in a normal individual in contrast to the increase in pressure in patients suffering from a fissure.

Diagnosis

This principally involves inspection, because nearly all fissures can be seen if sufficient care is taken. Perianal palpation quickly produces sphincteric spasm. It should be remembered that a squamous carcinoma of the anal canal or an adenocarcinoma of the rectum infiltrating the anal canal produce similar symptoms. Therefore, if the sentinel pile frequently associated with a chronic fissure feels hard the patient should be examined under an anaesthetic and appropriate biopsy material taken.

Surgery

1. The simplest manoeuvre consists of gentle *dilatation of the anal canal* under a general anaesthetic until four fingers can be admitted. Whilst this simple procedure relieves pain in the majority, the sentinel pile associated with the fissure remains.

2. *Internal sphincterotomy*. Not until 1952 was it shown by Eisenhammer that sphincterotomy resulted in division of the internal sphincter. Until that date surgeons had been under the mistaken impression that the operation they were performing for the treatment of fissure was division of the external sphincter.

Internal sphincterotomy may be performed in a number of ways. The original operation consisted of division of the sphincter in the midline posteriorly. Later, lateral subcutaneous sphincterotomy became popular. However, a recent paper from America, in which the results of over 1000 cases of both simple posterior division of the sphincter and lateral division were compared, showed that there was no difference in the frequency of the common complications, which include the inability to control the escape of flatus, soiling and accidental bowel movement. The first of these complications occurred in 35% of patients, the second in 22% and the third in over 40%.

Lateral subcutaneous sphincterotomy is performed in the following manner: under general anaesthetic a Parks' self-retaining retractor is inserted into the anal canal and a few ml of 1:200 000 adrenaline is injected into the intersphincteric plane and then between the anal mucosa and the sphincter. A 1.5 cm incision is made in the perianal skin to expose the lower border of the internal sphincter which is then divided to the level of the dentate line, the most medial fibres being broken down by pressure of the index finger. The external wound is then closed by three chronic catgut stitches after which the sentinel pile is removed.

NON-MALIGNANT CONDITIONS OF THE ANAL CANAL

FISTULA-IN-ANO

This is characterized by a track lined by granulation tissue leading from the anal canal or lower rectum to the exterior. Commonly there is only one internal opening, whereas there may be many external openings and occasionally no internal opening may be demonstrable.

Aetiological factors

1. Fistulae may be secondary to a variety of conditions, including:
   a. Ulcerative colitis, in which 3–6% of patients suffer from an associated fistula.
   b. Crohn's disease. Crohn himself reported this complication in 18 percent of patients and this incidence has subsequently been confirmed. In this disease fistulae are more common in colonic than in small bowel disease.
   c. Carcinoma of the lower third of the rectum and anal canal.
   d. Specific infections, including tuberculosis and actinomycosis.

2. The commonest cause of fistula is, however, the development of a pyogenic abscess which develops to such a degree that perforation of the anal canal or lower rectum has occurred, after which an external opening develops. Grace et al suggested that, when an abscess in the region of the anal canal was present, if gut-associated organisms were isolated in a high proportion of patients a fistula will be found, whereas if no gut-associated organisms were isolated the presence of a fistula was unlikely. The present concept is that infection begins in one of the 10–15 anal glands lying between the internal and external sphincters in the intersphincteric plane, leading to an intersphincteric abscess which tracks inferiorly in this plane to present at the anal verge as a perianal abscess, or penetrating the external sphincter at a variable level to form an ischiorectal abscess. At some point the abscess penetrates the mucosa again at a variable level (see below) to form a complete fistula with a variable relationship to the sphincter mechanism.

Anatomical classification of fistulae

Goodsall's rule

The position of the external opening should be noted. Goodsall observed that when the external opening of a fistula lies behind a transverse line drawn across the mid-point of the anus, the internal opening is in the midline on the posterior wall of the anal canal. In contrast, when the external opening is anterior to this line the fistula runs directly backwards into the anal canal.

An exception to this rule may occur when the external opening anterior to Goodsall's transverse line is further than 3 cm from the anus. In such cases that tract may curve backwards and end in the midline posteriorly.

Classification in terms of vertical plane

The most important issue in regard to the vertical height to which the fistula rises is in relationship to the puborectalis muscle. As a general rule the whole of the internal and most of the external sphincter can be divided, with the exception of the puborectalis muscle, without any serious loss of function. This is, however, true only for the younger patient. In an elderly person with a weak external sphincter even partial division of the internal sphincter may cause incontinence, hence the varying degrees of incontinence seen following haemorrhoidectomy.

The most simplistic way of considering fistula-in-ano is to consider them as high or low, depending on the relationship of the internal opening to the levator ani. All high fistulae open at or above this level and are rare, whereas low level fistulae open below. Parks and his colleagues, in their paper in the *British Journal of Surgery*, while recognizing the importance of the puborectalis, divide fistulae into four main types: intersphincteric; trans-sphincteric; suprasphincteric; extrasphincteric.

Fortunately for the practising surgeon, 90% of all fistulae open internally below the level of the puborectalis. The commonest variety is the intersphincteric followed closely by the transsphincteric. The risk, therefore, of incontinence following the surgical treatment of the great majority of fistulae is negligible.

Symptomatology

The majority of patients present with a history of recurrent attacks of perianal suppuration associated with an intermittent purulent or serosanguinious discharge. Few fistulae discharge continuously and there may be little to see or feel but when discharging, the external opening appears as a red elevated circle of granulation tissue.

Diagnosis

Examination normally confirms the diagnosis. Sigmoidoscopy and biopsy, if negative, rule out the presence of a neoplasm or proctocolitis but not necessarily Crohn's disease, since in this last condition fistulae may complicate small bowel disease. Inspection will normally rule out hyperhidrosis suppurativa which chracteristically presents with multiple discharging sinuses.

The most important step is to discover the relationship between the internal opening and the ano-rectal angle, the latter marking the level of the puborectalis. However, in approximately 50% of patients no detectable internal opening is present.

In low level anterior fistulae, a palpable tract may be felt or it may be possible to pass a probe through the fistula even without an anaesthetic. In most fistulae, however, initial delineation of the tract requires a light anaesthetic; light, at least initially because it is essential to be able to relate the path of an exploring probe to the puborectalis.

Treatment

The accepted method of curing all types of anal fistulae is a complete laying open of the track to allow subsequent healing to take place from the anal origin of the track towards the surface, i.e. making sure that the saucerized wound heals from its depth.

If the fistula is high, a two-stage procedure may be advisable. At the first stage a black silk seton is placed through the tract to act as a marker and to stimulate fibrosis adjacent to the sphincter muscle, so that in the second stage, which involves laying open the intersphincteric portion of the fistulous tract, the sphincter does not gape.

Hanley and Parks suggested that in complicated horse-shoe fistulae, as an alternative to deroofing, a posterior sphincterotomy should be performed and the lateral tracts should be curetted and drained. Curettage being repeated if healing does not take place.

Recently Mann and Clifton of St Mark's have described a rerouting operation for high anal and anorectal fistulae transposing the extrasphincteric portion of the tract into the intersphincteric position with immediate repair of the external sphincter. The newly positioned interspfinteric fistula is then dealt with at a later date when the external sphincter is soundly healed. They concluded after treating five patients in this manner that a colostomy was unnecessary, healing occurred rapidly and continence was preserved.

SECTION SIX

28. Chronic ischaemia of the lower limb: pathology, clinical features, and investigations

The chief causes of chronic ischaemia in the lower limbs are atherosclerosis and Buerger's disease.

ATHEROSCLEROSIS

The commonest cause of chronic ischaemia of the lower limbs is atherosclerosis, which was defined by the World Health Organization study group as a variable combination of changes in the intima and media of arteries consisting of focal accumulations of lipids, complex carbohydrates, blood products, fibrous tissue and calcium deposits.

The various factors that have been incriminated in the aetiology of the disease include:

1. *Age*. This is an important factor, since whilst early atherosclerotic changes are seen in young individuals, fully developed lesions are uncommon before the fourth decade, after which the frequency and severity of the disease increases.

2. *Sex*. In the female the pathological changes associated with atherosclerosis lag behind those in the male by about two decades. Death as a consequence of the complications of atherosclerosis is seldom seen in the female prior to the menopause, after which this marked difference between the sexes rapidly disappears. This difference between the sexes is considered to be due to oestrogen secretion by the female, which is known to depress serum β-lipoprotein.

3. *Smoking*. Epidemiological studies implicate cigarette smoking as a significant atherogenic factor.

4. *Haemodynamic stress*. Atherosclerosis does not develop in the low-pressure pulmonary system except in the presence of pulmonary hypertension or in peripheral veins, unless an arteriovenous fistula is present. Whilst many patients suffering from atherosclerosis have a normal blood pressure, in the presence of hypertension the disease

tends to develop at an earlier age and to be more severe than in normotensive individuals.

5. *Environment.* The death rate from the complications of this disease is much lower in developing countries than in the industrialized countries of the Western world. However, migration from the former to the latter results in the slow development of the same mortality as that of the host population. The question posed by this finding is whether diet or some other factor is at work.

6. *High serum cholesterol.* Certain conditions in man associated with a high serum cholesterol are related to an increased incidence of this disease. These include myxoedema, the nephrotic syndrome and certain types of familial xanthomatosis. However, in normal atherosclerotic patients the serum cholesterol is only slightly, although significantly, elevated above the accepted upper limit of normal. Extension of this work has led to the finding that particular lipoprotein fractions, with particular sedimentation constants, are significantly increased in the serum of patients suffering from advanced atherosclerosis.

7. *Social class.* Atherosclerosis appears to be more frequent in social classes I and II, especially in the males of these groups, possibly because of the type of diet eaten by these groups.

8. *Diabetes.* In this condition atherosclerosis begins at an earlier age, advances more rapidly, and is about twice as common as in non-diabetic controls. The condition is rendered more serious by the presence of neuropathic lesions as well as the vascular lesions, the former leading to neuropathic ulceration on the plantar aspect of the foot and the latter to failure of conservative measures to deal with the situation.

The relationship of diet and fat metabolism to atherosclerosis

The presence of cholesterol in atheromatous plaques was demonstrated in the middle of the last century. It has since been shown that atheroma can be produced in experimental animals such as the rabbit by means of a high-cholesterol diet. However, the applicability to man of these results is doubtful because, as well as atheroma, changes in other tissues occur in the rabbit which are not seen in man. In other animals, similar vascular changes to those observed in man can be produced but the serum cholesterol must be kept elevated for prolonged periods. Few, if any, of these experiments reproduce the 'normal' situation in humans and their validity is doubtful.

In the human, epidemiological studies have shown that high-calorie, obesity-producing diets rich in animal fats are associated with a high incidence of arterial disease, whereas diets low in calories and animal fats cause relatively few arterial changes. Also playing their part among the possible dietary causes are the source and quality of the protein, the type and quality of the carbohydrate, and the presence of a high content of cholesterol. The ratio of polyunsaturated to saturated fats is probably not critical. If a patient eats a diet containing only a moderate amount of unsaturated fats, the serum cholesterol falls. Studies in the human do not conclusively demonstrate whether such a diet will reduce the progress of established disease although in the experimental animal, if the diet is altered in this manner prior to ulceration of the atheromatous plaques, reversal can be induced.

Regardless of the source of the lipid, one of the central points of disagreement surrounding the pathogenesis of this disease is the manner in which lipid reaches the subintimal layer.

Mechanism of lipid accumulation

In 1852 von Rokitansky suggested that the lipid represented degeneration in small thrombi deposited on the arterial wall. The thrombogenic theory was revived by Duguid and Robertson in 1957, who proposed that the original thickening of the intima resulted from the deposition of small fibrin and platelet thrombi on the intimal surface, which were then later organized by fibroblasts and recovered by endothelium. The accumulation of lipid was considered a secondary phenomenon due to fat molecules diffusing into the intima from the circulating plasma, described as fat imbibition.

However, even if the above theory is accepted it still leaves unanswered the question of how or by what mechanism the thrombi form on the intima in the first place. Possible explanations are that there may be either an increased sensitivity of the coagulation mechanisms or, alternatively, a diminished fibrinolytic power of the blood. In support of the former mechanism, it has been shown that fatty meals cause shortening of the clotting time, probably an action of ethanolamine phosphatide, which is present in many animal and vegetable fats. In support of the latter, it has been shown that the fibrinolytic activity of the blood is increased by exercise and decreased by a fatty meal.

A second theory is that proposed by Texon, who suggested that the intimal proliferation is due to a suction effect on the arterial wall due to the fall in lateral pressure in the arterial system where the velocity of the blood increases as the arteries become smaller. This theory offers a possible explanation of the increasing incidence of atherosclerosis in the lower abdominal aorta and the common iliac vessels and also the manner in which the lesions progress once they have begun.

Yet a third theory has been put forward, the filtration theory, in which it is postulated that the lipids reach the deeper layers of the intima after being deposited on, and filtered through, the endothelium.

Whatever the precise aetiology of atherosclerosis the pathological changes in the affected vessels pass through a number of changes, although in a single individual all stages of the disease may be seen from the less severe to the gross changes of ulceration, calcification, dilatation, or stenosis of the affected vessels.

The development of the lesions

Clinically, atherosclerosis is only diagnosed when it has reached an advanced stage in pathological terms; thus the internal diameter of the superficial femoral artery must be reduced by 70% before claudication occurs. However, the disease slowly develops over a number of stages.

Stage I

The 'fatty' streak. This is the first naked eye evidence of disease. Such streaks can be found, even in childhood, most commonly in the aorta. They may be multiple extending from the arch downwards towards its bifurcation. The streaks seen under a hand lens appear as a row of 'fatty dots' tending to bifurcate and surround the ostia of the branches of the artery.

Microscopic examination at this stage shows that each streak is composed of a collection of large cells which can be identified by electron microscopy as smooth muscle cells stuffed with fat lying immediately beneath the endothelium.

There is, however, still disagreement as to whether these fatty streaks represent the earliest stages of irreversible disease or whether they may spontaneously resolve.

Stage II

This is the stage normally reached in the fourth decade but in familial disorders of carbohydrate metabolism when endogenous (hepatic) triglycerides are overproduced from the dietary carbohydrate, the arterial changes occur earlier.

At this stage an uncomplicated plaque appears as a smooth yellowish lesion several millimetres in diameter and slightly raised above the surrounding surface. This elevation is possibly an artefact since arteries are normally examined in an empty and collapsed condition. Depending on the severity of the disease the plaques may be few or plentiful in number; if the latter, they may be confluent. In severely involved vessels the whole artery may be lined by diseased intima.

Microscopic examination shows that the plaques consist of a mass of lipid. In the peripheral area of the plaque the lipid is still confined within the cells, but in the central zone it forms a structureless amorphous mass containing fat droplets among which may be found the typical boat-shaped cholesterol crystals. In paraffin sections, the last are seen as clefts since all fat is dissolved out. Deep to the plaque the internal elastic lamina is commonly fragmented and the media reduced in thickness. Superficial to the plaque, i.e. on the luminal surface, a layer of hyaline fibres gradually separates the plaque from the endothelium.

Stage III

At this advanced stage widespread proliferation of fibrous tissue occurs around and in between the plaques so that the intima becomes irregularly thickened. Small vessels derived from the vasa vasorum now extend through the media into the thickened intima, possibly because the diseased intima cannot be nourished in the usual manner by the diffusion of nutrients from the blood stream.

The endothelium over the thicker plaques then breaks down and the underlying lipid is exposed and may then be discharged into the circulation in the form of 'grummous' or gruel-like emboli. This leaves an atheromatous ulcer which is shallow, has ragged edges and lipid in its base. Once ulceration has developed mural thrombus rapidly develops on its surface, the thrombus chiefly consisting of fibrin which may later become covered by endothelium after which it is slowly organized to a limited extent.

Ulceration is considered to be a complication of atheroma, as are calcification and haemorrhage into a plaque. Calcification occurs especially in the aged and particularly in the distal aorta. Severe calcification converts the wall of the vessel into a brittle shell which may crack like an egg if roughly handled. Microscopic examination shows that the calcific deposits occur chiefly in the deepest layers of the intima and around the periphery of the lipid masses. Intramural haemorrhages may develop due to leakage from the new vessels derived from the vasa vasorum.

Whether the lumen of an affected vessel becomes occluded depends upon a number of factors including the degree of medial degeneration which by itself will lead to dilatation, and the degree of mural thrombosis and organization which alone lead to narrowing of the affected vessels. A further factor of importance is the systemic blood pressure, dilatation being common in the larger vessels in which the pressure is relatively higher. Stenosis, on the other hand, is commoner than dilatation in the coronary blood vessels. Regarding the last, a factor in coronary occlusion which is seldom, if ever, considered is the normal variation in calibre of the coronary arteries in different individuals. The situation is one of 'disproportion' since an individual in whom wide coronaries are present can tolerate a thick layer of atheroma while, conversely, the unfortunate person with healthy but narrow arteries is more easily compromised by slight atheroma.

THROMBOANGIITIS OBLITERANS (BUERGER'S DISEASE)

Although known as Buerger's disease, this condition was in fact first described by Winwarter in 1879. The disease as described by Buerger in 1908 consists of an inflammatory reaction in the arterial wall with involvement of the neighbouring vein and nerve terminating in thrombosis of the artery. Although considered a specific entity, some who have closely observed the pathological changes consider that they merely represent presenile atherosclerosis.

Whatever its relationship to atherosclerosis as a cause of obliterative arterial disease, it is fortunately much less common than atherosclerosis itself. When first described it was considered to be a disease confined to the Jewish race but epidemiological studies have disproved this. It is, however, predominantly a disease of white males between 20 and 40 years of age, and is uncommon in women. It is also a disease of heavy smokers although the exact mechanism of this association remains unclear.

Pathology

The gross features of Buerger's disease are characteristic of an inflammatory process. The diseased artery is usually surrounded by a dense fibrotic reaction often incorporating the adjacent vein and less commonly the nerves. The distribution of the lesions is entirely different from that of atherosclerosis in that smaller, more peripheral vessels are involved, usually distal to the brachial and popliteal arteries, often in a segmental fashion. Whereas atherosclerosis rarely involves the upper limbs this is quite common in Buerger's disease, in which condition the upper limbs are involved in 30% of patients.

Early in the course of Buerger's disease the superficial veins are involved, producing a recurrent superficial thrombophlebitis, although the deep veins are rarely affected.

Microscopic changes

The microscopic changes seen in the small thrombosed arteries are those of extensive proliferation of the intimal cells and fibroblasts throughout the arterial wall, although the basic architecture of the vessels is preserved. Lipid deposition and calcification, which are commonplace in atherosclerosis, are absent. Spaces within the thrombus are common but not characteristic since they are seen in any form of occlusive lesion.

SYMPTOMS OF ISCHAEMIA OF THE LOWER LIMB

The symptoms of ischaemia are due to the decrease in blood supply to the tissues supplied by the affected blood vessels. The dynamics of arterial flow are governed by numerous factors, including the peripheral resistance, turbulence, compliance, and rheological factors, but the chief determinant remains the size of the lumen as governed by Pouiseuille's equation:

$$\text{Flow} = \frac{\pi R^4 (P_1 - P_2)}{8 \eta L}$$

where R = radius, L = length, η = viscosity, and $(P_1 - P_2)$ = pressure difference between the two ends of the vessel.

Thus, a small increase in luminal reduction, say from 70 to 80% (70% being a clinically significant lesion) reduces the flow fivefold.

When the decrease is gradual, in the majority of individuals the disease must be symptomless, because quite gross atherosclerotic changes are seen in the blood vessels of the elderly at postmortem who are known to have been free of symptoms associated with arterial disease in life. In others the chief symptoms are as described below.

Intermittent claudication

This indicates a reduction, usually by more than 60%, in the blood flow to muscle groups undergoing exercise. Although it is most often a symptom of arterial occlusion it may also be apparent when there is a deficient oxygen supply to muscle, as can happen at a high altitude or in severe anaemia. The pain of claudication is usually typical; it is produced by muscular effort and it is relieved by stopping the exercise even when the limb remains dependent. This distinguishes claudication from the pain of venous stasis which may be felt on exercise but which can only be relieved by elevating the affected limb.

The precise algogen responsible for the pain of claudication is unknown. Lewis, in his original papers in the 1930s concluded that the factor responsible, the P factor, was a product of muscle metabolism.

If a patient continues to walk after the pain of claudication begins, the muscles gradually stiffen and tighten so that, regardless of the patient's pain threshold, he or she must eventually stop. Variations in the amount of exercise required to produce pain, 'the claudication distance', gives an approximate measure of the progress of obliterative arterial disease, and the site of the pain is an indication of the site of the block, which is always proximal to the area of complaint. Thus, claudication in the foot, often interpreted as 'foot strain' indicates occlusion at or above the ankle. Claudication in the calf indicates femoropopliteal disease whereas pain in the buttocks and thighs indicates occlusion of the aorta or iliac vessels (Leriche's syndrome).

Claudication is nearly always associated with absent peripheral pulses. If this happens not to be so, the usual explanation is the presence of an aortic block, in which condition the femoral pulses are absent but the popliteal and posterior tibial pulses are palpable. However, if clinical examination reveals that all the pulses are present, the patient should be asked to walk until claudication develops. Re-examination at this time often reveals that the previously palpable pulses have vanished, but as the pain disappears the pulses slowly return. The explanation of this phenomenon is the shift of the blood flow into the muscle bed.

Differential diagnosis

Symptoms superficially resembling claudication may be produced by many conditions including orthopaedic, muscular and neurological pathologies. In nearly all cases, however, the minutiae of the history, together with the obvious physical signs allow the diagnosis of occlusive vascular disease to be made with comparative ease.

A very similar pain, known as pseudoclaudication, may be experienced due to compression of the cauda equina. However, in this condition the distress may also be brought on by standing or bending, and it is usually associated with numbness or muscle weakness, which is relieved by sitting or lying down.

Constant limb pain

This is nearly always due to ischaemic neuritis, which may be felt after either a sudden or gradual occlusion of the arterial supply to the limb.

In this condition the pain is usually severe, diffuse, and bears no relationship to dermatomes. Typically, it is worse in bed at night. It may be associated with paraesthesiae, formication and a sense of numbness and coldness in the affected extremity. At some point the patient usually observes that putting the foot out of bed into a dependent position brings relief. Still later, the patient may begin to sleep sitting upright in a chair.

Because the pain of ischaemic neuritis is nervous in origin, physical examination may reveal reduced sensation to touch, pain and/or vibration. A similar pain, known as rest pain, which cannot be differentiated on clinical grounds from ischaemic neuritis, is sometimes experienced before the onset of gangrene. Both conditions indicate a serious deterioration of the peripheral circulation.

Occasionally, severe rest pain is felt in a limb that seems completely normal but in which the pulses are absent. In such a limb gangrene is inevitable.

Differential diagnosis

Once again, in the presence of physical signs the diagnosis of ischaemic neuritis or rest pain is simple. However, it must occasionally be distinguished from causalgia, which follows injury to peripheral nerves and any type of peripheral neuropathy.

In aged people, even in the highly developed countries, there is a syndrome known as the burning feet syndrome. This is probably caused by dietary deficiencies since the majority of people are cured if given a good diet with vitamin supplements. The major symptoms of this disease are intense burning in the foot associated, often, with shooting pains. Some patients obtain relief by sitting out of bed with their feet in cold water.

Diabetic neuropathy, which is relatively common in older people, often gives rise to gross sensory changes together with pain in the presence of relatively normal motor function.

PHYSICAL SIGNS OF ARTERIAL OCCLUSION

The major physical signs associated with *gradual* occlusion of a limb artery are those associated with atrophy. The affected limbs are wasted, the toe pads disappear, and the hair vanishes.

In addition, there are always significant colour and temperature changes in any limb in which the arterial supply is in danger. In general, the skin becomes cyanotic when the limb is dependent because the rate of blood flow is so slow that a longer period is allowed for the reduction of oxyhaemoglobin. When the limb is elevated it usually becomes pallid because the blood pressure in the diseased limb cannot overcome gravity. Because the skin temperatures is determined by both the blood flow and the heat loss, the affected limb nearly always feels cooler to the examining hand; coldness may, indeed, be a cause of bitter complaint by the patient.

Following inspection of the limb a search is made for other appropriate physical signs, which include the following:

1. *Absent pulsations.* The pulses normally palpable in the lower limb include those of the common femoral artery, the popliteal artery, the posterior tibial and the dorsalis pedis. If it appears that there is an element of vasospasm associated with absent pulses a sublingual tablet of glyceryl trinitrate will release the spasm and the pulses will become palpable, if the arteries are patent, within a few minutes. When the lower femoral and popliteal arteries are blocked, pulsation may be felt in the medial and lateral geniculate arteries.

2. *Bruits.* Arterial murmurs develop in partially occluded arteries due to turbulence of the blood flow. Bruits can be made louder and more obvious by exercising the limb, because this increases the rate of proximal blood flow and dilates the artery distal to the block, so increasing the rate of 'run-off'. This increases the velocity of the blood flow across the stenotic segment and a louder systolic bruit is heard. As an affected segment narrows, the bruit may be apparent

even under resting conditions. Any bruit is usually conducted peripherally so that a partial occlusion at the bifurcation of the common iliac artery may be heard in the thigh.

3. *Venous changes* As arterial occlusion progresses and the blood flow to the affected limb diminishes so the veins lie empty and collapsed, forming grooves rather than elevations under the skin.

4. *Ulceration.* Ischaemic ulcers most commonly develop on the heel and digits but may be found elsewhere on the leg below the level of the knee joint. Ischaemic ulcers thus occur in areas in which venous ulcers may develop but they are distinguished clinically by the fact that they are usually more painful and often invade the deep fascia, tendons and bone. They are also associated with the signs of circulatory insufficiency, including pallor, dependent cyanosis, dystrophic nails, reduced skin temperature, sluggish venous filling, poor capillary return, and absent peripheral pulses. Such ulcers have, of course, to be distinguished from other causes of limb ulceration, including:

   a. *Stasis ulceration (venous ulceration).* Venous ulceration is the commonest cause of leg ulcers in the Western world. They are usually seen in the 'gaiter' region near the medial malleolus or adjacent to the lateral malleolus, and when the condition is severe they may involve the whole circumference of the leg. Venous ulcers have a shallow base with a flat margin and the surrounding skin shows evidence of venous hypertension, i.e. pigmentation, atrophe blanche, eczema and lipodermatosclerosis.

   b. *Neurotrophic ulcers.* These occur in patients suffering from a peripheral neuritis, whatever the underlying cause, and in patients suffering from syringomyelia. Such ulcers usually occur on the toes, often under the first metatarsophalangeal joint, and are indolent, painless and penetrating. Other less common causes of ulceration of the lower leg include:

   c. Blood dyscrasias such as haemolytic anaemia, sickle cell anaemia, leukaemia, and polycythaemia.

   d. Specific infections such as syphilis, when gummatous ulceration may appear on the legs and Kaposi's sarcoma.

   e. Basal cell carcinoma or epithelioma, the last sometimes complicate longstanding causes of chronic ulceration such as venous ulcers, burns, osteomyelitis, when they are known as Marjolin's ulcers.

   f. Melanoma.

   g. Pyoderma gangrenosum complicating agammaglobulinaemia, and ulcerative colitis.

h. Disease of small blood vessels, diabetes, rheumatoid arthritis, and autoimmune disease.

A complete history and physical examination is one of the most important parts of the evaluation of a patient thought to be suffering from chronic ischaemia in the lower limbs. The history will most probably establish the cause. The diabetic patient, in addition to claudication, may have a typical history of increasing thirst and polyuria due to the osmotic diuresis caused by the raised blood glucose, loss of weight in the presence of a normal or increased appetite, and fatigue; in women, pruritis vulvae is common due to infection with *Candida albicans*. The diagnosis of diabetes is easily confirmed by performing a fasting blood sugar, which in diabetes should exceed 8 mmol/l. Buerger's disease is relatively easy to exclude due to the age of onset and the associated phlebitis.

The possible site of the vascular stenosis is indicated by the site of claudication: pain in the buttocks indicates an aorto-iliac block; pain in the calves, femoro-popliteal block; and constant pain in the legs, severe stenosis below the level of the popliteal artery.

Concomitant cardiac and pulmonary disease should also be looked for.

INVESTIGATIONS

Following history-taking and clinical examination, special investigations may be used to establish.

a. The precise level of the block and its extent.
b. Possible course of action.

In most patients nothing active need be done (see Ch. 29). Non-invasive methods of investigation are now available which are easy to perform and have no complications. Those now seldom used include:

1. *Gravimetric plethysmography.* This investigation has the disadvantage in that it will only indicate the cumulative effect of the disease rather than demarcate a specific lesion. The method is designed to estimate the whole lower limb blood flow calculated from the increase in weight of the limb following a period of arterial occlusion by an inflatable cuff.

2. *Radioisotope imaging.* In this technique a bolus of ^{99m}Tc is injected and the rate of advance is measured by a series of gamma cameras placed at intervals over the limb.

Ultrasound

Ultrasound is the most commonly used non-invasive technique. Doppler ultrasound is based on the shift in ultrasound frequency, the Doppler effect, which occurs when an ultrasound beam is transmitted to and reflected from the moving blood cells. The frequency shift is proportional to the velocity of the blood flow. This may be analysed audibly by listening to the intensity, pitch and phasic nature of the sound, or may be recorded graphically – for example, over a normal femoral artery a characteristic triphasic sonographic pattern is seen in which the first deflection corresponds to forward flow during systole, the second to reversed flow during diastole, and the third to the return of forward flow. Using a non-directional Doppler, all deflections occur above the zero line, whereas using directional equipment the reversed flow phase appears below the line. In the presence of obstruction proximal to the probe the first phase becomes shallow and the second and third phases are abolished.

The Doppler effect can also be used to determine the systolic blood pressure. The probe is used as a sensitive stethoscope over an artery distal to a pressure cuff. When the cuff is inflated to occlude the artery the Doppler signal disappears, only to return as the cuff is released. Pressures obtained by this method are compared to pressures in the arm or the unaffected extremity and recorded as a ratio of the normal systolic pressure. When the arm pressure is 120 mmHg and that in the dorsalis pedis 40 mmHg, the ankle : arm pressure ratio is 0.33. In healthy individuals the ankle : arm ratio is 1 or higher, whereas in advanced degrees of lower limb ischaemia complicated by claudication the ratio may fall to 0.5, and in patients suffering from rest pain the ratio may be as low as 0.05. The Doppler probe is a useful tool in the follow-up of patients who have undergone arterial surgery.

Arteriography

In vivo angiography was first performed in 1920, but it was not until the 1950s, when safer iodine-containing contrast media were introduced, that the method came into general use. Further advances have followed: the introduction of low osmolarity compounds; the development of percutaneous catheterization; and, lastly, digital subtraction angiography which, although providing less resolution, is wholly adequate for the examination of the vessels of the lower limb. One of the great advantages of the latter technique is that contrast medium can be given intravenously, thus avoiding the hazards of arterial puncture.

The radiological signs of atherosclerosis include:

1. Diffuse narrowing of the affected arteries.
2. Irregularity of the vascular contour.
3. Variations in the density of the opaque column. If there are variations they give a clue to the presence of plaques and mural thrombi. Unfortunately there can be large plaques even in the absence of any radiological abnormality.
4. Tortuosity of the vessels indicating fragmentation of the internal elastic lamina.
5. Aneurysm formation.
6. Frank occlusion.
7. Decrease in the magnitude of the 'run-off' following a narrow segment.

Interestingly the surgeon nearly always finds a greater degree of luminal compromise, intimal degeneration, mural thrombosis and calcification than is apparent on the aortograms or arteriograms.

Arteriography is not without its complications, which include:

1. *Local complications:*
   a. Bleeding from the puncture wound, leading to haematoma formation.
   b. Arterial occlusion from the dislodgement of atheromatous plaques or by embolization from catheter clot formation, a complication requiring immediate surgical intervention.
   c. Arteriovenous fistula formation due to faulty needle placement.
2. *General complications:*
   a. Contrast reactions, causing hypotension and tachycardia.
   b. Vagal inhibition, causing hypotension and bradycardia.
   c. Allergic reactions, resulting in rigors and fever.

By the use of translumbar, direct femoral or retrograde catheterization the precise site of obstruction and the degree of stenosis can be accurately assessed.

Biochemical changes in peripheral atherosclerosis

Investigations have shown that the mean serum total cholesterol and triglyceride levels are higher in patients of both sexes suffering from peripheral vascular disease than in control subjects, although the only significant difference is in respect of the triglyceride level in males. This difference is not, however, associated with a significant reduction in the high density lipoprotein cholesterol concentration although there is some difference in the levels of this fraction between the sexes.

In ischaemic heart disease due to coronary artery disease there is an increase in the very low density lipoproteins (VLDL) and low density lipoproteins (LDL) and this is thought to promote atherosclerosis by enhancing the rate of deposition of cholesterol in the arterial wall.

In contrast it has been suggested that increased levels of high density lipoproteins (HDL), which are known to be associated with a decreased risk of coronary artery disease, counteract the accumulation of cholesterol either by promoting its removal from the arterial wall or by preventing the uptake of low density lipoprotein.

One way of expressing these contrasting effects of serum lipoproteins is to calculate the ratio of 'protective' HDL cholesterol to the sum of atherogenic VLDL and LDL cholesterol. The HDL ratios are reduced in boith male and female with peripheral vascular disease but in males this is partly due to an increase in VLDL and LDL whereas in females a decrease in HDL is probably more important.

ACUTE OCCLUSION (See Tutorial 30)

In any patient suffering from artherosclerosis acute occlusion of the affected vessel may suddenly occur due to subintimal haemorrhage or thrombosis. If either of these events occurs, sudden pain develops in the affected limb associated with a feeling of coldness, numbness and tingling. Depending on the site of the lesion such a catastrophe may be followed by gangrene. Gangrene occurring in atherosclerosis is, however, more usually precipitated by injury or by interdigital fungal infections which macerate the skin in patients in whom progressive deterioration has been occurring. The gangrene is usually dry; the tissues involved are at first purple, later black, and in the absence of infection or oedema the affected part in due course becomes dry and shrunken with a line of demarcation developing between the affected part and the viable tissues.

29. Chronic ischaemia of the lower limb: management

In the majority of patients suffering from ischaemia of the lower limbs with associated claudication no intervention is necessary. Boyd in 1960 published a classic paper in which he reviewed the life expectancy and the risk of amputation in patients already suffering from claudication over a period of time. His chief findings were as follows:

1. So far as life expectancy was concerned, 73.5% of patients were still alive at 5 years; 38.5% at 10 years; and 22.0% at 15 years.
2. So far as the risk of amputation was concerned, the chance of amputation was 7.2% during the first 5 years and 12.2% within the first 10 years, although the risk of amputation was shown to rise with the age of onset of the disease.

Thus it is apparent that it is the minority rather than the majority of patients suffering from claudication who require intervention of any sort. Obviously other factors come into play, e.g. the occupation and pastimes of the patient, and the presence of coexisting disease.

LIFESTYLE MANAGEMENT

In those patients in whom non-intervention is considered the best management, the following may assist:

1. *If the patient is a smoker, he or she must be persuaded to stop.* The risk of claudication in smokers is some 15 times higher in male smokers than in non-smokers and 7 times higher in females, a risk which appears to increase according to the number of cigarettes smoked. In patients already claudicating, the treadmill walking distance has been shown to improve after ceasing to smoke and the ankle : brachial blood pressure ratio increases. The cessation of smoking is especially important in Buerger's disease.

2. *Regular exercise.* Larsen and Lassen found that by progressive treadmill exercise the walking time before the onset of claudication could be increased from 2.9–8.2 minutes.
3. *Weight reduction.*
4. *Attention to the diet.* The chief concerns are:
   a. A division of the total calorie intake more evenly throughout the day.
   b. A reduction of the total fat, increasing the intake of non-saturated fats as compared to saturated.
   c. Reducing the intake of high-cholesterol foods such as eggs and liver. Although human studies do not indicate for certain that such dietary restrictions will reduce the progress of the disease, animal experiments have shown that it is clearly possible to influence non-ulcerating atherosclerotic lesions for the better by these means.
5. Care to avoid injury to the skin of the feet, which is particularly liable to happen in the older person when attending to the toenails, or in minor gardening accidents.

MEDICAL TREATMENT

1. *Hypolipidaemics.* In patients in whom the fasting cholesterol exceeds 7 mmol/l, the drug clofibrate (ethyl-α-(p-chlorophoxy) isobutyrate) will reduce the circulating level of cholesterol, serum triglycerides and serum phospholipids. In atherosclerosis affecting predominantly the coronary arteries, the Newcastle Study Group found that the number of deaths and non-fatal infarcts was significantly less in a clofibrate treated group as compared to a matched group of controls treated with corn oil. Assessed angiographically, other workers have found that intensive hypolipidaemic therapy was associated with a two-thirds reduction in the rate of progression of atherosclerosis involving the lower limbs.

2. *Vasodilators.* The use of vasodilators is highly controversial because in ischaemic areas of the limb vasodilatation is already at a maximum due to acidosis and accumulation of metabolites.

3. *Haemodilution.* Limb blood flow is directly related to the perfusion pressure and inversely proportional to vascular resistance. Perfusion pressure cannot be altered because of the fixed arterial resistance, but vascular resistance is a product of the diameter of the vessels through which the blood is flowing and its viscosity. Again, the diameter of the vessels cannot be altered but theoretically the viscosity can be reduced by haemodilution. The effect of haemodi-

lution is of course to reduce the oxygen-carrying capacity of the blood as well as reducing the viscosity. The former obviously reduces the efficacy of this mode of treatment. Some investigators have, however, found that beneficial effects can be demonstrated in some but not the majority of patients by: blood letting and retransfusion with plasma, low molecular weight dextran or hydroxethyl starch solutions; or oxpentifylline, which apparently alters the deformability of the red cells enabling them to pass through the capillaries at the low flow rates which are encountered in these vessels in atherosclerosis.

SURGICAL TREATMENT

Indications for direct arterial surgery

1. *Claudication.* This is a relative indication for direct arterial surgery because the degree of disablement with similar claudication distances will be different in each individual owing to various factors such as work, hobbies, and age. The individual degree of disablement is, therefore, important.

2. *Rest pain.* This may be regarded as an absolute indication since it always leads to general deterioration in the patient's general condition, because of interference with sleep and the depressive effect of chronic pain. Furthermore, this type of pain is difficult to control with non-addictive analgesics of low or intermediate potency.

3. *Ischaemic ulceration of the leg: incipient or actual gangrene.* Ischaemic ulceration, incipient or actual gangrene are an indication for arterial surgery assuming that the radiological findings indicate that some benefit will be achieved. If, however, investigation shows only small vessel disease or occlusion below the trifurcation it is unlikely that any benefit will accrue from direct arterial surgery. However, an operative or chemical sympathectomy will sometimes prevent incipient gangrene from becoming a true necrosis of tissue.

Sites of occlusion

The common sites of occlusion producing lower limb symptoms are:

1. Adductor region of the femoral artery in 70%.
2. Aortoiliac area, 50-60%.
3. Popliteal artery, 12%.
4. Popliteal bifurcation, 12%.

The proximal parts of the superficial femoral artery, and the popliteal artery below the level of the knee joint are relatively uncommon sites of occlusion. In recent years it has also been realized that the artery of supply in the thigh, the profunda femoris or deep femoral artery, is seldom involved along its length but only at its junction with the common femoral and along its first few centimetres.

It is also important to recognize that a considerable proportion of patients suffering from aortoiliac disease also have disease in the femoropopliteal segment and that this can dramatically alter the results of surgical interference if this is deemed necessary, about 25% of such patients presenting with intermittent claudication progressing to severe ischaemia.

Surgical treatment methods

Grafts

These are of many types and new prosthetic grafts are constantly being introduced.

Synthetic grafts. An ideal graft should not excite a chemical, inflammatory, allergic or foreign-body cell reaction. They should be capable of withstanding the mechanical strains imposed upon them and they should have a low thrombogenic potential, a biological porosity of 10 000 ml/H_2O per minute at 120 mmHg, and a low implant porosity of less than 50 ml/cm^2 per minute. Lastly, they should have easy handling properties.

Many synthetic grafts have been introduced, only to be withdrawn when their adoption by the clinician shows that their practical properties do not live up to their theoretical expectations. Currently one of the most popular synthetic grafts is made of woven or knitted Dacron (polyethylene terephthalate), which possesses sufficient porosity to ensure that the neointimal lining is firmly fixed in place by fibroblasts growing through the interstices of the material from the host tissues. Knitted Dacron has such a degree of porosity, however, that a new graft, exposed immediately to a normal arterial flow, leaks in an alarming fashion; to overcome this the graft must be 'preclotted' before insertion by allowing it to lie in the recipient's blood, and then prior to insertion flushing it free of clots. Approximately 1 year after implantation, examination shows that a new pseudointima, 0.5–1 mm thick, has formed from the components of the arterial blood. Electron microscopy shows that this layer consists of interlocking fibres in which are enmeshed all types of blood cell.

Two graft materials which have been recently introduced are:
1. *Polytetrafluoroethylene (PTFE) (otherwise known as Gore-Tex)*. This was introduced into the UK in 1976 and is a prosthetic graft made of fibrillated PTFE. It is of low thrombogenicity and the thin, flexible fibres allow tissue ingrowth and hence the formation of a satisfactory neointima which is much thinner than the pseudointima forming within a Dacron graft, being only 5–35 μm in thickness. The grafts are 6 mm in diameter and are anastomosed to the recipient vessel with a continuous polypropylene suture. The graft has the advantage of flexing without kinking and does not require preclotting, no extravasation occurring even in a fully heparinized patient, because of the high PTFE–blood surface tension.

2. *Glutaraldehye-stabilized umbilical vein grafts* were introduced in the mid-1970s by Darlik et al as an alternative to the use of autogenous saphenous grafts. They are part natural and part synthetic – the most commonly used variety has an outer layer of Dacron mesh in order to increase its tensile strength. Its protagonists claim that it is useful in replacing small vessels such as the peroneal and tibial arteries. However, the thick wall of the graft makes it difficult to sew, and the Dacron mesh with which it is surrounded makes it more difficult to pull through tissue tunnels. The graft is made of the venous channel of the cord, which is first dilated with a glass madril and treated to denature the Wharton's jelly, so reducing antigenicity and, by causing cross-linkage in the proteins, greatly strengthening the graft.

Natural grafts. These include:
1. *Homologous arterial grafts.* These are difficult to procure and were gradually abandoned in the early 1950s as the use of autologous vein grafts and synthetic grafts became popular.

2. *Autogenous vein grafts.* Autogenous vein grafts were introduced into vascular surgery by Kunlin in 1949, although the concept had been previously explored by Carrel and Guthrie in the experimental animal as early as 1905. Most commonly used is the saphenous vein, which should not be varicose and should be of at least 4 mm in diameter. It is carefully dissected from the thigh from the level of the saphenous opening to the lower end of the thigh. Each tributary is carefully identified and ligated, and care should be taken to mark the upper end of the graft to make certain that the graft is reversed before making the proximal anastomosis. If an unreversed in situ vein graft is used the valves must be carefully destroyed either through open venotomies or by the use of special strippers.

It is also possible to construct composite grafts using 6 mm thin-walled Gore-Tex to which is sutured a vein graft. This type of graft is used when extra length is required, as for example when anastomosing the superficial femoral to the anterior tibial artery. The aim of the composite graft is to avoid taking the Gore-Tex across the knee joint.

Endarterectomy

In the latter part of the 1940s Dos Santos described the operation of thromboendarterectomy. The technical efficiency of this operation depends on the presence of a plane of cleavage between the adventitia and the media of the diseased artery. This plane is between the external elastic lamina and the media so that in performing an endarterectomy the entire intima and media are removed. Endarterectomy is only technically possible because calcification rarely extends into the external layer of the artery. The dissection can be accomplished under direct vision by using multiple arteriotomies or by dissecting instruments such as the Cannon loop or by the injection of gas. The advantages of endarterectomy are that it avoids the transplantation of tissue or materials and that it preserves all major branches of the segment of the artery which has been disobliterated.

The method does, however, have certain limitations:

a. The need for an adequate run-off from the disobliterated segment in order to prevent early thrombosis.
b. Technical difficulties, which usually occur when the atherosclesclerotic lesion is calcified or extends deeper than usual into the media.
c. The difficulty of its application to arteries in which the disease has caused contraction of the total diameter, a difficulty usually overcome by the use of an autogenous vein patch.

Autologous arteries themselves are now used as grafts although not in the lower limbs. Experience has shown that internal mammary artery grafts used for coronary artery bypass surgery have a better patency rate that vein grafts.

Transluminal angioplasty

In 1964 Dotter and Judkin described transluminal angioplasty, in which they produced progressive dilatation of an atheromatous vessel by passing a series of co-axial catheters through the affected segment of the vessel, dilating the strictures to a diameter of 4 mm. In 1974 the method was transformed by the invention by Gruntzig and Hopff of a non-elastic balloon which provided a safer and more effective radial dilatation force. This allowed a much greater luminal diameter to be produced after the insertion into the affected artery of a much smaller instrument, thus reducing the incidence of local complications.

It is somewhat ironic that experimental studies indicate that angioplasty produces benefit by injuring the affected vessel when one of the theories put forward to explain the development of atherosclerosis is that it represents a response to vascular injury.

The dilatation of the atheromatous segment causes:

1. Compression and longitudinal redistribution of the atheromatous plaque.
2. Desquamation of the endothelium.
3. Cleaving of the atheromatous plaque. The resulting roughness of the surface of the vessel, which can be seen on radiographs taken immediately after the procedure, does not appear to represent a problem, and follow-up radiographs show that remodelling occurs, leaving the artery with a smooth wall some weeks later.
4. Stretching of the medial layer.

This controlled injury causes platelet aggregation, a foreign-body reaction, and retraction of the protruding atheroma, later followed by the formation of a fibrous neointima.

The most critical manoeuvre in angioplasty is to cross the lesion with a guide wire, which must be kept in place throughout the procedure. Prior to dilatation the stricture must be visualized by angiography. The catheter is then advanced to the site of the obstruction, an injection of 5000 units of heparin is given, and the guide wire, if possible, is advanced through the lesion, which is then dilated by inflating the balloon to a pressure of 6–8 atmospheres for 30–60 seconds. The early efficacy of angioplasty in peripheral vessels can be judged by the measurement of the intra-arterial pressure above and below the lesion.

The complications of angioplasty are:

a. Local dissection due to the catheter or guide wire passing subintimally.
b. Perforation of the affected vessel by the guide wire.

c. Spasm of the vessels distal to the stenotic segment after passage of the guide wire, which can usually be overcome by an injection of lignocaine.
d. Rupture of the balloon.

The fact that an emergency may arise as a consequence of this procedure means that it should not be carried out unless a competent vascular surgeon is available at all times.

Adverse factors affecting the results of angioplasty include:

a. Cases referred for limb surgery rather than intermittent claudication.
b. Lesions longer than 5 cm or the presence of multiple lesions.
c. The presence of tibial vessel disease.

Various modifications of balloon angioplasty are now under investigation. These include:

1. The Blosa catheter, in which a heated element is placed into the stricture.
2. The Kensey catheter, which drills out the atheromatous plaque, the debris been removed by suction.
3. Laser angioplasty. The advantage of the laser technique is that the lesion need not be crossed by a guide wire and, according to the innovators, it is therefore possible to deal with longer lesions.

RESULTS OF SURGERY

In disease confined to the aorta and common iliac vessels endarterectomy is the treatment of choice. This operation has the advantage over bypass grafting that the operation itself is of lesser magnitude and avoids the use of expensive graft materials. In addition the results are equal to bypass grafting. Cotton found that the patency rate was 90% in a follow-up study of 6 months to 9 years (average 2.5 years); mortality, once the 'learning curve' had been overcome, was 3%.

However, in approximately 50% of patients suffering from aortoiliac disease atheromatous changes are also present in the superficial femoral arteries, in which case a Dacron Y graft can be inserted, placing the distal anastomosis at the level of the common femoral artery and performing a profundoplasty, either over a short or longer distance in the deep femoral artery, repairing the defect with a vein patch (see below).

In some patients, long grafts are taken from the axillary artery to the femoral, and in others transfemoral cross-over grafts are used for unilateral iliac stenosis where a good run-off exists in the vessels below the groin in the asymptomatic limb.

Where the disease is limited to the iliac vessels, percutaneous angioplasty is an acceptable alternative. Patency rates in excess of 90% have been achieved by this means over long periods.

In femoropopliteal disease the 'gold standard' by which all other treatments have to be compared is the autologous vein graft. Followup studies have shown that autologous vein grafts in patients suffering from severe claudication alone have patency rates in excess of 78% at 5 years, whereas using prosthetic grafts the 5-year patency rate was only 58%. Similarly, when used for limb salvage the corresponding patency rates are 70% when using autologous vein grafts as compared to 24% using prosthetic grafts.

The status of the arteriographically determined run-off, defined as 'good' if two or three branches of the popliteal artery are patent and 'poor' if there is only a single outflow vessel, does not appear to affect the patency rate of vein grafts but has a significant effect on prosthetic grafts.

As an alternative to femoropopliteal reconstruction Martin and his colleagues suggested the use of profundoplasty, endarterectomizing the profunda femoris artery and closing the arteriotomy by means of a vein patch. The theoretical basis for this operation is the recognition that the deep femoral artery is an artery of supply rather than of conduction, and as such is relatively free from atheromatous disease except at the ostia and at its proximal end. Profundoplasty is especially indicated when the femoropopliteal segment is occluded and there are no distal run-off vessels suitable for the distal anastomosis of a bypass graft. It can also be used as the distal limb of an aortofemoral graft in the presence of femoropopliteal occlusion.

The use of profundoplasty as an alternative to bypass surgery, although originally described by Martin and his colleagues in 1968, was developed by Cotton and Roberts, who reported the use of an extended type of profundoplasty in 72 patients, in 69% of whom femoropopliteal reconstruction would have been possible. They reported that by performing this operation they were able to abolish intermittent claudication completely in approximately 50% of patients and produce an extension of the walking distance to an acceptable 200 m in the great majority of them. Extended profundoplasty, however, means that the profunda artery, having been dissected free from its attachment, is incised along its length until its wall is found to be supple. Following endarterectomy the subsequent defect is closed by an extensive vein graft. In a series of patients in whom bypass surgery would have been impossible they achieved a success rate of only 33% and if distal gangrene was present only 25%. Similar results have been reported by other authors even when the operation has been limited to a curved arteriotomy from the common femoral to the first major branch of the profunda, together with a local endarterectomy if the mouth of the profunda is found to be blocked at its origin.

The largest series of limited profundoplasty is that described by Martin and Bouhoutsos in 1977, in which they were able to review 112 patients in whom, in some, the operation had been performed at least nine years previously. In this series operative failure was deemed to have taken place if amputation was required prior to the patient leaving hospital, whereas a limited success was claimed if amputation was required within four years. In their entire series, satisfactory results were achieved in 68 patients out of a total of 107, in whom no amputation was required within 9 years.

In femoropopliteal disease angioplasty also produces very acceptable results as long as the stenosis is of limited extent; patency rates of 70% at 5 years and 60% at 7 years have been reported. Most recurrences take place within the first year, and some investigators have found that better results are obtained if the stenosis is concentric rather than eccentric.

Early failure of direct artery reconstruction is nearly always due to technical difficulties and late failure to occlusion of the graft itself or the natural progression of the disease.

LUMBAR SYMPATHECTOMY

In patients suffering from severe chronic ischaemia of the lower limb in which investigations have shown that direct arterial surgery is impossible or, alternatively, such methods have failed, ischaemic rest pain, ischaemic ulceration or gangrene is almost inevitable. In such patients lumbar sympathectomy is indicated, even though the results of such treatment are unpredictable.

The sympathetic innervation of the lower limb arises in the spinal cord from T10–L2. The fibres pass via the anterior nerve roots to the paravertebral sympathetic chain to synapse in ganglia opposite the nerve roots of the femoral, obturator or sciatic nerves. These nerves distribute the sympathetic fibres to the leg. Complete sympathectomy of the calf and foot can be achieved by excising the 2nd and 3rd lumbar ganglia. In the past this was commonly achieved by open surgical means, but this relatively major procedure has now been replaced by chemical sympathectomy using phenol.

The technique is performed with the patient lying on his side, the side for injection being uppermost. The table is broken to angle the upper and lower halves of the body at 20°. The skin is then marked to indicate the site of insertion of the needles, which should be 10 cm lateral to the spinous processes opposite the spaces between L1-2, L2-3 and L3-4. The skin is suitably prepared and the areas infiltrated with a local anaesthetic agent, after which the skin at the points marked is punctured with the point of a scalpel; three needles, each 15 cm in length and marked at 12 cm, are then introduced and carefully advanced towards the posterior midline. When the body of each vertebra is reached the needle is withdrawn several centimetres and then advanced again in a more forward direction in order to clear the body of the vertebra. In the average patient the depth of the needles should now be at the marked level, i.e. at 12 cm. Each needle is aspirated to make sure that neither the cava nor the aorta has been entered, after which 4 ml of phenol is slowly injected along each needle.

The results of this procedure are extremely variable, many patients coming to amputation within months especially in the presence of existing gangrene.

30. Acute ischaemia of the lower limb

The common causes of acute ischaemia of the lower limb are:

- Arterial emboli.
- Subintimal haemorrhage or thrombosis in a pre-existing atheromatous plaque.

A distinction between these two major causes is of supreme importance, since attempted embolectomy in the presence of thrombosis occurring in an already diseased artery not only fails but may lead to worsening of the situation.

EMBOLISM

The word 'embolus' is derived from the Greek word meaning 'peg' or 'stopper', and the generally accepted definition of an embolus is an abnormal mass of undissolved material that is transported from one part of the circulation to another. Emboli may of course travel in the arterial, venous or lymphatic vessels and they may be solid, liquid or gaseous. The commonest emboli are composed of thrombus or clot, debris from atheromatous plaques, tumour cells, bacteria, fat or oil, air, or nitrogen.

Effects

The effects of an embolus depend upon its composition, its size, and the tissue supplied by the vessel in which impaction has occurred.

Thus solid emboli of even small dimensions produce gross disturbance of function when impaction occurs in the coronary or cerebral circulation, whereas the same emboli lodging in the pulmonary vessels may cause neither symptoms nor signs. The effects also depend in part on the blood supply of the organ in which impaction has occurred. The lungs are supplied not only by the main pulmonary artery but also by the branches of the bronchial arteries; and the liver, whilst receiving its major supply via the portal vein, is also supplied by the hepatic artery.

Embolization to the lower limb

Ninety percent of all emboli reaching the lower limb arise in the heart from one of three causes: mitral stenosis, atrial fibrillation or myocardial infarction.

Mitral stenosis

The embolus arises from a thrombus forming in the left atrium because of the restricted blood flow through the stenotic mitral valve. At first the thrombus is mushroom-shaped, but ultimately it may lie free in the lumen as a ball thrombus. Many patients suffering from mitral stenosis have associated atrial fibrillation, although the latter can arise in the absence of valvular disease especially in older patients.

Atrial fibrillation

The chance of an embolus is seven times greater in patients suffering from atrial fibrillation than in individuals in normal sinus rhythm. The clot forms in the left atrium due to incomplete emptying of the chamber caused by the feeble contractions of the atrial wall. The resulting clot may then enter the left ventricle to be propelled into the bloodstream by ventricular contraction. In some patients embolization occurs at the moment the regular normal cardiac rhythm is restored, at which point the atrial appendix presumably expels the thrombus.

Myocardial infarction

Mural thrombosis occurs in at least one-half of fresh infarcts which have extended to involve the endocardium. In some 10–20% of affected individuals, pieces of thrombus break loose and enter the peripheral bloodstream, usually within 2–3 weeks of the initial episode. If a severe infarct of the myocardium occurs, an aneursym of the left ventricle may develop, which eventually becomes the site of thrombosis and clot formation.

A rare form of embolus is the so-called paradoxical embolus arising on the venous side of the circulation and passing through the heart via a congenital atrial or ventricular septal defect to lodge in the peripheral circulation.

Other causes of solid emboli endangering the circulation to the lower limb include:

1. Emboli originating in aortic or iliac atheromatous plaques. Small emboli from these sites may cause sudden and complete occlusion of a digital vessel in the foot, with little or no impairment of the pulses in the leg as a whole.
2. Thrombi originating in aortic, femoral and popliteal aneurysms.
3. Thrombi originating on prosthetic heart valves.
4. Atrial myoma.
5. Bacterial endocarditis.

Sites of impaction

Emboli usually lodge at the bifurcation of major arteries, at which point the diameter of the vessel abruptly diminishes. Common sites are:

a. At the bifurcation of the aorta, 10%, producing the so-called saddle embolus in which both lower limbs are affected.
b. In the common iliac artery, 10%.
c. At the bifurcation of the common femoral artery into its superficial and profunda branches, 40%.
d. In the superficial femoral artery, 30%.
e. In the popliteal artery at the trifurcation, 10%.

CLINICAL PRESENTATION

Symptoms

The chief clinical manifestations of acute occlusion are:

1. *Pain and paraesthesia.* The pain may initially be felt over the site of the impaction; thus in the presence of an embolus impacted in the aortic bifurcation there may be pain in the back and in the suprapubic region, whereas when the embolus impacts in the common femoral artery pain and tenderness may be first felt in the thigh. Apart from local pain, abrupt and unremitting pain develops in the muscles distal to the site of the impaction. As the duration of anoxia increases so the pain usually increases in

severity until a point is reached at which the peripheral nerves become non-functioning, at which time a sense of numbness replaces the pain.
2. *Coldness* of the affected limb or limbs.
3. *Loss of function.*

Physical examination

Inspection reveals pallor and cyanosis and, later, mottling from alternate areas of cynanosis and pallor. After some 24–36 hours the limb is usually brownish-black in colour as gangrene develops.

Palpation reveals possible tenderness over the site of impaction and absent pulses distal to the block. As time passes, increasing firmness of the muscles becomes apparent which, for a time at least, become increasingly tender on pressure.

Obviously the severity of the symptoms and their progression depends on a variety of factors, including the general condition of the patient, the site of impaction and the possible presence of an already established collateral circulation.

Pathology

After impaction, stasis results in the formation of propagated thrombus both proximal and distal to the embolus, such thrombosis occluding the ostia of the collaterals which in turn causes further stasis and in situ thrombosis of the collaterals.

Differential diagnosis

The chief concern is to distinguish embolism from thrombosis in an already diseased artery. The principal points in favour of thrombosis as opposed to embolization are:

1. A history of intermittent claudication prior to the acute event favours a diagnosis of arterial thrombosis.
2. The absence of acute or chronic heart disease also favours thrombosis.

Other conditions which occasionally mimic the effects of an embolus are:

1. *Phlegmasia caerulea dolens*, a condition associated with extensive deep venous thrombosis in which arterial spasm occurs. Unlike

arterial occlusion, however, massive venous thrombosis is normally accompanied by severe swelling of the affected limb.
2. *Dissecting aneurysm*, in which there is no obvious site of origin of an embolus and the femoral pulses, although present, may be of different magnitude in the two limbs.

Investigations

In the great majority of cases the diagnosis is made solely on the clinical history. An electrocardiogram may confirm the presence of cardiac disease if this is indeed present. If doubt exists an arteriogram should be performed.

TREATMENT

The first duty of the surgeon is to relieve pain.

In the presence of overt cardiac disease, digitalis, diuretics and anti-arrhythmic drugs are administered and the patient is heparinized. However, if the limb is to be salvaged, embolectomy should be performed within 4–6 hours, otherwise irreversible changes take place in the muscle. It has now been appreciated that the more proximal the embolus the less chance there is of limb survival. Thus if aortic, iliac or common femoral emboli are treated conservatively, gangrene develops in approximately 50% of affected limbs. Below the common femoral artery, gangrene develops in about 30%. However, when a distal embolus is treated conservatively the limb thereafter suffers from the effects of chronic ischaemia causing claudication. In general terms therefore, assuming that the condition of the patient is satisfactory the treatment of all emboli above the level of the popliteal trifurcation is embolectomy.

The development by Fogarty of the balloon catheter has considerably increased the number of limbs saved, although because of the poor general condition of many of the patients the mortality remains high – up to 40%.

Technique

The operation is normally carried out using only local anaesthesia. One or both limbs are prepared along their whole length, depending on whether one is dealing with a saddle embolus which demands exploration of both groins.

The skin of the whole limb or limbs is prepared using a colourless chlorhexidine solution so that changes in the colour of the skin are immediately apparent and the pulses can be easily palpated. An X-ray cassette is placed beneath the limb or limbs before commencing the operation.

A vertical skin incision is made over the common femoral artery and the wound deepened to afford access to the common femoral, the superficial and the profunda femoris arteries, each of which, after isolation, is controlled by a silastic loop. A transverse or vertical arteriotomy is then made. In dealing with thrombus lying proximal to the incision this is dealt with first; a Fogarty catheter No. 6 is inserted and passed proximally, the balloon is inflated and the catheter withdrawn, and with it the thrombus. Several 'passes' are made until a good forward pulsatile flow is obtained, after which 40–60 ml of heparinized saline is injected proximally using a bell-ended cannula, after which the vessel is controlled.

A No. 3 or 4 Fogarty is then passed distally, being careful to measure the limb so that it is possible to appreciate the position of the catheter tip in the limb. At the desired point the balloon is inflated until slight resistance is felt as the balloon reaches the diameter of the vessel. The catheter is then withdrawn, keeping gentle and gradually increasing pressure on the balloon so that it remains in contact with the vessel wall. One practical way in which clot can be forced out of the smaller arteries of the leg is to bind the leg with a sterile Esmarch bandage. Following several 'passes' and the possible use of the bandage technique, an arteriogram is performed before closing the arteriotomy, which may require a vein patch. If the arteriogram reveals the presence of residual clot in the leg, the popliteal artery is exposed and either a Fogarty catheter passed from above is guided distally, or a separate arteriotomy is made in the popliteal artery and a small-diameter catheter introduced distally. After a successful embolectomy the colour of the limb should rapidly return and the pulses become palpable once again.

Complications

1. Bleeding due to heparinization, which might require reversal.
2. Re-occlusion, which may result from thrombosis, pre-existing chronic atherosclerosis or technical failure caused usually by producing intimal flaps at the site of the arteriotomy.
3. Post-revascularization swelling, which is normally mild if the operation is performed early but which may require fasciotomy if

the affected muscles are enclosed in a rigid compartment, e.g. the anterior tibial compartment.

Treatment following surgery is aimed:

1. At preventing a recurrence, which normally means that the patient must remain anticoagulated.
2. Treatment of the underlying cause, e.g. the cardiac complaint.

Treatment of acute atherosclerotic occlusion

Many patients in whom thrombosis occurs on an atherosclerotic lesion do not appear for treatment but, assuming that the condition is serious enough to bring them to a physician at an early date, a decision must be made as to whether or not the condition demands intervention. Papers have appeared in the surgical literature suggesting that such blocks, even if seen late, can be lysed by means of streptokinase or urokinase, but even after lysis has been achieved the underlying lesion must be dealt with by either angioplasty or reconstructive surgery.

31. Varicose veins and the postphlebitic limb

Varicose veins are defined as dilated, tortuous and elongated veins involving the lower limb. In the vast majority of patients they are caused by valvular incompetence causing increasing pressure on the veins of the superficial venous system of the lower limb. The condition is commonly familial, commoner in females than males, related to parity in the female, and also related to body mass. There appears to be little or no relationship with prolonged standing. Very occasionally varicose veins appear as a result of an arteriovenous fistula caused by trauma, a stab wound and, even more rarely, they are found in Klippel–Trenaunay syndrome, where they appear in childhood and are associated with hypertrophy of the affected limb.

The symptoms of uncomplicated varicose veins apart from their cosmetic appearance are non-specific, the patient complaining of heaviness of the legs or aching after standing, relieved by sitting.

ANATOMY OF THE VENOUS SYSTEM OF THE LOWER LIMB

The venous system of the lower limb is composed of the superficial system lying in the skin and subcutaneous fat, and the deep system in which the veins usually lie in relation to the arterial tree: in the calf as the vena comitantes, which join together at the level of the knee to form the popliteal vein, which then passes through the adductor hiatus to become the femoral vein.

The chief named superficial veins are the long and short saphenous veins. The former begins in the medial end of the dorsal venous arch of the foot and passes approximately 2.5 cm anterior to the medial malleolus, and then crosses the lower third of the tibia to ascend along the medial border of the tibia close to the saphenous nerve to finally terminate by penetrating the deep fascia at the saphenous opening, which lies approximately 4 cm below and lateral to the pubic tubercle. Just before passing through the saphenous opening the long saphenous receives tributaries from the medial aspect of the thigh, the lower abdominal wall and the scrotum via the superficial epigastric, circumflex iliac and external pudendal veins.

The short saphenous vein commences at the lateral end of the dorsal venous arch and, passing behind the lateral malleolus, passes upwards in a vertical direction accompanied by the sural nerve, to pierce the deep fascia behind the knee to enter the popliteal vein.

In addition to the communicating veins which carry blood from the superficial system to the deep, there also exists a third system which was first described by Cockett in the mid-1950s. Cockett's contribution was to describe the so-called perforating veins, vessels draining the skin on the medial and lateral aspects of the leg which pass directly into the vena commitantes surrounding the posterior tibial artery; these veins normally have only a minimal communication with the superficial system. Thus, any alteration in pressure in the deep system can be, and is, immediately transmitted to the skin and subcutaneous tissues drained by the perforators. Normally all three systems are protected from undue increases in pressure by a series of valves that also impose the following pattern of venous return.

Blood in the deep system normally flows upwards, pumped by the compression caused by the contracting calf muscles acting within the ensheathing layer of deep fascia; this system has been called the 'peripheral venous heart'. Blood from the skin on the medial and lateral aspects of the leg flows inwards to the deep system and blood from the superficial system can move either upwards or centripetally; in all, about 85% of the blood from the legs is returned to the vena cava via the deep veins.

VENOUS PRESSURE IN THE LOWER LIMB

The venous pressure in the lower limb has been investigated under different conditions by many workers in this field. The normal pressure in the foot in a standing person is equal to the pressure of a column of blood extending from the heart to the point on the venous system at which the vein has been cannulated, i.e. from the heart to the ankle, 90 mmHg. If the venous system is normal this pressure falls to approximately 20 mmHg within a few moments of commencing active exercise.

When uncomplicated varicose veins are present, although the pressure falls it does not do so to the same degree as in a normal limb but the return to normal values is speedier. However, if the varicose long saphenous vein is occluded by extrinsic pressure at the level of the knee, there is an additional fall in venous pressure provided the communicating veins are functioning normally. This physiological measurement parallels the clinical test attributed to Perthes, who described how the superficial varicosities below the knee emptied on walking if the superficial veins were occluded at the level of the knee joint by a tourniquet. When the deep venous system is blocked or incompetent, there is little or no reduction in venous pressure on exercise and occlusion of the long saphenous vein makes no difference, a state of affairs called by Linton, 'ambulatory hypertension'.

TREATMENT OF UNCOMPLICATED PRIMARY VEINS

In some female patients small dilated venules appear on the lower limbs during pregnancy or the menopause, which are known as thread veins or spider bursts, somewhat resembling the spider naevi seen in advanced cirrhosis of the liver. Aggressive treatment of these is highly unsatisfactory and the best advice is to use a camouflaging cream or wear a suitable stocking.

In many aging patients the most appropriate treatment for primary varicose veins, if symptomatic, is the use of elastic stockings which, if worn when the patient is active, will conceal the veins and relieve the usual symptoms of heaviness and aching in the limbs. Such stockings as now manufactured exert a graded pressure on the lower limb, the calf pressure being not greater than 75% of that exerted on the ankle, and the thigh pressure not more than 50%.

Sclerotherapy

Sclerotherapy alone can be used for varicosities below the knee joint. The technique most commonly used is that popularized by Fagan, who pointed out that to be successful the sclerosant should be injected into a vein emptied of blood and kept empty after the injection by persistent pressure, thus preventing the formation of a thrombus in the 'injured' vessel. With the walls of the vein in apposition an aseptic inflammatory response develops, which results in adherence of the walls of the vein and hence obliteration of its lumen. Sodium tetradecyl 3% is injected into the varices, after these have been marked on the skin, with the patient in the erect position, after which the patient assumes the recumbent position, the leg is raised and small quantities of the sclerosant is injected into several sites; compression is then exerted before the patient stands, and is maintained for a period of 2 weeks.

Surgical treatment

Prior to the commencement of the operation the varices should be carefully marked.

Surgical treatment consists of a flush ligation of the long saphenous vein. According to Royle, who investigated the site of the saphenous opening in 167 patients, the most adequate incision for this part of the operation is one made 1 cm above and parallel to the inguinal crease, centring the incision at a point 4 cm lateral to and level with the pubic tubercle. It is essential that the three main tributaries are tied off and divided, and also that a few centimetres of the long saphenous itself are sacrificed, otherwise anastomoses will develop between the divided vein and its tributaries. Following division of the saphenous vein, attention is paid to the varicosities of the thigh and leg. Small punctate incisions are made over the individual varices and the thin-walled varices carefully teased out of the subcutaneous tissues. With patience, several centimetres of vein can normally be avulsed from each incision. A question to which no clear answer has yet been provided is whether or not it is necessary to strip out the long saphenous vein itself. Often this vein, being thick-walled, is not varicose at all but merely dilated. Hence it is frequently very easily removed, sometimes to the detriment of the patient, who at some future date may require a vein graft.

COMPLICATIONS OF SIMPLE VARICOSE VEINS

Thrombophlebitis

This condition is not infrequently precipitated by trauma. The patient knocks a varix and then notices that the area has become painful with localized swelling along a variable length of the affected vein. In the past this condition was treated by bed rest but it has now been appreciated that this is totally unnecessary and the patient should be kept mobile. A suitable non-steroidal anti-inflammatory agent is prescribed; normally indomethacin and a firm bandage is applied to the limb.

Haemorrhage

Occasionally a varix may bulge out through atrophic skin and be easily damaged by mild trauma. If this occurs and the wound is external, profuse haemorrhage will occur. The immediate first-aid treatment is to ask the patient to lie down and elevate the affected limb above the level of the hip. A tight bandage can then be applied and in due course the matter dealt with by sclerosants or by surgery.

THE POSTPHLEBITIC LIMB

The belief that the postphlebitic syndrome is due to a previous deep vein thrombosis stems from the work of Bauer, who popularized the use of venography. However, recent investigators have cast doubt on the validity of this hypothesis. For example, Browse and his colleagues in 1980 found little correlation between the phlebographic severity of the thrombosis and the later symptoms and physical signs in limbs examined some 5-7 years after the event; they therefore concluded that the development of the classical symptoms and signs indicated by ankle oedema, lipodermatosclerosis and cutaneous ulceration could not wholly depend on the extent of the initial thrombosis, and that such a complaint can apparently arise in the absence of a thrombotic episode. Burnand in 1990 came to a similar conclusion, since in only 40-50% of ulcerated legs did he find changes compatible with a previous deep vein thrombosis.

From the statistical viewpoint, when a patient develops a severe thrombosis extending to involve the femoral vein or the inferior cava, such a patient has a 25% chance of escaping any post-thrombotic complications, a 35% chance of developing mild symptoms and signs, and a 40% chance of developing moderate to severe symptoms and signs. Linghagen also examined the long-term outlook in patients in whom the development of a deep vein thrombosis had been confirmed by fibrinogen uptake studies. After 5 years he was unable to detect any significant differences between limbs in which the test had been positive and those in which the test had been negative.

A positive conclusion cannot be reached from the above data but it would suggest that neither phlebography nor fibrinogen uptake will accurately foretell what will happen in a limb following a thrombotic episode, and that possibly some additional, as yet unidentified, factor is required to precipitate the development of the syndrome.

Symptoms and signs

Pain

One of the major symptoms may be pain, although it is remarkable how painless the postphlebitic limb can be. The pain of severe venous insufficiently develops with exercise and is felt as a bursting sensation in the calf. Unlike intermittent claudication, cessation of activity does not produce relief, which can be obtained only by lying in a recumbent position with the leg elevated. Such pain can be disabling and may occasionally follow walking as little as 100 metres.

Dermal changes

In the course of time, dermal changes appear in the skin areas drained by the perforating veins, the incidence of such changes increasing with the passage of time. The first change is usually the development of multiple small tortuous veins under the skin in the ankle region in the absence of any demonstrable abnormality in the superficial veins. At the same time, the patient may note that the foot and leg are oedematous, particularly after standing. As time passes, the pitting oedema gives way to an indurated pigmented area. The induration is produced by a low-grade inflammatory reaction which is probably chemical in origin, possibly stimulated by the haemosiderin liberated into the subcutaneous tissues from red blood cells escaping by diapedesis from the dilated venules. Eventually, the indurated area forms a large plaque which involves nearly the whole circumference of the lower leg. Once in this condition the leg itches and the subsequent scratching may lead to an extensive eczema involving the whole area. If there should now be a bacterial infection cellulitis follows, and many patients give a history of repetitive attacks controlled by intermittent bed rest and an appropriate antibiotic.

Ulceration

Local trauma frequently precipitates ulceration, but the thesis that failure of the calf muscle pump leads to ulceration – the old concept of stasis – was refuted when it was found that the O_2 tension in the venous blood of the affected limb was higher than that of the unaffected limb and that the blood flow through an area of lipodermatosclerosis was increased fivefold. There therefore appears to be a significant reduction in oxygen extraction. This has been explained by the finding of pericapillary fibrin deposition in the dermis, which suggests that fibrin and other macromolecules cause a diffusion block.

Yet another theory advanced by Thomas and his colleagues in 1988 is that of the disappearing white cell. They found that more white cells disappeared from the vascular bed in dependent limbs of patients suffering from chronic venous insufficiency than from normal limbs and therefore suggested that leucocytes trapped in the capillaries caused occlusion and tissue ischaemia.

Treatment

The initial treatment of a varicose ulcer is by conservative management. This involves general measures, such as dieting to reduce weight, and local measures.

First, the ulcer should be cleaned, either by the use of a scapel if much slough is present, or, less severely, by the use of Eusol (Edinburgh Universal Solution) or by hydrogen peroxide. This may be required for several days, but once clean granulation tissue is present in the base of the ulcer it can be dressed with paraffin gauze cut to the shape of the ulcer crater, and then covered with a medicated bandage, e.g. cotton impregnated with ichthammol and zinc oxide. Antiseptics as such should only be used for a short time, and topical antibiotics should be avoided in case sensitivity develops. Most important of all is adequate support, which is provided by graduated-compression below-knee stockings exerting a pressure of 20–25 mmHg at the ankle or, if the patient finds this intolerable, by the use of two layers of Tubigrip, as well as a well padded paste bandage. In a recent article Gilland and Wolfe claimed that 90% of ulcers can be healed using such a regime; others have reported similar results, and yet others somewhat poorer. Once the ulcer is healed continuous support is required to prevent recurrence.

Skin grafting

The speed with which some larger ulcers heal can be increased by applying split-thickness grafts so long as infection has first been eliminated.

Specific surgical measures

These are usually reserved for severe intractable ulcers or for patients who are unable to comply with the rigid conservative regime necessary to achieve healing.

Special investigation before surgery

Before operation, venography can be helpful in defining the deep system and demonstrating the incompetence of both the communicating and perforating veins. It is performed either by the injection of 30 ml of opaque water-soluble medium into a superficial vein on the dorsum of the foot, or by an intraosseous injection into the calcaneum. In the former method, which is less hazardous, the superficial veins are occluded prior to the injection by a tourniquet at the ankle. The presence of tortuous leashes of veins which have no valves in the deep circulation, or trunks with irregular outlines demonstrates that the deep system is abnormal.

Surgical techniques

The surgery of varicose ulcer owes much to Linton and Cockett. Linton originally described an operation that consisted of the following steps:

1. Excision of the ulcer and the underlying deep fascia; this, he stated, severed the communications between the deep and superficial veins.
2. Removal of all large superficial varicosities, especially in the lower leg.
3. Ligation of the superficial femoral vein at its junction with the profunda, the latter being preserved.

Once Cockett had demonstrated the existence of the perforating veins, Linton's operation was placed on a sounder physiological basis although Cockett modified the operation by leaving the femoral vein untouched. Cockett's operation involves removing the incompetent perforators, the subcutaneous plaque of thrombosed venules and fibrofatty tissue, and the ulcerated area. The latter is then allowed to granulate, and when the base of the ulcer is clean and healthy in appearance a split-thickness skin graft is used to close the defect. The patient should be kept in bed with the leg elevated until the first dressing at 6 days. After this, the graft can be supported by a foam dressing and elastic bandages, although there is always a little separation at the line of junction with the abnormal skin.

Management following surgery

Even when the graft has firmly healed, continuous support is usually required and, if possible, the patient should avoid long periods of standing.

Treatment of venous pain

Deep bursting pain in the limb represents an almost insoluble problem. One operation described in the literature is to divide the deep fascia from the level of the knee to the ankle. The author has used this with complete lack of success and little has appeared in the literature following the initial reports, which again suggests that the operation carries little hope of success.

32. Amputation

INDICATIONS

- Tumours of bone, soft tissue, muscles, blood vessels or nerves.
- Rarely in
  a. Extensive infections not responding to conservative treatment.
  b. Extensive trauma.
  c. Irremediable paralysis.
  d. Congenital deformities.
  e. Cosmetic deformity.
- Peripheral vascular disease.

SITES OF LOWER LIMB AMPUTATION

The sites at which lower limb amputations are performed are: distal amputation through a single toe; the toe together with the respective metatarsal; Syme's amputation through the ankle joint; below knee; through knee; transcondylar; above knee; hip disarticulation; and, lastly, hind-quarter amputation.

The commonest cause of amputations involving the lower limb in western societies is peripheral arterial disease, estimated to account for 70% of the total, amputation being the end-point in treatment of approximately 14% of sufferers from this disease. The usual indications are: severe rest pain alone; rest pain associated with ulceration; or overt gangrene, which in this disease is usually dry unless occurring in the diabetic.

When considering the possible site of an amputation, two opposing philosophies are at work. Occasionally, the site is mandatory, particularly when it concerns the treatment of malignant disease. Otherwise the site of amputation is governed by the following:

a. The desire of the surgeon to achieve a low mortality together with primary healing of the wound.

b. The patient's aspiration to become mobile following operation.
c. The age of the patient.

In childhood, in general, so far as the femur is concerned, disarticulation through the knee joint is better than amputation through the shaft because the distal epiphysis is thus preserved and, therefore, the growth of the stump continues at a normal rate. Mid-thigh amputation in a child of 6 years may result in an extremely short stump at 14 years because of the elimination of the distal femoral epiphysis. In contrast, a below-knee amputation with a short stump in a 5-year-old child produces a satisfactory stump in the adult because the growth rate at the proximal tibial epiphysis has continued. The age of the patient is also important at the other extreme of life: old age may lead to learning difficulties and difficulty with balance, making the successful use of a prosthesis doubtful without prolonged and enthusiastic aftercare.

As a general rule, the more distal the amputation the more easily the patient attains mobility. Whilst only about half of all patients in whom an above-knee amputation has been performed regularly wear a prosthesis and walk unaided, approximately three-quarters of all unilateral below-knee amputees are able to mask their disability.

LOWER LIMB AMPUTATION IN PERIPHERAL VASCULAR DISEASE

When an amputation is performed in the lower limb for the complications of peirpheral vascular disease, if it is found that the blood supply is compromised at the site chosen this site should be abandoned and a more proximal site chosen since a failed amputation is a severe psychological blow to any patient. So far as primary healing is concerned, above-knee amputation has found most favour in atherosclerotic gangrene because the rate of primary healing of the stump is high. However, below-knee amputation is gaining in popularity because it has been shown that if a long posterior flap is fashioned without detaching it from the underlying muscles a high primary rate of healing can be achieved, and the protagonists of the below-knee amputation maintain that as many as 60% of patients suffering from atherosclerotic gangrene could undergo a below-knee amputation.

Clinically, if a below-knee amputation is planned, the following points must be considered:

1. The femoral pulse should be present.

2. There should be no flexion deformity at the knee joint.
3. The skin and subcutaneous tissues should not be affected by the ischaemic lesion at the site of skin flap construction.
4. There should be good bleeding at the site of amputation.

Tests designed to indicate whether success or failure will follow a below-knee amputation have been described. Those which have been recommended include:

a. Estimations of the Doppler ultrasound blood pressure, which should exceed 40 mmHg at the chosen site.
b. Pretibial xenon clearance, which should be greater than 2.7 ml per 100 ml per minute.

In general, if the blood supply to the skin flaps appears to be sufficient to allow primary healing the muscle blood flow is also adequate and primary healing of the stump will occur. If at all possible a below-knee amputation is preferred to an above-knee because preservation of the knee joint means that most amputees may walk on a patellar tendon-bearing prosthesis. Furthermore there is a marked difference in the mortality between above- and below-knee amputations, the mortality of the former being variously reported as 22–42%, and of the latter between 10 and 15%.

TECHNIQUE OF ABOVE-KNEE AND BELOW-KNEE AMPUTATIONS

Both above- and below-knee elective amputations are usually performed by a myoplastic technique originally promoted by Dederich and Mondry.

The site of election for above-knee amputations is 25–30 cm below the greater trochanter, and in an adult the stump must terminate 10–12.5 cm above the axis of the knee joint in order to provide room for a movable prosthetic device.

The advantage of a long femoral stump is that the newer suction sockets can be used, rather than waist bands and shoulder straps. The hinge mechanism at the knee can be fitted with friction devices which arrest flexion when weightbearing.

Below the knee the site of election is 14 cm below the tibial plateau, and this amputation is rarely effective if the stump is less than 9 cm long.

In an above-knee amputation the adductors are stitched to the abductors over the bone end, following which the flexors and extensors are sutured together. The advantage of this technique is better adherence of the stump to the socket, and the prominent bone end is eliminated.

When the same technique is applied to a below-knee amputation a transverse skin incision is made on the anterior surface of the limb 11.5 cm below the knee joint, extending for one-third of the circumference of the leg. The incision is then carried distally along the axis of the limb on each side for a distance of 15 cm. The two limbs of this incision are then joined to make a long posterior flap.

A recently described modification to the traditional skin flaps of a below-knee amputation is the use of skew flaps. The advantage claimed for this method is that a durable stump with parallel sides and a hemisperical end is produced onto which a patellar tendon-bearing socket can be fitted at an early stage, usually within four weeks. Regardless of the skin flaps the tibia is divided 14 cm below the knee joint and the fibula 2.5 cm proximal to this. The soleus and gastrocnemius are dissected from the tibia, after which the bulk of the muscle is reduced by an oblique slice, using a Syme's amputation knife cutting through the muscle in a downwards and backwards direction.

In both amputations the nerves are divided proximal to other tissues in an attempt to prevent neuromas developing.

Particularly with above-knee amputation, preoperative training, if possible, greatly shortens the period required for rehabilitation. In the early postoperative period both stumps should be carefully bandaged to ensure that they are moulded into a conical shape, and postoperative exercises should be performed in order to prevent the development of contractures and deformity.

Alternative procedures

From time to time, two other major types of amputation have been strongly advocated. The first of these is the Stokes–Gritti amputation, first described by Gritti in 1857 when he performed the operation on a corpse. It was not, however, until 1870 that Stokes began to perform this operation on the living. Essentially, this amputation is performed through the level of the femoral condyles. In the initial description the patella was preserved after shaving the articular cartilage from its posterior surface, following which the raw surface of the two bones were opposed. This amputation never gained general acceptance because non-union between the lower end of the femur and the patella, which leads to the latter slipping out of position, can cause a painful stump and difficulty in fitting a prosthesis. However, a modification has been described which obviates these difficulties. The femur is transected at the supracondylar level with the angle of the cut surface sloping backwards and upwards from the anterior aspect of the femur. The patella minus the articular cartilage is then approximated to the cut end of the femur by absorbable sutures placed between the joint capsule and the soft tissues on the posterior aspect of the femur. According to Martin (1967) who performed this modified operation on 237 limbs, only 10% of patients required revision to an above-knee amputation, a healing rate of 87% being achieved with an operative mortality of approximately 10%. Such an amputation is best fitted with a No. 2 Modular Assembly Prosthesis (Blatchford & Sons) although in a few cases in this series the patient was content to use his original walking pylon.

The second alternative major amputation is the through-knee. The advantages claimed for this type of amputation are that it gives an end weightbearing stump, that it is relatively bloodless, and that the resulting limb is powerful because the majority of muscles are left intact.

The disadvantages of a through-knee amputation are:

a. That the stump is bulbous, and hence difficult to fit with a convenient and cosmetic prosthesis.
b. The excessive length prohibits the use of a swing phase controlled prosthetic knee mechanism.
c. It requires as much skin for coverage as the short below-knee stump, which provides a better functional result.

The advantage of a long stump achieved by both a Stokes–Gritti or through-knee amputation is that the long stump gives extra weight and leverage, allowing the bilateral amputee to sit up in bed and turn unaided.

DISTAL AMPUTATIONS

Syme's amputation

The indications for Syme's amputation, which basically involves section of the tibia and fibula 0.6 cm proximal to the ankle joint, are:

1. Destruction of the forefoot by trauma.
2. Small vessel disease causing ischaemia of the foot.

Functionally it maintains the length of the limb, and the tough durable skin of the heel flap provides normal weightbearing skin. When this amputation heals well it is extremely satisfactory, but complications – chiefly necrosis of the skin flap – may require amputation at a higher level. This complication is normally due to too vigorous trimming of the inevitable 'dog ears'. A major objection to this amputation is cosmetic because of the flaired end of the distal tibial metaphysis.

In the classical Syme's amputation a single long heel flap is used. The incision is begun at the distal tip of the lateral malleolus and passes anteriorly across the ankle joint at the level of the distal end of the tibia to a point one-finger's breadth inferior to the tip of the medial malleolus. It then extends directly plantar-wards and across the sole of the foot to end at the starting point.

In order to preserve the blood supply to the heel flap the dissection involved in removing the calcaneum must be kept as close to the bone as possible and when stitching the wound together the temptation to remove the dog ears must be resisted.

A Syme's amputation can be fitted with an immediate prosthesis in which some of the weightbearing is transferred to the patellar tendon and the flares of the tibial condyles, it not being necessary to immobilize the knee joint. Unfortunately the prosthesis is difficult to fit because it is bulky and because of this a below-knee amputation is preferable in women.

In the foot, single digit amputations may be performed, or 'ray' amputations in which the gangrenous toe together with the appropriate metatarsal are excised. Such amputations are never justified in atherosclerotic gangrene in which the major vessels are involved, but may be applied in patients suffering from diabetic gangrene in whom all the peripheral pulses are present. In this type of patient, if there is considerable soft tissue infection, the wound can always be left open and delayed primary or secondary suture performed.

AMPUTATIONS OF THE UPPER LIMB

The majority of amputations involving the upper limb are performed for trauma, much less commonly for malignant disease, and even less commonly for peripheral vascular disease such as Buerger's disease or peripheral embolization.

The common amputations involve the hand, and only these will be considered in detail.

In every case treatment is directed at conserving as much viable tissue as possible and, in distal amputations involving the hand, maintaining the function of the hand as a grasping organ which involves preservation of the intrinsic muscle–tendon systems and the more powerful flexors and extensors which have their origins in the forearm.

All skin flaps, particularly of the hand and fingers, should be designed so that the scars avoid injury at work or in a domestic environment; thus, in amputating a digit, the volar flaps should if possible be longer than the dorsal so that the scar is always away from the trauma to which the fingers are subjected in normal everyday living.

Digital amputation

In amputations involving the distal phalanx a long volar flap should be fashioned if at all possible. When less than half of the nail has to be removed the nail bed should be preserved, but if more than half of the nail requires removal the nail bed should also be excised and replaced by a skin graft.

Disarticulation through the distal interphalangeal joint should include the removal of the cartilage from the head of the middle phalanx and transection of the flexor digitorum profundus tendon.

Amputations through the middle phalanx will result in no reduction in extension, assuming that only the more distal portion of the dorsal expansion of the extensor digitorum communis tendon is cut and also assuming that the central slip of the extensor tendon attached to the base of the middle phalanx is intact. If the latter has been damaged a buttonhole deformity develops and the proximal interphalangeal joint becomes flexed.

In contrast, the tendon of the flexor digitorium sublimis has an extensive insertion along the margins of the middle phalanx and, if a significant part of this cannot be preserved, disarticulation through the proximal interphalangeal joint may be necessary. Whenever possible an amputation through the proximal phalanx is preferable to disarticulation at the metacarpophalangeal joint because, however short the stump, provided it is active it retains at least some function. If more than one finger must be removed, attention must be paid to the long-term consequences to the hand as a whole. If both the middle and ring fingers are removed, the index and little fingers may deviate towards one another, weakening flexion. If either the middle or ring fingers are removed alone, the head of the appropriate metacarpal should be removed to allow the adjacent metacarpals to approximate to each other. This tends to prevent the adjoining fingers from rotating and crossing towards one another. An alternative technique if the middle finger is removed is to resect the metacarpal through the proximal third of the shaft and move the index finger medially; alternatively, if the ring finger is amputated one can excise the distal two-thirds of the metacarpal and move the little finger laterally. If the index finger is removed the head of the metatarsal should be partially removed to improve the appearance of the hand.

COMPLICATIONS OF MAJOR AMPUTATIONS

Many of the complications of major amputations result from lack of clinical judgement, for example:

a. Flaps are produced from skin which cannot survive.
b. Misjudgement to the relative lengths of the skin and bone.
c. Preserving skin lacking in sensitivity.
d. Placing the scar awkwardly and allowing the peripheral nerves to become caught up in it.

Specific complications include:

1. *Those related to the skin.*
   a. Delayed healing due to ischaemia.
   b. Chronic ulceration. This may be caused by underlying osteomyelitis which may lead to the development of sinuses, or adherence of the scar to the underlying bone resulting in tension on the skin when the stump is in use; both these conditions call for a surgical revision.
   c. Staphylococcal infection of the stump.
   d. Dermatitis, eczema and intertrigo.
   e. Sebaceous cysts.

2. *Tension on the soft tissues.* Tension on the soft tissues over a prominent bone end is a particular problem when an amputation is performed through growing bone, when epiphysical growth proximal to the amputation causes a conical stump to develop which may give rise to considerable pain and deformity.

Alternatively it may be due to a poorly shaped bone end, which may result in osteophyte formation.

3. *Conditions of the bone.*
   a. Cross-union between two bones. This is of no importance in the lower limb but should it occur between the forearm bones loss of function develops.
   b. Spur formation, leading to pain and adventitious bursae.
   c. Osteomyelitis, leading as described above to chronic ulceration beneath which a classical 'ring' sequestrum may form.

Conditions of muscle: contractures leading to deformity and inability to wear a prosthesis. In an above-knee amputation the commonest deformity of the stump is fixed flexion of the hip with associated abduction, because the adductors and the hamstring muscles have been divided. In below-knee amputations a fixed flexion deformity can develop.

Phantom limb

This condition occurs in nearly all patients at some time, but is less common in the young. A sensation of tingling is present in the non-existent fingers or toes and the patient may feel that the rest of the limb is missing altogether. As the months pass so the phantom shortens whilst the hand and the foot may appear to be the same size, merely getting closer to the stump. Whilst in the upper limb the fingers and thumb remain identifiable to the patient, in the foot the distinction between the digits diminishes. If the sensation does not fade with the passage of time the stump may begin to feel tender and the patient may begin to complain of aching, burning, or a lancinating or causalgic type of pain which may be of great severity. In 1948 Russel suggested repeated percussion for this syndrome; nowadays transcutaneous nerve stimulation may have the same beneficial effect.

In some patients the pain has organic basis – a neuroma may have developed on the divided nerve or nerves. Relief from this syndrome may occur if the neuroma is removed, but in all patients suffering from stump pain the surgeon must take care not to be too optimistic otherwise the psychological blow already present as a result of the loss of a limb will merely be magnified if treatment fails.